THE NURSE MANAGER'S
PROBLEM SOLVER

THE NURSE MANAGER'S PROBLEM SOLVER

edited by

TIM PORTER-O'GRADY

RN, CS, EdD, CNAA, FAAN

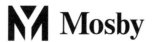 Mosby

St. Louis Baltimore Berlin Boston Carlsbad Chicago London Madrid
Naples New York Philadelphia Sydney Tokyo Toronto

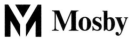

Dedicated to Publishing Excellence

Senior Vice President and Publisher: Alison Miller
Executive Editor: N. Darlene Como
Assistant Editor: Barbara M. Carroll
Project Manager: Patricia Tannian
Senior Production Editor: Ann E. Rogers
Senior Designer: Gail Morey Hudson
Cover Designer: Teresa Breckwoldt

Printed in the United States of America

Composition by The Clarinda Company
Printing/binding by Maple-Vail Book Manufacturing Group

Mosby–Year Book, Inc.
11830 Westline Industrial Drive
St. Louis, Missouri 63146

Library of Congress Cataloging in Publication Data

The nurse manager's problem solver / edited by Tim Porter-O'Grady.
    p.   cm.
    Includes bibliographical references and index.
    ISBN 0-8016-7945-1
    1. Nursing services—Administration.   I. Porter-O'Grady, Timothy.
    [DNLM: 1. Nurse Administrators.   2. Nursing, Supervisory—
organization & administration.   3. Personnel Management.
4. Nursing Care—organization & administration.   WY 105 N9715 1994]
RT89.N75   1994
362.1'73'068—dc20
DNLM/DLC
for Library of Congress   94-2184
                                                CIP

94 95 96 97 98 / 9 8 7 6 5 4 3 2 1

References to gender and the pronouns in this book are often feminine. While the authors recognize that there are nurses who are men, they also acknowledge that a great majority of nurses are women and defer to that reality. In so doing, no offense to either gender is implied or intended.

Contributors

Gregory A. Adams, RN, MN

President and Chief Executive Officer
St. Bernadine Medical Center
San Bernadino, California

Mary Adlersberg, RN, MSN*

Nursing Practice Consultant
Registered Nurses Association of British Columbia
Vancouver, British Columbia

Margaret Alderman, RN, DNSc, CNAA, FNS

Assistant Hospital Health Plan Administrator
Nursing Division
Kaiser Permanente
San Francisco, California

Judith W. Alexander, RN, MBA, PhD, CNAA

Associate Professor, College of Nursing
University of South Carolina
Columbia, South Carolina

Joan Ellis Beglinger, RN, MSN

Vice President, Nursing
St. Mary's Hospital Medical Center
Madison, Wisconsin

Suzanne Smith Blancett, RN, EdD, FAAN

Editor-in-Chief
Journal of Nursing Administration
Bradenton, Florida

Carol Bradley, RN, MSN

Vice President, Nursing Services
Huntington Memorial Hospital
Pasadena, California

Ann Marie T. Brooks, RN, DNSc, MBA

Senior Director and Director of Nursing
Strong Memorial Hospital
Associate Dean for Nursing Practice
School of Nursing
University of Rochester
Rochester, New York

M. Laurel Brunke, RN, BScN, MSN*

Nursing Practice Consultant
Registered Nurses Association of British Columbia
Vancouver, British Columbia

Jill Blake Coltrin, RN, BA, MN*

Director, Professional Services
Registered Nurses Association of British Columbia
Vancouver, British Columbia

Gregory L. Crow, RN, EdD

Associate Professor and Specialty Director
Nursing Administration Program
Sonoma State University
Rohnert Park, California
Administrative Nurse Specialist
Kaiser Permanente Medical Center
Oakland, California

Brenda H. Dugger, RN, CRNI

Director of IV Therapy and Nursing Consultation
St. Joseph's Hospital of Atlanta
Atlanta, Georgia

Sister Mary Finnick, RN, EdD

Assistant Professor, School of Nursing
State University of New York at Buffalo
Buffalo, New York

Sharon A. Finnigan, RN

Senior Partner and Systems Consultant
Affiliated Dynamics, Inc.
Atlanta, Georgia

*Five members of the Registered Nurses Association of British Columbia collaborated on answers to selected questions. This collaboration is noted after the answers to these questions in the book as "JB COLTRIN ET AL."

Beth Foster, RN, MSN, CNAA

Vice President, Nursing
Community Hospitals of Central California
Fresno, California

Donna D. Giles, RN, BSN, CCRN

Unit Director, Cardiac Care Unit
Carondelet, Saint Mary's Hospital
Tucson, Arizona

Rosalinda M. Haddon, RN, MA

President, Deltacare, Inc.
Dover, New Jersey

Mary C. Hansen, RN, PhD

Assistant Professor, Division of Nursing
Drake University
Des Moines, Iowa

Robert G. Hess, Jr., RN, MSN, CCRN, CNAA

Editor, *Nursing Spectrum*
Independent Consultant
Voorhees, New Jersey
Doctoral Candidate, Nursing Administration
School of Nursing
University of Pennsylvania
Philadelphia, Pennsylvania

Jan Hixon, RN, MS

Coordinator of Congress and World Conference
    Programs
Center for Perioperative Education
Association of Operating Room Nurses, Inc.
Denver, Colorado

Jennifer E. Jenkins, RN, MBA, CNAA

President, Jenkins & Associates
Memphis, Tennessee

Lois M. Johnson, RN, MA

Former Vice President, Nursing/Patient Care Services
Former Clinical Chair, Nursing
Rose Medical Center
Denver, Colorado

Karlene Kerfoot, RN, PhD, CNAA, FAAN

Executive Vice President, Patient Care
Chief Nursing Officer
St. Luke's Episcopal Hospital
Houston, Texas

JoEllen Koerner, RN, PhD, FAAN

Vice President, Patient Services
Sioux Valley Hospital
Sioux Falls, South Dakota

Vicki D. Lachman, RN, PhD, CS, CNAA

President, V.L. Associates
Philadelphia, Pennsylvania

Sheila Lenkman, RN, MHCA, CNAA

President and Senior Consultant
Lenkman & Associates, Inc.
St. Louis, Missouri

Laura M. Lentenbrink, RN, MSN, CNA, JD

Vice President, Nursing Services
Borgess Medical Center
Kalamazoo, Michigan

Cindy C. Campbell Levens, RN, MSN

Chief Operating Officer
Memorial Hospital at Gulfport
Gulfport, Mississippi

Catherine E. Loveridge, RN, PhD

Associate Professor, School of Nursing
San Diego State University
San Diego, California

Valerie Mancini, RN, EdD

Vice President, Division of Nursing
Saint Vincent Hospital
Worcester, Massachusetts

Pamela Maraldo, RN, PhD, FAAN

President
Planned Parenthood Federation of America
New York, New York

Kathryn J. McDonagh, RN, MSN, CNAA

President
St. Joseph's Hospital of Atlanta
Atlanta, Georgia

Jean M. McMahon, RN, MA, CNAA

Senior Vice President
Morristown Memorial Hospital
Morristown, New Jersey

Margaret Murphy, RN, PhD

Nurse Consultant, Empowering Change
Wauwatosa, Wisconsin

Joan O'Leary, RN, EdD

President and Chief Executive Officer
O'Leary and Associates, Inc.
Port Jervis, New York

James O'Malley, RN, MSN

Vice President, Nursing
The Allegheny General Hospital
Pittsburgh, Pennsylvania

Pamella Ottem, RN, BScN, MSN*

Nursing Practice Consultant
Registered Nurses Association of British Columbia
Vancouver, British Columbia

Marilyn E. Parker, RN, PhD

Associate Professor of Nursing
Florida Atlantic University
Boca Raton, Florida

Marjorie Peck, RN, PhD

Assistant Administrator
Salt Lake Valley Cluster of Hospitals
(LDS, Cottonwood, and Alta View Hospital)
Salt Lake City, Utah

Tim Porter-O'Grady, RN, CS, EdD, CNAA, FAAN

Tim Porter-O'Grady, Inc.
Atlanta, Georgia

Donna Sheridan, RN, PhD

Director of Nursing and Chief Nurse Executive
Saint Francis Memorial Hospital
San Francisco, California

Linda J. Shinn, RN, MBA, CAE

Deputy Executive Director
American Nurses Association
Washington, DC

Mary Therese Sinnen, RN, MSN

Nurse Manager, St. Michael Hospital
Coordinated Care Specialist
Nursing Systems Consultant
Milwaukee, Wisconsin

Sandra H. Smith, RN, CNA, CPHQ

President and Consultant
Comprehensive Resources, Inc.
Baton Rouge, Louisiana

Sheila F. Smith, RN, MSN

Assistant Vice President, Nursing
Children's Hospital Medical Center
Cincinnati, Ohio

Mary Ann Sorenson, RN, MS

Director, Nursing Resources
Saint Joseph's Hospital of Atlanta
Atlanta, Georgia

Carolyn St. Charles, RN, MBA

Senior Vice President, Patient Care Services
Overlake Hospital Medical Center
Bellevue, Washington

Jaynelle F. Stichler, RN, DNSc, CNAA

Vice President, Sharp Healthcare
Executive Vice President
Stichler Design Group, Inc.
San Diego, California

Sharon A. Stone, RN, BScNgEd, MSc (Health Services Planning and Administration)*

Nursing Practice Consultant
Registered Nurses Association of British Columbia
Vancouver, British Columbia

Barbara Volk Tebbitt, RN, MS

Consultant in Nursing and Healthcare Administration
Shoreview, Minnesota

Jolene Tornabeni, RN, MA, CNAA

Senior Vice President, Hospital Operations
Mercy Hospital and Medical Center
San Diego, California

Joan Trofino, RN, EdD, CNAA, FAAN

Vice President, Patient Care
Riverview Medical Center
Red Bank, New Jersey

Laura Gasparis Vonfrolio, RN, MA, CEN, CCRN

Publisher, *REVOLUTION—The Journal of Nurse
  Empowerment*
President, A.D. Von Publishers
President, Education Enterprises
President, Power Publications
Staten Island, New York

Cathleen Krueger Wilson, RN, PhD

Senior Partner, Specialty Applications
Scottsdale, Arizona

Karen Zander, RN, MS, CS

Principal and Co-owner
The Center for Case Management, Inc.
South Natick, Maine

Preface

Welcome to *The Nurse Manager's Problem Solver*, a resource designed to help you as a nurse manager as you face the myriad issues confronting leaders in today's transforming health care system. This book addresses those issues that are critical to your role by answering the questions most frequently asked by nurse managers. All of the questions posed in this text were generated by nurse managers struggling with current management issues in the clinical setting. Although it would be impossible to address every problem in health care leadership in one book, we have attempted to include the most challenging situations and most complex issues confronting the nurse manager in her or his daily work experience.

While we wanted to remain practical in our responses to timeless nurse manager concerns, we also wanted to address some of the more challenging issues of the day. By including some of the newer challenges to managers, we hope to prepare you to address many of the changes occurring as the health care system continues to be redefined and restructured.

We are fortunate to have many of the best minds in nursing management addressing the questions and topics contained in this book. Through assembling the experts, we have provided the guidance of the best thinkers and problem solvers in one reference, with easy access to their responses to critical management issues. Some of their responses describe tried-and-true processes for specific problem solving and others indicate newer creative strategies to address some old as well as new nursing management issues.

This book is a handy reference to help solve problems. It is not meant to be read from cover to cover like most books. However, the situations and challenges described are both enlightening and interesting. You should keep *The Nurse Manager's Problem*

Solver readily available to address real issues in the exercise of your management role. We have tried to maintain a broad focus to ensure that the many real issues that managers face would be addressed. Some responses to questions are specific to the issue addressed, yet others can be applied to a number of management situations.

You will note that there is an assumption made in this book that the move to leadership is a primary shift in the function of the manager. The responses to issues in this text suggest that the manager already recognizes that the style of leadership that is appropriate to the management role today is highly involved and committed to staff participation in owning and resolving their own issues. The manager at the threshold of the twenty-first century can no longer use strategies or styles that suggest maternalism, parochialism, or dependency roles to confront issues and to solve work-related problems. The enlightened manager is empowering in applying strategies for problem solving and solution seeking to the full range of issues having an impact on all the players in the work environment.

As with all books of this kind, this book can be helpful only if it is used and shared with others. We know that not every issue or circumstance can be contained in any work of this sort. There are many problems and issues that are specific to a setting and don't fit general or universal responses. We hope, though, that this book will serve as one of a number of resources the manager will use in the pursuit of clinical excellence and in the resolution of issues that can affect the delivery of care. The authors hope most of all that this book will serve as a resource that increases the options and information of the manager in leading the health care enterprise into the twenty-first century.

Tim Porter-O'Grady

Contents

Absenteeism

◆ WHAT SHOULD I SAY TO A NURSE WHO OFTEN CALLS IN SICK?

Q When I was counseling an employee regarding her absenteeism, she responded that she was "really sick" and that I must want her to work when she is ill. How should I respond?

A The response made by your employee indicates a lack of understanding relative to the absenteeism policies in your organization. It also appears that your expectations have not been clearly stated or are not clearly understood by this individual and possibly by others.

1. Begin by making a personal commitment that you will treat all employees fairly and equally. In this way the individual will not feel singled out.
2. Schedule a formal meeting with this employee to review your expectations rather than responding to the remark casually. This individual requires firm action and is looking to you to provide that leadership.
3. Begin the meeting by reminding the employee that each employee provides a critical service and that when one member of the team is out sick, everyone else must work harder. Also, unplanned absences are costly when they require replacement. As a manager, you are committed to providing high-quality service and you expect your staff to participate in that endeavor.
4. Review the organization's basic philosophy with this individual. Tell the employee that sick-leave policy is not a time-off benefit but an insurance in case of illness.
5. If you have requirements in your policy, for example, a physician's note, review these requirements with the employee.
6. Try to have an open dialogue about the work environment. Ask the individual if the work schedule is problematic and inquire about subjects such as working conditions, wages, benefits, and control over work. Your willingness to discuss these issues will indicate that you are sincere about helping your staff to succeed.
7. Since personality and life-style issues often influence our behavior at work, attempt to assess emotional maturity and see if there are personal concerns affecting work performance. If it seems appropriate, suggest an employee assistance program. Or if a change in scheduled hours would help and you can accommodate the change, offer this flexibility; 10- or 12-hour shifts may be just the answer.
8. If this employee has been counseled before, you may want to formalize the disciplinary process in the following way:
   ◆ Meet to discuss the problem of absenteeism *privately.*
   ◆ Provide a list of all sick-call occurrences and previous counseling sessions. If there is an apparent pattern, like calls just before a weekend or holiday, point this out.
   ◆ Ask for explanations.
   ◆ Delineate the change in behavior that you expect, for example, there will be no sick-calls for the next 3 months.
   ◆ Specify if this is a verbal or written warning.
   ◆ Schedule a follow-up meeting.
   ◆ End on a positive note, perhaps by telling the individual that you appreciate the contributions she makes to the team when on duty.

Remember that others will be watching to see if you really do follow through.

In addition, supply data to your staff on a regular basis about the number of call-ins. Don't be afraid to openly discuss how other employees feel about no-shows. If you have the ability to promote motivational or reward programs in your organization, do so. Wellness pay, lotteries, or time-off programs may help all of you in the long run. And remember, in dealing with any staff member, be objective.

V MANCINI

Advance Directives

◆ WHAT ARE MY OBLIGATIONS REGARDING ADVANCE DIRECTIVES?

Q Our hospital is required to provide our patients with advance directives. What are advance directives, and what is my obligation as a nurse manager in meeting the requirements of this new law?

A Advance directives are documents that are used to guide the provision of care when an individual is incapacitated. Specific types of advance directives and their scope are defined by state law and may vary significantly from state to state. Examples of advance directives include Living Will, Durable Power of Attorney for Health Care, Directive to Physicians, Natural Death Act Directive, and Values Statement.

To understand your obligation as a nurse manager regarding advance directives, it is first important to understand the basic components of the federal Patient Self-Determination Act (PSDA). The PSDA was passed on December 1, 1991, and requires hospitals, skilled nursing facilities, home health agencies, hospice organizations, and health maintenance organizations (HMOs) serving Medicare and Medicaid patients to provide written information to adults to whom they provide care regarding the following:

1. An individual's rights, under state law, to make decisions about medical care, including the right to accept or refuse medical and surgical treatment.
2. An individual's rights, under state law, to formulate advance medical directives, such as a Living Will or a Durable Power of Attorney for Health Care, to guide the provision of care when the individual is incapacitated.
3. The policies and procedures that the institution has developed to honor these rights, including the commitment not to condition the provision of care on whether the patient has an advance directive.

The law further requires that

1. Institutions provide education regarding PSDA legislation to the community, staff, and physicians.
2. The patient's medical record indicates whether the patient has an advance directive.

As a nurse manager, you are responsible to ensure that

1. Staff receive appropriate education and are knowledgeable regarding PSDA legislation and the requirements of state law regarding advance directives.
2. Staff receive appropriate education and are knowledgeable regarding your institution's specific policies and procedures and that those policies and procedures are followed.

3. Care provided to an individual will not be conditional or otherwise discriminatory based on the presence or absence of an advance directive.
4. Staff know whom to contact, 24 hours a day, if they have questions about how to interpret the hospital policies and procedures in any given situation.

C ST CHARLES

Agency Use

♦ WHO SHOULD CHOOSE SUPPLEMENTAL STAFFING AGENCIES?

Q Should the choice of supplemental staffing agencies be delegated to a hospital purchasing department or to the staffing coordinator?

A The choice of which supplemental agencies for a hospital to use can have profound or minimal impact on a hospital's bottom line depending on the usage of agency staff. However, the choice of which agency to use should be made by the nurse executive rather than either the staffing coordinator or the purchasing agent. The ultimate responsibility for the competency of the agency staff, as assured by departmental quality checks and appropriate management, lies with the nurse executive. Liabilities ensuing from the use of the agency staff and failure to meet standards for quality care also rest with the nurse executive. Yet the actual execution of the contract(s), billing practices, and staffing needs can be handled by both or either the purchasing agent or staffing coordinator. The purchasing department should have a good understanding of negotiating for price, contract terms, and other contract issues, whereas the staffing coordinator knows what skills and experience are essential, must keep all records related to orientation and evaluation, and must observe all licensure requirements. Use of a tripartite committee in which all three members review previous and predicted usage requirements, the evaluations on record, and financial constraints seems to be the best course to take. The nurse executive would then make recommendations, and the staffing coordinator and purchasing department would request proposals from the final vendors. All three would review proposals. The awarding of the contract would be handled by the purchasing office. All technical and professional documentation would be managed by the staffing coordinator. The committee could meet quarterly to review satisfaction with performance. If the purchasing department is not aware of the obligations of the nursing department to ensure competency of all agency staff, the nurse executive should intervene to establish the roles as defined above.

S LENKMAN

◆ WHAT INFORMATION SHOULD A STAFFING AGENCY PROVIDE?

Q What kinds of screening processes do supplemental staffing agencies administer to agency nurses?

A The type of screening varies somewhat from agency to agency, but the key to having some control over the skill base and qualifications of the candidates is to have a clear, specific nursing policy that defines the screening responsibilities of the providing agency. These screening processes should include

1. An application and skills checklist that highlights the background of the potential candidate.
2. Evidence of the clinical experience necessary to qualify the individual to work in your institution. Often this means the RN must have 1 year of practice in medical/surgical nursing and 2 years in critical care.
3. Satisfactory work references. Your standard could be two positive work-related references.
4. Current licensure in your state.
5. Current CPR certification. ACLS certification may be your requirement if the nurse is to work in critical care or on a telemetry unit.
6. Documentation of a satisfactory health assessment including a chest x-ray or TB skin test.
7. Documentation of annual in-service training on fire, safety, and infection control, including in-service training on blood pathogens.

8. Passing scores on written exams (clinical and pharmacology).

If your institution is using local agencies for supplemental staffing, it may be possible to do a personal interview. For those using traveling nurses, a phone interview including specific clinical questions as well as questions to determine the flexibility of the candidate may enhance the screening process.

MA SORENSEN

◆ ARE CONTRACTS REQUIRED BY JCAHO BETWEEN A HOSPITAL AND A SUPPLEMENTAL AGENCY?

Q Does JCAHO require a contract between a hospital and a supplemental staffing agency? What should be covered in a contract or written agreement with an agency?

A JCAHO does require that a contract exist between each supplemental staffing agency and the hospital. These contracts should be reviewed annually to remain current. The contract or written agreement should include statements about the responsibilities and obligations of the staffing agency as well as those of the hospital. A written agreement should include the following items:

1. The hourly rates to be paid by the hospital for the supplemental staff.
2. The requirement that each nurse demonstrate evidence of current registration in the state.
3. Evidence of professional liability insurance (although the hospital is liable for the nurses' actions while on duty).
4. Current CPR or life-support certification.
5. A skills roster for each clinical specialty to which the nurse will be assigned.

In addition, the hospital should require that supplemental staff be oriented to specific units within their hospital before their engagement. This orientation may include review of current documentation forms, nursing care maps or care plans, and orientation to the physical unit. The agency is also required to provide evidence that each of their supplemental staff has had tuberculin skin tests or chest x-rays. The hospital may have additional requirements related to drug screening, immunization against rubella, or other requirements extended to the usual staff members.

JF STICHLER

◆ DOES JCAHO REQUIRE AGENCY NURSES TO BE ORIENTED?

Q Does JCAHO require agency nurses to be oriented to each hospital where they may work?

A The Joint Commission refers to agency nurses as outside contract staff and expects compliance with minimal competency checks to protect patients (Nursing Care Standard 2.4; JCAHO, 1992). Specifically these staff must be oriented before providing patient care and must have documented evidence of licensure and current clinical competence in assigned patient care responsibilities. To ensure consistency in achieving compliance with these standards, the mechanisms or systems and procedures governing this practice are usually centralized. This means that the policy and procedure for use of agency nurses is defined by the department of nursing and not by the individual unit. Thus every nurse manager should be using the same uniform methods for monitoring, reporting, and managing agency nurses. If you cannot find a centralized department of nursing policy for how all the nursing units handle this task, you need to raise this issue with your supervisor or nurse manager colleagues to propose drafting such a policy.

MC ALDERMAN

AIDS

◆ WHAT SHOULD I DO WHEN STAFF DO NOT WANT TO TREAT HIV-INFECTED PATIENTS?

Q We recently admitted an HIV-positive patient to our department. I am having difficulty getting

staff to care for this patient. What alternatives do I have to ensure proper patient care?

A Patients have the right to expect and receive appropriate care regardless of their diagnosis. Nursing staff have the responsibility, as a condition of employment, to provide care regardless of the patient's diagnosis. The hospital or the nurse manager should not allow any staff member to refuse to provide care for an HIV-positive patient.

Ideally, as the nurse manager you should have an open conversation with staff to discuss any fears or concerns they may have regarding providing care to HIV-positive patients before any issues arise about caring for a specific patient. Your commitment to the staff should include ensuring that appropriate protective equipment is available, as well as providing any education or ongoing support they may require. Education may include having staff meet with the hospital infectious disease physician or infection control nurse on a regular basis as they work through their concerns. And most important, you should make it very clear that all nursing staff are expected to provide care to HIV-positive patients in a professional manner.

C ST CHARLES

◆ SHOULD PREGNANT NURSES BE EXCUSED FROM TREATING CONTAGIOUS PATIENTS?

Q As nurse manager, I am frequently confronted by expert nurses who are pregnant and refuse to care for HIV patients. What is the best and fairest way to handle this situation?

A This is a situation that, at one time or another, every nurse manager will face, whether in relation to the risk of HIV infection or with more common diseases such as hepatitis and herpes. However, when HIV infection is the center of the controversy, emotions can run very high.

The first step is to review the most current literature regarding modes of transmission and techniques to decrease exposure to HIV. Currently, universal precautions are the most effective method to prevent transmission of HIV and hepatitis. You may wish to start with federal guidelines available through the

Centers for Disease Control (CDC) and Occupational Safety and Health Administration (OSHA). In addition, review your agency's guidelines to ensure that they are congruent with state and federal guidelines. This is recommended because agency guidelines sometimes exceed those of the state and federal policymakers.

After reviewing the guidelines, meet with experts in your agency from nursing, medicine, human resources, and occupational/employee health departments to review the documents to ensure that your agency standards are, in fact, the ones you wish to implement as guidelines and that they are uniformly used throughout your agency. Further, ensure that all required and suggested equipment is available in quantities that are sufficient to meet requirements of the job. The staff must be able to trust that the agency will always have the necessary equipment available to care for patients with communicable diseases. It is also the agency's responsibility to ensure that all personnel know how to properly use equipment; this includes storage, operation, and proper disposal of all associated materials.

Now you are ready to meet with the staff. It is suggested that you first listen to their concerns in order to fully understand their fears. Often the act of listening provides a major step toward resolution. You may find that the process of vocalizing fears and concerns lends the opportunity for meaningful dialogue and mutual understanding regarding the issue and proposed solutions.

Because universal precautions are the accepted method for reducing the risk of transmission of HIV and other communicable diseases, personnel must be educated in how proper implementation of these precautions will provide for their safety. Dealing with the fear of HIV infection is an ongoing process and must be carried out in a factual and open manner.

GL CROW

♦ **SHOULD NURSES INTERVENE IN A LIFE PARTNER'S CARE OF A DYING AIDS PATIENT?**

Q We have a person in the final stages of AIDS on our unit. His life partner stays all evening and through the night to assist in his care. The nursing staff is not always sure that he is using the best technique or doing things that are right for the patient. He also appears to be very possessive of his relationship. How do I help the staff deal with this situation?

A Compassion is perhaps the most important aspect of caring for a dying patient. Supporting the presence of a partner to assist both the patient and partner in the grieving process is a true demonstration of compassion and of addressing a priority need of this patient. Perhaps to improve techniques, some one-to-one patient and partner education would be helpful. An overall plan would be best designed at an interdisciplinary conference with the patient and partner and selected health care team members present.

D SHERIDAN

Assertiveness

♦ **HOW CAN I BE MORE ASSERTIVE AND IMPROVE MY COMMUNICATION SKILLS?**

Q Many of my colleagues have told me that I am not very affirmative in my management style. They claim that I appear to be more passive than I should be. How do I deal with my own passivity and become more self-directed?

A Assessing management styles is a complex process. Receiving constructive criticism from peers and supervisors along with self-assessment can be very helpful.

Initially you should explore further what is meant by "not very affirmative." Specific examples from peers and supervisors will give you a better understanding of the preception of others. If available, management assessment tools such as the Myers-Briggs inventory can offer more information and clue you in to your vulnerable areas.

Some areas to consider in assessment are:
1. Do you deal with conflict directly?

2. Do you resolve issues and problems in a timely manner?
3. Do you make firm decisions?
4. Are you self-directed or do you wait to be told or asked before acting?

If the answer to most of these questions is *no,* then you do need to develop your conflict-resolution, decision-making, and self-direction skills. You should initiate a development plan by investigating resources such as books, articles, and conferences. You also should seek assistance from your immediate supervisor who can assist you with a development plan.

If the answer to most of these questions is *yes,* then perhaps the perception is based on your communication style. *How* you communicate, as well as *what* you communicate, influences how you are perceived. Your body language, voice tone and quality, and inflection affect others' perceptions of you. It is important to assess the communication style of the person you are talking to and adjust your style based on this perception. You should also analyze the words you use that may not accurately reflect your actions, intentions, or abilities.

SF SMITH

◆ WHAT DO I SAY TO A STAFF NURSE WHO WANTS TO TAKE CREDIT FOR WORK SHE DIDN'T DO?

Q We have a staff nurse who gets others to do work for her and then takes all of the credit herself. What can I do to remedy this?

A Behavior problems such as this require straightforward approaches. This is a situation in which the staff knows what is going on but does not want to confront the offender. This lack of response enables the nurse to continue the behavior while others remain frustrated and unrecognized. The collective reaction of the staff is a form of victim behavior, since no one feels adequately empowered to deal with the situation.

As the manager, you need to discuss this behavior with the employee but should not take the issue away from the staff. They need to be part of the solution on

an ongoing basis. In addition, you should take the following steps:
1. Meet with the staff nurse and describe the behavior you have observed. From your management perspective, discuss how it affects unit functioning.
2. Identify what behavior changes need to occur and how they will be evaluated.
3. Meet with individual staff members who have recently been on the receiving end of this behavior. Discuss how they might have handled the situation to let their feelings be known. If the staff members need coaching, role-play possible approaches. Encourage the employees to discuss the issue with the offending nurse.

Acknowledge the efforts of all staff members in their work. If the situation arises again, openly acknowledge the contribution of other staff as well. Be consistent in your response to each incident but see that staff also participate. Assertiveness training might be helpful as a group activity.

B FOSTER

◆ HOW DO I MANAGE A JEKYLL-HYDE STAFF NURSE?

Q How do I deal with a passive-aggressive staff member whose behavior is exemplary in my presence but is reported to be quite the opposite when I am absent?

A Dealing with "reports" from others regarding a staff member's behavior is a challenge. While the information should be taken seriously, as a nurse manager, you must go beyond merely listening to others before making any judgment requiring action. Labeling of behavior is not helpful and can create a stereotype related to an individual's performance that is unfair or misrepresents the actual situation.

You should create opportunities to observe the individual's behavior with other staff, patients, and families. Are there other individuals who could provide another perspective in understanding the situation? Data related to the staff member's performance can be helpful in assessing the situation. Stepping back and processing what is happening on the unit is also an important part of evaluating the situation.

If you cannot observe or collect objective data to help you understand the situation, then meet privately with the staff member. This interaction could be over lunch or a coffee break, but it needs to be a private conversation that focuses on how others perceive the staff member. The staff member's reaction may range from one of surprise to one of distress because of its unexpected nature. The nurse manager should reassure the staff member that the meeting is informal and intended for dialogue and exchange.

The nurse manager should prepare for the meeting by reviewing all past annual performance appraisals, anecdotal notes, patient or staff letters, and other supporting documentation. This will allow the nurse manager to discuss past activities and involvement in role expectations. If the discussion during the informal meeting does not seem to support the reported perception regarding the staff member, then the nurse manager should identify several opportunities to involve the specified staff member in unit activities. It is important to share with the individual that other staff need to see that genuine collegiality and partnership are shared values and that inconsistencies in performance are detrimental to unit operations.

Clarifying expectations and holding an individual accountable for consistent behavior are helpful and contribute to enhanced team functioning. However, it is important for the nurse manager to assess the situation and take action on *objective* data and not on second-hand information that is not necessarily based on fact.

AMT BROOKS

Assignments

◆ ARE ACUITY-BASED ASSIGNMENTS FAIR?

Q How can I get RNs to move beyond the pressure from staff to assign everyone the same number of patients and start basing assignments on acuity?

A A valid and reliable acuity system can determine the appropriate professional and nonprofessional staff needed to meet the care needs of patients. Most of the accepted "acuity systems" require input from the registered nurses on the unit. This input is usually translated via a computer into work-hours required. Nursing administration should support the results of the data gathered. The RNs on the unit should be informed as to required staffing, and they also should be told the level of care required and hours needed to meet those care needs. There are significant differences in the nursing care required for a high-acuity patient. The RNs need to be educated about the benefits of an acuity system. Once they understand the acuity system, they should more readily accept the fact that everyone does not have to have the same number of patients for an assignment.

JG O'LEARY

◆ HOW SHOULD I DEAL WITH A NURSE WHO REFUSES A PATIENT ASSIGNMENT AND WALKS AWAY?

Q As the head nurse of a medical unit, one morning I recently made patient assignments. One of the RN staff refused her assignment and also refused to give me a reason why. I stood by my decision but she left the ward to find "someone with more authority." Is this abandonment of patients? How should I deal with a situation like this?

A You have much work to do. First consider the assignment. Could *you* have managed that assignment? What did you base the assignment on? Do you have a reliable patient classification system, and would you consider the assignment fair for an average employee? Was this individual a new employee who required additional orientation or support? Were you in any way showing bias or favoritism within your staff? Did you assign your friends a lighter caseload? Did this employee have difficulty yesterday with a specific patient and truly feel that she could not properly care for that individual? How much time have you as a manager spent with this employee understanding his or her role? Is this individual having personal problems? If so, what are they?

I would not even consider the question of patient abandonment until I had answered the above questions. Also, once the employee voiced her concerns, I would have suggested that we do that assignment together, and that she in turn help me with my responsibilities.

JG O'LEARY

◆ HOW CAN I BALANCE ASSIGNMENTS EQUITABLY?

Q On our managed-care team we have a couple of staff members who are continually at odds with regard to work load and patient care. No matter what the issue is, I can't seem to balance assignments. Do you have any insights that can help me?

A The two types of case management, in-house and community based, lend themselves to different ways of balancing work load. In-house case management assignments can be balanced utilizing an acuity tool to measure intensity of service. Assignments can then be made accordingly. Community-based case management lends itself to a professional group practice. In our system, a group of case managers are assigned to cover a group of zip codes. The case managers are responsible for screening referrals and adding to their caseloads within these zip codes. The individual nurse as case manager is then responsible for letting his or her peers within the zip code group know when help is needed with a caseload.

DD GILES

Bonuses

◆ SHOULD BONUSES BE OFFERED?

Q Some hospitals offer bonuses for recruitment, retention, or productivity enhancements. Should our hospital be doing this?

A Financial rewards such as bonuses and paid vacations have been used as enhancements for both the new recruit and occasionally for the nurse who served as the recruiter. Usually these methods have been used during periods of extreme staffing shortages and crisis within the organization. However, unless a satisfying professional practice model exists for nurses in the organization, new recruits will generally seek other employment as soon as their obligations at the current agency are complete.

The new emphasis must support cost-effective models that retain nurses, encouraging them to build their knowledge base over the long term within the same organization. In organizations committed to professional models of nursing practice, accountability for goal achievements by all professionals is an expected cultural norm of the system. Gain sharing or bonus rewards are more closely aligned with performance, productivity, and actual quality of patient care outcomes.

Gain sharing as defined by Belcher (1991) refers to

. . . a compensation system that is designed to provide for variable compensation and to support an employee involvement process by rewarding the members of a group or organization for improvements in organizational performance. Gains, as measured by a predetermined formula, are shared with all eligible employees typically through the payment of cash bonuses.

Gain sharing, pay for performance, and incentive and bonus plans describe performance-based monetary rewards. Generally, these incentives have been limited to executive-level compensation in most hospitals (Bell & Bart, 1991).

However, there is an increasing awareness by progressive health care organizations of the valued contributions made by "expert" professional nurses who are "knowledge specialists" in their various areas of clinical practice. Such visionary organizations have moved to include other professional nurses in their incentive programs (Bell & Bart, 1991).

Gain sharing, which is directed toward productivity and quality outcomes, tends to reward members of an organization as a group for their contributions to improved achievements. This serves as a perfect incentive in those organizations that stress staff participation, team building, and empowerment.

J TROFINO

◆ **MUST BONUSES BE AWARDED TO EVERYONE ON A UNIT?**

Q Is it really necessary that bonuses be given to everyone on every service and unit, even though units are becoming more specialized, customer driven, and self-directed?

A The simple answer to this question is, "No." It is unnecessary to give bonuses to everyone; however, the concept of rewarding performance is significantly more complicated than just giving bonuses. Today more than ever, nurse managers are challenged to design systems for compensation that reward achievement, performance, and contribution, but unit specialization, in and of itself, is not a good criterion for giving bonuses. Bonuses today should be based foremost on the outcome needs of the organization.

Every good organization should have in place a merit pay increase system designed to reward employees for their expertise, performance, and output. Such a system should have clear and definable objectives. In my experience, all too often institutions have poorly organized and poorly administered merit pay systems that lead to the creation of *additional* reward systems to accomplish what was intended with the merit system.

Initiation of a bonus system should be directed at accomplishing more for the organization and its employees than what should be expected from a merit pay system. In today's health care environment where we are challenged to do more with less and where survival is being determined by our ability to reshape not only our organization but our paradigm of health care delivery, opportunities exist to reward nurses who improve productivity, redesign delivery systems, and generally improve outcomes.

The following points might be useful in developing a bonus system:

1. Understand the needs and priorities of your organization.
2. Determine if your goal is to reward individuals or a group for improved outcomes. Rewarding the group can promote team development and overall group cohesiveness.
3. Identify the organizational need you wish to have addressed within the bonus system and state it as a clear, measurable objective.

4. Develop a mechanism for measuring performance outcome. The measurement process should be defined before beginning any activity and must be objective and quantifiable. For example, if your objective is to develop an orthopedic service strategic plan, before initiating the objective you must document and have agreement on (a) what your organization or superior defines as a service strategic plan, (b) what particular needs or issues are expected to be addressed, and (c) what level of financial analysis or projection is acceptable.
5. It must be clear who will be evaluating the outcome.

Truly effective bonus systems can be quite challenging to develop; however, when properly developed and administered, they may contribute significantly to the organization's accomplishments. In addition, they provide incentives for employees to significantly improve performance in specifically targeted areas. Generally speaking, if applied loosely throughout an organization, a bonus system will have a short-term impact on morale, and one should not expect any significant impact on organizational performance.

GA ADAMS

Budgeting

◆ **HOW CAN I MANAGE BUDGET VARIANCES?**

Q What are the criteria for analyzing budget variances? What is a normal or acceptable budget variance? What variances need justifications and to whom?

A The first question you need to ask is what is considered a budget variance within your institution. Do you have an FTE (full time equivalent) variance or a total dollar variance?

If you have an FTE variance, you need to ask what the standard FTE budget is and how it was determined. Do you have a reliable and valid acuity system that determines the number of professional and nonprofessional staff required to meet your patient care needs, or was your budget developed based on stan-

dard nursing hours required for your patient population? If your budget was developed on dollars received, take the time to understand the formulas. You
may be in a no-win situation. You may have some
non-paying clients. If this is the case, you may have a
negative balance to begin with.

If your variance is significant (I consider anything
over 10% significant), you may have to ask why. If
you have fewer patients on your unit than usual, you
could have a variance at the end of the month. Remember, you do not need the same number of staff if
you have 50% fewer patients. Next year you should
become involved in determining the acuity of your
patients and develop your own budget. Do not let
someone else determine the number of staff members needed to provide quality care.

Eliminating overutilization and nonproductive
time is another way of managing budget variances.
Consider this scenario. Two staff members call in sick
(your hospital pays them for sick time), and you replace them with two agency nurses, who cost you
one third more in salary. These costs go against your
cost center and result in variances. Everyone is entitled to "sick time," but abuses do occur. Track and
follow those individuals who abuse what really is a
privilege in a job. Also watch overtime. Frequently an
overtime abuser clocks out late, and in many institutions any time over 8 hours a day or 40 hours a week
is considered overtime. Overtime can really eat up
dollars fast. Scheduling some part-time employees
who are paid at an hourly rate would be better than
having your full complement of staff as full-timers at
any given time on your schedule.

JG O'LEARY

Burnout

◆ WHAT CAN I DO TO KEEP FROM BEING OVERWHELMED WITH WORK PROBLEMS?

Q How can I keep from becoming discouraged
when so many things seem to be beyond my
control, and the management's and staff's expectations of me are so high?

A These are difficult and confusing times for
nurses and others in the health care arena. We
are in the midst of the most rapid and significant
change we have ever experienced. Uncertainty
abounds and is a powerful influence on everyone and
every situation. In the midst of such change, it is
helpful to get back to basics by honestly examining
our situations and the expectations we experience in
light of who we are as a person and a nurse. These
times urge us to step back and reflectively examine
the values, beliefs, and expectations that form our
personal and professional grounding.

Facing up to reality is an important first step in not
becoming overwhelmed. In truth, many factors affecting practice today are beyond our control. It is also true
that expectations of nurses and nursing are greater
and more complex than ever before, and many of
these requirements are inappropriate. In addition,
some of the expectations we impose on ourselves are
greater than we can manage and may be out of step with
our individual interests, talents, and preparation.

The nurse who is best prepared for today's world
and its expectations is one who is on solid footing
personally and professionally and who can tolerate
continuous uncertainty. The nurse who can tolerate,
if not thrive on, ambiguity is one who knows himself
or herself and is in touch with a central source of
insight that enriches life, connects with others, and
guides his or her being. The nurse who has a clear
focus for nursing and for his or her practice is able to
examine aspects for which nursing has legitimate accountability and explore practical ways to develop
helpful influence in practice settings.

Ask yourself the following questions and write about
your responses. What values are most important to me
as a person? What are my most basic beliefs about
nursing? What is the central purpose of nursing? As a
manager, how can I best support this purpose? How
can I become more caring for myself and more helpful
to others? What can I do to be more in touch with what
is important to me and to nursing? How can I support
myself and others in these difficult times?

ME PARKER

◆ HOW DO I COMBAT DISSATISFACTION AND WEARINESS WITH MY JOB?

Q I'm tired of being a nurse manager, but I believe
that if I leave my position I will never be able to

find another role that gives me as much freedom or pays as well. What should I do?

A Career decisions are difficult to make. By identifying the components of the position that are causing you to want to leave the position, you will help to determine if these are issues that may be addressed and improved. In many situations, responsibilities continue to be added to the point of unrealistic expectations. The expectations are often self-generated. When work begins to affect one's personal life to the point of frustration and thoughts of leaving, it is definitely time to reassess the role, your personal goals, and your expectations. The following points may be considered:

1. Review your current job description to determine if the job has expanded to include added responsibilities.
2. Keep a time log for at least a week to assist you in defining how you are spending your time.
3. Assess the time log to identify areas that may need to be addressed. (What activities are preventing accomplishment of the things that are important?)
4. List your options, with advantages and disadvantages of each option.
5. Identify those areas that need to be addressed and schedule an appointment with your director to discuss possible alternatives.

You must reassess the reasons you want to be a manager. Money and freedom are important factors. However, to be an effective manager and leader one must be committed to the principles of management and leadership.

A vacation in a peaceful setting is often helpful when one needs time to think and plan.

SH SMITH

◆ IS IT EFFECTIVE TO HAVE ONE MANAGER OVER SEVERAL UNITS?

Q My hospital is planning to decrease the number of nurse managers. Then each manager will be responsible for several units. Is this effective, or can it lead to burnout?

A There are a number of issues that need to be resolved before this can work:
1. Both the staff and the manager need to be very clear on the role of the manager. They all need to

know that she is a manager, that managing is her priority, and that she is not the clinician. Many head nurses who have played a clinician's role along with a coordinator's role find the transition very difficult, and so do their staff.
2. Changes in the role of the staff nurses need to be clearly articulated, and the nurses need to be educated to help them make the change. The new role must be explained to other health professionals so they can adjust their expectations.
3. A good clinician must be in place to take on the role that the head nurse had previously filled. The staff need the clinical support to learn new skills and maintain old ones.
4. To be successful, the manager must be educated to do the job. Many promotions occur with no background, training, or in-service instruction for the new role. An ongoing leadership program and peer support are very helpful, as are role models and mentors.
5. The manager needs to be able to communicate readily to both her staff and her supervisors and to have immediate access to the resources that are required to manage her units.

Reducing the number of unit managers becomes a problem when one manager is expected to fill several positions with no other supports. There is only so much work that one person can do, and only so much work that can be delegated to the staff nurses. If too much work is delegated to the staff in addition to their existing work load, and if senior management has not replaced the unit managers whose positions have been eliminated with other types of nurses or workers, the unit manager and the staff nurses are primed for burnout.

JB COLTRIN ET AL.

◆ WHAT CAN I DO TO BOOST MORALE?

Q My medical/surgical unit is chronically short staffed. The nurses are overworked and tired and display low morale. Hospital administration states there is a budget crisis and a hiring freeze. What can I do to boost morale and create a healthier environment?

A The situation described in this scenario is one of the most difficult for the manager to handle.

B

The following list of suggestions may work in some situations and not in others, depending on the actual work environment.

1. *Dealing with reality.* Given that nothing can be done to increase staffing and that this is the reality of the situation, discover how much worse the situation is being made by absenteeism, poor teamwork, disorganization, and other issues that are under the control of the staff and manager. In any situation, determining what you can change, what you cannot change, and how much impact your changes will have is the most important first step.

2. *Redesigning the work.* Is there any activity (e.g., telephone calls, interruptions, or documentation) that if altered would give staff more time? Rather than large increments of time, look for small amounts of time that can be salvaged on a constant basis. Are volunteers used as much as possible? Can a volunteer staff a visitor desk closer to the unit elevator to handle all deliveries and visitor information and requests? Can volunteers deliver patient education materials to patients' rooms or give them to families for nurse follow-up? Can unit clerk job descriptions be revised to give them more decision-making authority than they currently have? Can time needed for documentation be reduced by using a checklist charting system at the bedside, using problem-oriented charting, and removing all duplication? Can physician communication forms be placed on all charts when nurses need to ask nonurgent questions? Are there pull-down wall charting desks outside each patient room? Can each fifth or sixth room be made into a miniature nursing station complete with limited narcotics supplies, ice box, and computer to decentralize the nurses to where the patients are?

3. *Dealing with low morale.* Although it is very difficult to deal with low morale when a unit is chronically short staffed and nurses are tired, a caring manager can often work wonders. When there are no alternatives and decreased staffing is the reality, the sense of achievement gained by recognizing reality and working as a team to make the situation bearable is a great morale booster. When all other issues (absenteeism, poor organization, and work redesign) have been taken care of by the manager and staff working together, teamwork and collaboration can thrive. Crucial to success is the ability to reward, praise, and have fun. The manager will need to foster comraderie, perhaps with competitions

such as "recognize that baby" and "clinical whiz of the month," or birthday and service recognition on a consistent basis. The manager must recognize every example of team building and collaboration that occurs. The values of the unit and its culture must become matched; the attitude should be, "United we can handle anything; we are the best." Jokes, cartoons, and posters need to be positive and demonstrate ability to work together to achieve success.

S LENKMAN

◆ HOW CAN I HELP MY STAFF ACCEPT CUTBACKS THAT WILL INCREASE THEIR WORK LOAD?

Q Whenever there is a budget crunch at my hospital, nurse managers are expected to reduce spending by eliminating overtime, reducing agency usage, or cutting staff. Care expectations, however, do not change. Staff go home exhausted and dissatisfied. How can I help the staff cope with the pressure, this increased work load, and the feelings of frustration?

A First and foremost, *you* must be comfortable with the administrative decisions to cut back on resource allocation. From your question, I am not sure that this is the case. It is important to evaluate organizational directives that you receive as a manager and to determine if they fit with what you believe is ethical. Kenneth Blanchard and Norman Vincent Peale (1988), in *The Power of Ethical Management,* provide managers with an ethical checklist to use when evaluating organizational decisions:

1. *Is it legal? (Existing standards)* Will the decision to cut back violate civil or regulatory standards, your hospital's policies, or your nursing practice standards?

2. *Is it balanced? (Sense of fairness and rationality)* Is the implementation of cutback decisions equally fair to all groups involved? Are some of my nurses suffering more than others? Are some hospital departments suffering more than others? Are the decisions part of an overall strategy for survival or an automatic, "quick-fix" approach to the situation? Is there a balance between a short-term

strategy and the long-term view? Are the decisions implemented in a win-win manner?

3. *How will it make me feel about myself? (Personal values)* Will my management of these decisions make me feel proud? How would I feel if my method of implementation were published in a professional journal? Would I feel good telling my friends and family about it?

If your ethical audit reveals that you are comfortable with the decisions, then you will be able to support your staff. By creating a climate of open dialogue and debate, and by setting a positive example, you can create opportunities for individual and group problem solving. Staff can be coached in problem solving around difficult issues. With your guidance, they can make their own decisions about how to preserve certain programs, or how to redesign patient care on a temporary basis in order to avoid fatigue and frustration. You are the role model for turning problems into opportunities.

On the other hand, if your ethical audit reveals to you that you cannot support the policies as laid down, then you must take what Warren Bennis calls the "leadership imperative" (Bennis, 1989b). You *must take a stand* and actively work to change the approach to resource management. You cannot accept the argument, for example, that "every hospital in town is doing it." If the decision is wrong, the only way to make it right is to change it. Unfortunately, the reality may be that some administrators lack the courage to change their approach to resource management or to stand up to directives that jeopardize patients and their caregivers. In such a situation, you need to consider if you can continue in a management position within that particular organization.

The ethical audit is a powerful tool for the middle manager who is caught between senior management and the staff. Applying it to troubling management challenges is sure to lessen some of the stress in middle management roles, as well as point to the direction for needed changes.

CK WILSON

♦ **HOW DO I CREATE SUPPORT FOR STAFF WHO ARE WORRIED ABOUT BURNOUT?**

Q How can I create a support network for new staff worrying about feeling overwhelmed and worried about burnout?

A A preceptorship program is an effective approach for successful competence building and retention of new staff. If such a program isn't in place in your institution, changes in the characteristics of patients in the past few years (increasing acuity, increasing percentages of surgical interventions, and earlier discharge) make the development of a staff peer support system vital.

The peer support groups are ideally unit based. If there are not sufficient numbers of new staff nurses, it may be necessary to bring together staff from several units. Initially, the group should meet once a week for an hour, with gradually diminishing frequency as time goes on. A facilitator who is not in a position to evaluate the participants ensures a safe environment and structures the experience to enhance group development.

In the group meetings, the new staff have the opportunity to vent their frustrations, compare notes, gain insight into working within the system and affecting it, explore authority relationships, and understand and solve problems. Members offer suggestions to each other. There is an opportunity to share situations that were handled especially well, as well as those that were problematic.

Such groups are well worth the investment. The competence and self-esteem of new staff are increased, and retention is more likely.

J HIXON

Career Advancement

♦ **IS AN ADVANCED DEGREE NECESSARY TO GET AHEAD?**

Q I have heard that an advanced degree in nursing is required for career advancement. Is this true? Are there any alternatives available to me other than a master's in nursing that would help me advance in the nursing profession?

A The only thing that is and will continue to be required for career advancement in nursing management is the acquisition of certain skills and

C

knowledge bases. The route you choose to gain that information is becoming less important than your ability to demonstrate integration of those new skills into your daily work challenges. With that said, don't be misled into thinking that no formal graduate education is expected. The fact of the matter is that some type of master's degree, whether in nursing, business administration, or health administration, is expected and considered a minimal requirement for significant advancement opportunities in nursing management and administration. The volume and complexity of the knowledge and skills needed to be a good manager in today's challenging health care world are increasing. A master's degree will provide you with a solid foundation that you will continually need to update—through both formal post-graduate courses and challenging continuing education offerings. Experience is a wise educator also, but the days are gone when we can afford to always learn lessons through experience. We need to be "ahead of the curve," and that means that we must learn to anticipate the challenges that managers will face and try to develop and implement strategies that will prevent problems before they occur.

In choosing an educational track to pursue, consider what your current strengths and weaknesses are. Attempt to match a curriculum to your specific needs. There are some general areas of management that everyone will need to learn, but there are also unique challenges and issues that are faced only within a health care setting. As you already know, health care is different in many ways from other industries. We need to expose ourselves to the lessons learned and ideas generated in these other industries, but we need to balance that exposure with specific knowledge and information generated in our field. That balance has historically been achieved through the acquisition of a master's degree in nursing with generous numbers of electives in business, finance, and general health care administration. It is possible to achieve a similar balance through other combinations such as a master's in business administration with elective focus in health care and nursing-related courses. What is most important is the acquisition of a broad-based education that addresses both general and specialist management needs and complements your personal achievements to date.

CCC LEVENS

◆ WHAT SHOULD A GOOD RESUMÉ CONTAIN?

Q What are the fundamental elements of a good resumé for a nurse manager who wants to move into a new leadership role?

A A good resumé usually has four distinctive parts: a clearly stated job objective, a career summary or highlights of qualifications, a chronologic work history, and a listing of relevant education and training. Personal style or taste may dictate other entries, but these four are essential.

As an interviewer who has seen hundreds and hundreds of resumés, I value simplicity, clarity of purpose, and readability. A quick look should tell the reader that you have the right educational background—or a defensible equivalent. The second inspection would be for a work history written in a way that focuses attention on strong points and accomplishments. In your efforts to exhibit your leadership, versatility, or energy, you may wish to show participation in both work and community environments.

There are many good books on the market to guide you in preparing a resumé. Find the style that best suits you. Avoid wordy jargon. Keep it simple, and look forward to the interview!

MA SORENSEN

◆ IN PREPARING MY RESUMÉ, WHOM SHOULD I LIST AS REFERENCES?

Q I am writing a resumé for possible advancement in my institution. Should I consult the people I want to use as references before listing them? How many references are appropriate? How many past jobs should I have references for?

A First, it is presumptuous to take for granted that others will be delighted to speak in your behalf. Second, it is a matter of courtesy to allow the people you expect to eloquently describe your talents the opportunity to think about what they want to say before they get the phone call, the letter, or the visit from your interviewer. It is also a good idea to let them know something about the position you are applying for, how you have prepared yourself for the advancement, and what you could bring to the position.

If you are seeking advancement in your own institution, most likely you are known by a number of people with whom you interact daily. Your skills, attitudes, and behaviors speak for you. But choose your additional references with an eye toward what the position is, how these people know you, and· what abilities, aptitudes, and talents they have witnessed in you. Committee work may have provided excellent exposure.

If your tenure in your present environment is very short, you will need to provide references from a previous environment. I recommend the same guidelines: someone you have worked with, someone you have worked for, and someone who has witnessed your performance as a leader, facilitator, educator, or whatever role you are aspiring to. Very old references will probably have relevance only if you have not worked for a long time or have not had the opportunity to use a skill for a long time. Specific additional references may be needed, but these should be defined by the interviewer.

MA SORENSEN

♦ **HOW DO I CHOOSE BETWEEN TWO CANDIDATES WHO SEEM EQUALLY DESERVING OF PROMOTION FOR THE ONE POSITION THAT IS AVAILABLE?**

Q I have two equally qualified candidates for promotion to assistant manager on my unit. They are both excellent practitioners, have wonderful leadership skills, and are well respected by staff and management. My challenge is making a choice. This is an extremely difficult decision, and I do not want to disadvantage either of these candidates. Are there any insights to help me in this decision?

A Perhaps one of the greatest contributions we can make as managers and as leaders is to assist those who aspire to grow and develop into new or expanded roles. Your question suggests a sensitivity to the valuable role you can play in helping to shape the careers of these individuals. By your comments it

is clear that you have gone through a process of identifying the skills, abilities, and mind-set required to be successful in the assistant manager's position. As a result of this process and your experience with the candidates, you have concluded that they are equally qualified. At this point it is important for you to know and fully understand the policies of your institution regarding employee selection for advancement. Your human resource director should be of assistance.

An institution's promotion policies are generally very specific on this issue. In unionized organizations, seniority is most often the determining factor for selecting which individual would fill the position. A standard consideration would be whether both employees are employed full time. Although you will probably find your human resources policies very specific, the answer may be somewhat limiting.

Based on your desire not to disadvantage either of the candidates, you may choose to expand your options beyond those normally proposed and yet remain within the parameters of the policies. Consider the following possibilities.

Assuming your organizational policies are not opposed, you may wish to consider sharing the assistant manager's position between the two candidates. Such direction would require that the assistant managers and yourself operate as a management team and that you all establish very clear means of communication. Depending on the needs of your staff and unit, this may be an effective way to advance both individuals and also model team development for the staff.

In the event one candidate is selected over the other, the individual not selected does not necessarily have to be disadvantaged. In your role as nurse manager you may choose to establish a mentoring program, under a collaborative or shared governance model, to assist in developing the careers of those individuals on your staff who aspire to advance. Implementing a shared governance model on the unit should not only involve members of your staff in decisions but also assist them in developing skills and experiences that will better prepare them for advancement.

Finally, although you have only one assistant manager position available on your unit, there may be other positions available in your organization. Work with other nurse managers to assist in placing one of your candidates outside of your unit. Your seeking opportunities for the individual and speaking out forcefully about her abilities and contributions

C

should help that person to be considered for other opportunities in the organization.

GA ADAMS

♦ WHAT EXPERIENCE, ACTIVITIES, AND EDUCATION WILL HELP ME TO BECOME A NURSE EXECUTIVE?

Q I am currently a nurse manager. I like the management process and am looking forward to moving toward the nurse executive role. What mix of experience, activities, and education will help me in this process?

A A nurse executive's education, experience, and background are often as diverse as the personalities of the individuals chosen to take on this extremely challenging and demanding role. To reorient your career direction to assist you in becoming a successful nurse executive, you might explore the attributes of the successful nurse executives you know. There should be many highly visible, acknowledged nurse executives you might observe to determine what attributes they possess and use in the role.

Clearly and foremost, the successful nurse executive is called on to be a leader. Many technically competent individuals have failed in the position because they were not versed in leadership skills. As leaders, nurse executives must have a strong commitment to the profession of nursing and be capable of articulating that commitment through their overall, unbiased vision for the institution's nursing organization. They must have the ability to communicate this vision and to gain support from the nursing organization as well as other important constituents within the organization. As with all leaders, the nurse executive must be persistent and consistent. The ability to remain focused and to maintain the course toward both institutional and organizational goals and objectives is absolutely necessary for anyone who is responsible for leading large numbers of people. Finally, as a leader the nurse executive must be capable of developing the appropriate environment to empower the staff and to tap and harness the energies and abilities of the members of the nursing organization.

As administrators, nurse executives must have a framework for incorporating the practice of nursing into their administrative role. In other words, they must continue to understand the components of care delivery and professional practice as they influence or make administrative decisions at the senior level. Like all senior administrators, they should possess strong skills from other disciplines, including finance and business. A successful nurse executive should also be adept in managing change, selling, negotiating, and public relations, as well as having a sense of entrepreneurship.

In addition, the following recommendations should assist you in planning a career in nursing administration:

1. Seek experiences and opportunities that will allow you to develop and optimize your leadership abilities. Successful leaders must be willing to take risks. Prepare yourself to take risks as you take on each new job opportunity or assignment.
2. Focus on being a good communicator. Endeavor to constantly improve your oral and written communication skills.
3. Identify yourself as a change agent. Changing for the sake of change is disruptive and, at the very least, costly; however, in today's world and within the current health care environment, we are called on to be authors of change. Any successful leader or administrator must be skilled in managing change and minimizing any negative impact on the organization.
4. In choosing a graduate education program, it is important to choose one that provides a solid education in nursing and nursing administration. However, it is equally important for the program to offer access to rigorous training in business, public health, and health care administration.
5. Work now to develop your skills in conflict management, negotiation, and sales. For some individuals these skills seem to develop through their cultural and life experiences. For others, mastering them requires a very defined and conscious effort.
6. As a nurse manager, now is the most opportune time for you to begin developing a variety of strategies for getting involved in the practice and management of nursing. Experiment with different models. As you examine what works for you in managing a clinical unit, evaluate your current nursing administrator. Do you perceive this person as an advocate for nursing? Is this individual in touch with the clinical needs of the nursing organization? Assuming that the individual

is, what structure or model has she created to operate within a clinical and management framework?

GA ADAMS

Career Ladders

◆ CAN CLINICAL LADDERS BE ESTABLISHED IN SMALL HOSPITALS?

Q I work in a small hospital (fewer than 80 beds). Is it possible to establish a clinical or career ladder program in a hospital this small?

A Clinical ladders are generally viewed as a method to recognize clinically proficient nurses who wish to remain in the bedside practice while still receiving professional advancements and financial enhancements. In many settings this vertical ascension method for caregivers has been successful. In others some cautions have been advanced.

There is a plethora of literature available on this topic. Multiple models and variations have been described: models that incorporate all caregivers, such as RNs and LPNs; those that encompass other professional disciplines within a hospital; and those that reference particular hospital capacities.

The core concept within a clinical ladder system is recognition with financial remuneration of the staff's clinical competence at the bedside. Ask the staff if this is the recognition and reward system they would like to see implemented. What is the fiscal impact of this approach? Does it respond effectively and appropriately to the previously identified program objectives and outcomes?

Newer concepts are emerging on the national agenda for professional nursing; these include differentiated practice and financial models that include gain sharing, incentive pay, criterion-based performance with financial adjustment, and patient-centered or patient-focused models. These are worthwhile exploring as part of your decision making. Each of these has specific components for recognition of the caregivers. In addition, they influence the roles of nurses and nursing in alternative ways

that should be considered when making a fully informed program determination.

LM JOHNSON

◆ WHAT ELEMENTS SHOULD BE IN A CAREER LADDER FOR NURSE MANAGERS?

Q What should a career ladder for nurse managers include?

A Nursing management is both an art and a science. Numerous management texts list traditional instrumental management functions such as budgeting, hiring, and evaluation processes. All of these are good foundational pieces for a career ladder; they all address the science of management.

However, moving individuals and systems into the twenty-first century requires other skills that make up the art of management. Interpersonal skills are essential to assist managers with communication, problem solving, and inspiring others to become their own best selves in a changing time. Imaginal or creative skills help to create new and innovative systems and responses to issues that arise in the changing context of contemporary society. And finally, comprehensive systems skills assist the manager to see whole–part relationships, anticipate problems before they occur, and accurately judge the impact of a strategy on the entire system. Thus a comprehensive career ladder for nurse managers must assess and reward instrumental, interpersonal, creative, and systems skills if transformation leadership is your goal.

JE JENKINS

Case Management

◆ WHAT ARE THE FUNCTIONS AND BENEFITS OF CASE MANAGEMENT?

Q What is case management? How is it different from primary nursing? What are the benefits of case management? What are the general functions of the nursing case manager?

C

A Case management is a clinical system (rather than a care delivery system) that focuses on the accountability of an identified individual or group for coordinating a patient's (or group of patients') care across a *continuum* of care; ensuring and facilitating the achievement of quality, clinical, and cost outcomes; negotiating, procuring, and coordinating services and resources needed by the patient and family; intervening at key points (and/or at significant variances) for individual patients; addressing and resolving patterns in aggregate variances that have a negative quality–cost impact; and creating opportunities and systems to enhance outcomes.

In contrast, care delivery systems refer to the staffing and assigning of direct patient care. Care delivery systems tend to be unit based, whereas case management covers transitions across units and beyond acute care. A CareMap system greatly facilitates direct care delivery systems in the following ways identified by Kathleen Bower (1992):

1. Standardized critical path or CareMap tools can be developed for approximately 60% to 80% of a patient population.
2. The system represents an approach to achieving *continuity of plan.*
3. It represents the integrated plan projected by the various disciplines providing care to patients.
4. The system is part of a clinical process that begins with assessing a patient's needs, issues, and strengths; proceeds through developing desired outcomes and a plan to move toward them; and continues on through evaluation and revision.
   a. Critical path or CareMap tools must be revised to reflect the needs of individual patients and situations.
   b. The tools strengthen the evaluation portion of the process.
   c. They provide a communication vehicle within and between disciplines.
5. The system implies a mind-set shift from staff nurse as clinician to staff nurse as clinical manager of care. Critical path/CareMap tools are not a substitute for clinician judgment.
6. Such a system must be integrated with other organizational strategies to manage the care of patients and evaluate the effectiveness of that care. Critical path/CareMap tools cannot be dropped into an otherwise unchanged environment.

7. Critical path/CareMap tools are *not:*
   a. Case management.
   b. A nursing care delivery system.
   c. A substitute for a well-developed accountability system.
8. Patients deserve, need desperately, and have a right to expect that the nursing care delivery system provides a registered nurse who will do the following:
   a. Coordinates their care, both within nursing and with other disciplines.
   b. Has continuity with them, and as a result
      ♦ Develops a therapeutic long-term relationship.
      ♦ Identifies subtle as well as obvious changes in condition (including physical and psychosocial or spiritual changes).
      ♦ Evaluates the plan of care and its effects and then modifies it.
      ♦ Does not need to constantly catch up with the patient, only to then leave the case.
9. In nursing, unit-, area-, and discipline-based care coordination plays out in four ways:
   a. It does not happen.
   b. The nurse manager or head nurse takes the responsibility.
   c. Primary nursing is used.
   d. A patient care coordinator is assigned.
10. Today, the real challenge is to develop nursing care delivery systems that provide at the patient–nurse level:
    a. Accountability.
    b. Coordination.
       ♦ Within nursing.
       ♦ Between disciplines.
       ♦ Throughout the unit or area based on length of stay.
    c. Continuity.

All patients need to have their care managed, but not every patient needs a case manager.

1. Case management is a strategy for *specific patient populations,* in general less than 20% of the total population.
2. Patients who are within high-cost and/or high-risk populations are often identified for case management. Priority *patient populations* for case management include:
   a. Patient receiving high-cost treatments.
   b. Predictably unpredictable or unpatternable patients.

c. Chronic repeated admissions.
d. Patients whose cases manifest significant variances.
e. Patients with high-risk socioeconomic factors.
f. Patients who are part of an institutional strategic mission (e.g., proposed or actual centers of excellence or product lines).
g. Patients who have multiple physicians or in whose cases other disciplines are involved.

3. It is sometimes useful to distinguish between *acuity* and *complexity* in selecting patients for case management. In general, the needs of patients admitted to a case management service are complex but not necessarily acute.

4. General case manager role functions:
a. Establishes target populations for the caseload, in conjunction with other members of the team and with institutional administrators and managers.
b. Establishes a system for coordinating each caseload patient's care throughout the entire episode of illness, spanning each geographic area in which care is provided.
c. Introduces self to the patient and/or the patient's family, explains the role of the case manager, and provides a business card.
d. Contacts other key members of the team when needed.
e. Establishes a means of communicating and collaborating with the physicians involved in the caseload.
   ◆ Shares and develops assessments, goals, and usual patterns of care for the patients in the caseload.
   ◆ Reviews aggregate variance and determines a path of action.
f. Establishes methods for tracking patients' progress through the system within each episode of illness.
g. Develops and reviews standard critical paths (CareMaps) for each stage of illness.
h. Analyzes patterns of variance from the standardized critical path/CareMap and implements strategies to resolve them. Requests the assistance of managers, administrators, and peers as needed to resolve each variance.
i. Participates in regular peer review regarding the management of the caseload.
j. Explores strategies to reduce length of stay and resource consumption within the case-

managed patient populations, implements the strategies, and documents the results.

5. What makes case management *different?*
a. The focus is on individual patients and patient populations whose care presents exceptional challenges for coordination.
b. Work is with patients across care areas and settings. Case management is episode based and continuum based.

6. A case management service is designed around three major factors:
a. The needs and characteristics of the patient population.
b. The actual and potential resources within the organization.
c. The goals for case management in general and for the specific patient population(s).

7. Case management services can be organized by:
a. Diagnoses or procedures.
b. Major diagnostic category (MDC) or major body system.
c. Age.
d. Insurer.
e. Geographic area.
f. Physician.
g. Other criteria.

8. Multiple factors will influence the size of a case manager's caseload:
a. Complexity and/or acuity of the patient population.
b. Role definition, for example, how much direct care is to be provided by the case manager.
c. The number of geographic areas or the size of the geographic area in which the case manager works.
d. Whether critical path/CareMap tools are used in the work.

K ZANDER

◆ WHO IS BEST QUALIFIED TO BE THE CASE MANAGER?

Q In a collaborative case management model, which profession do you think best prepares a person to be the case manager?

C

A Based on educational preparation and core curriculum for health professionals, the key skills and knowledge required for case management may be found within the nursing and social work disciplines. The case manager role may be viewed as a combined nurse–social worker role. However, unless the social worker has the clinical knowledge required, it is often easier for nurses to supplement their knowledge regarding the social and regulatory implications of patient care.

A college degree is viewed as valuable for case management since it proves experience in written and verbal communication, planning, organization, and analysis. Potential employers will seek individuals who demonstrate ability in assertiveness and problem solving, creativity, resource knowledge, and planning (Lowery, 1992). They will be interested in professionals who are able to collaborate, seek consensus building, and empower others. Case managers will also be expected to offer compassion and advocacy to patients while supporting them through the care process.

Regardless of the case management model implemented, the skills and knowledge needed to ensure consistent, high-quality outcomes must be comparable (Lowery, 1992).

J TROFINO

◆ IS A CASE MANAGER'S JOB MORE AKIN TO THAT OF A DIRECT CAREGIVER OR A NON–LINE MANAGER?

Q Is the role of the case manager more applicable to that of a direct caregiver or to a non–line manager such as a clinical nurse manager?

A The role of the nursing case manager has been described as a specific set of elements that constitute a process of care delivery. Because it is a process, there is simply is no "best way" to implement case management. What is important to keep in mind is the unique characteristics of the patients whom you serve and the nature of your organization, including its resources. Therefore we see case management operationalized today in the direct caregiver role, as well as in a staff position.

The American Nurses Association has outlined characteristics of case management systems and core components and role functions of case managers, along with educational preparation requirements and sample models of case management currently in practice (Bower, 1992). This is a good resource to guide decision making about the configuration of the role in your organization.

Many of the characteristics of case management systems are found in the direct caregiver role. For example, patients and their families are the central focus of case managers, who consider their clients' needs, advocate for them, and create a strong relationship with the patient and family as they move through their health care episode. The process also is strongly based in a cornerstone of professional nursing practice: collaboration with all of the disciplines involved in care as well as active work to engage them in the achievement of both quality and cost outcomes.

There are new role characteristics, which may be both unfamiliar to your bedside nurse and a challenge to your organizational resources. These include the definition of case management as episode based. That is, the case manager is focused on care provided in all areas during the health care episode, not just on a specific unit in your hospital, and must be able to move along through the system with the patient. Also, because case management focuses on putting the pieces together, the case manager must have a whole view, not just a shift focus or unit focus. This requires exposure to and education about the services available in your organization as a whole, as well as more global thinking than is required when a nurse is unit based. A third significant characteristic distinguishing case management from other systems is the emphasis on both quality and fiscal outcomes. Case managers are accountable for the procurement of and access to services for patients, as well as managing the cost of these services. They must be familiar with your hospital utilization issues, managed care contract requirements, and the problematic practice patterns of all disciplines. This information is not commonly available to the bedside nurse.

The advent of critical paths has greatly aided programs that attempt to integrate the case manager role into the staff nurse role. However, if you are considering integrating case management into the staff nurse role, you must be prepared to allocate the resources necessary for education. Also, staffing patterns must be examined so that they free the case

C

manager from nonnursing activities. Unit or team coordination responsibilities are very important for the case manager role to be effective. In addition, the organizational authority and the accountability for case management must be placed in the hands of the bedside nurse. The achievement of this outcome will be based on the degree to which you achieve consensus and role negotiation among key departments, including social services and utilization review.

CK WILSON

♦ **HOW DOES THE NURSE MANAGER SUPPORT THE NURSE CASE MANAGER?**

Q What is the nurse manager's role in relation to providing support for the nurse case manager?

A The nurse case manager in the acute care setting is relatively new, and the role will vary somewhat from one institution to another. A question of how the unit manager supports this role is important since the manager will be the key to successful implementation. The two roles should be seen as complementary: the nurse manager is accountable for managing the resources of the unit and the case manager is accountable for managing the full course of an illness within the constraints of available resources.

Care throughout an entire episode requires different support than care that is unit focused. The unit manager provides the operational support necessary for this change to occur. The following activities should provide a basis of support for the nurse case manager:

1. Integrate the case manager into the unit structure. This reinforces the case manager as a unit resource rather than an individual who functions external to the other caregivers. Encourage staff to consult with the case manager about patients requiring complex care.
2. Engage staff in actively changing the unit environment to support the principles of case management. Rather than looking at patient care in the usual shift-to-shift basis, the prehospital and posthospital care required must be considered.

Outcome planning should be far broader than what is accomplished on a single acute care unit. Integrate the nurse case manager into this educational process for the staff.
3. Understand the resources required across departments. Concentrate on those diagnoses that frequently occur in your unit. Share this information openly and routinely to facilitate the staff's knowledge-building in this area.
4. Develop close, productive relationships with other disciplines and departments. This will enhance the nurse case manager's ability to provide leadership in the interaction of these groups.
5. Provide necessary resources for education and development of staff to acquire managed care skills. Encourage attendance and participation in the development of case management plans and other organizational tools. This should include financial and contract information, which will generally be unfamiliar. Much of this work will occur in conjunction with the nurse case manager.
6. Identify resources to access or develop information regarding prehospital and posthospital status of patients, variance in practice patterns, and individual and population outcomes. Involve staff and the case manager in the use of these resources.

Without the necessary management support at the operational level, development of a successful case management program will be inhibited. Work within the quality improvement process to evaluate and audit the program's outcomes. A successful program can make a significant contribution to the hospital's success.

B FOSTER

♦ **HOW SHOULD THE CASE MANAGER INVOLVE THE NURSE MANAGER IN PLANNING AND IMPLEMENTING CRITICAL PATHWAYS?**

Q The vice president of nursing of our hospital decided that our institution should institute product line case management. We have been working on implementing this system for the past year. Our hospital now has eight case managers. They have been meeting frequently with one another but have

C

not involved the nursing managers very much. Now they arrive on our units and demand that the staff nurses follow these critical pathways. How do you suggest handling this?

A Product line case management is a clear, reasonable method to define and organize a case manager's role and responsibilities. Unfortunately, your question shows how the process of implementation (and trying not to make mistakes) can backfire. Your question can be addressed in two ways, first as to the communication style within the nursing department and the second as to what to do with the current situation.

The vice president of nursing needs to realize that case management models create a matrix model for nursing. In other words, patients need to be managed both *across* the continuum, such as across all units involved in the care of an MI patient, and *within* each unit. Therefore, in your model, the formation of the role includes several nurse managers who coordinate nursing resources for direct care around the clock, and case managers who manage the coordination of all departments across an episode of care (from entrance to exit from your hospital's system). Case managers cannot function effectively in a vacuum, and nurse managers cannot facilitate the goals of case management without knowledgeable participation in the design of the model.

The communication pattern sounds like one of passivity on the part of the nurse managers, and lack of participative management techniques on the part of the vice president. However, it is not too late to involve all the constituencies. Try addressing these questions:

1. What are the goals of *our* case management program?
2. What do the case managers add as far as continuity, accountability, and outcomes management that nursing staff currently cannot provide?
3. How are the critical pathways meant to work? Can they replace or streamline any current nursing documentation? How will they be used around the clock, 7 days a week? How will variance be handled?
4. What would be the most positive way for case managers to work with staff nurses, nurse managers, and members of other disciplines?
5. Where are the gray areas that will need some experimentation before we have final answers?

A few closing ideas. It may be time to consider getting a hospital-wide multidepartment executive-level steering committee for the case management project, and a nursing department task force for roles and responsibilities within nursing. The concept of collaboration wasn't meant for just RNs and MDs; it applies to interdepartmental communication as well. Case management is a strategy for specific patient populations for specific goals. As a structure it must remain responsive to needs and flexible to new demands. Nurse managers can provide invaluable feedback to the program.

K ZANDER

♦ **HOW CAN I EDUCATE PHYSICIANS TO UNDERSTAND CASE MANAGEMENT?**

Q Some of our physicians are still having difficulty referring patients for nurse case managers to follow. They see this as a means for nurses to control their practice. How can we help physicians understand our role?

A "The role of the professional nurse/case manager is multidimensional; however, the key components are the elements of the nursing process . . . " (Ethridge & Rusch, 1989). Physician referral to case management is not unusual, although not necessary within our institution. As the nurse case manager communicates specific nursing care issues with the physicians, this in and of itself tells the physician that her individual practice patterns are not being controlled, but that the nurse is attempting to have the physician's directives followed by the patient. In addition, as the nurse case manager cares for patients who were referred by someone other than the physician (such as staff, social worker, dietitian), communication with physicians may become necessary. In many cases, physicians who at one time were reluctant to utilize nurse case managers begin to appreciate the contribution and support that this role offers for their practice. They have come to realize that important issues such as teaching, counseling, brokering, and coordination of services can be achieved by the nurse case manager, thereby enhancing physicians' practice. This has become increasingly important since health care delivery systems are changing, with the focus on outpatient service and decreased length of stays.

DD GILES

◆ HOW CAN I HELP OTHER DEPARTMENTS BECOME INVOLVED WITH CASE MANAGEMENT?

Q Our pharmacy department is interested in our case-managed approach to delivering community-based care. They would like to become involved with us in the process; however, we are not sure how to manage this. How do we join with the pharmacy and other departments to build an integrated case management team?

A Ancillary departments can be a valuable part of the case management team. The expertise of pharmacists, dietitians, physical therapists, and respiratory therapists can be used to educate patients, as well as counsel them regarding their health care practices. A pharmacist who will make prescription deliveries to the home of a client can review the new medications with the client, as well as review what other medications the client may be taking, prescribed or not. Dietitians can work with the diabetic client at home to teach proper diet management. In our experience working with a population of clients with multiple sclerosis, exercise was found to be extremely beneficial. A physical therapist now runs the exercise class. The nurse case manager may also use these health care professionals as consultants to enhance her own practice.

DD GILES

◆ HOW CAN I HELP CASE MANAGERS COPE WITH JOB FRUSTRATIONS?

Q I work in an urban hospital that provides case-managed services to an underserved and very poor population. We have a difficult time with compliance, and our nurses are becoming very frustrated. As a manager, what can I do to help them deal with their frustration?

A The role of a nurse case manager is a supportive role that consists of brokering services for clients, rendering care, and assisting with coordination of services in the community. As a manager, you need to provide a forum for the nurse case managers to identify and discuss their personal beliefs and experiences that have led to their philosophic perspective of nursing. According to Newman, Lamb, and Michaels (1991), "The nurse case manager does not attempt to control or manage the client situation. On the contrary the nurse case manager works to build the patient's self-reliance by respecting her or his decisions and facilitating informed choices." Nurses in this role need to be taught how to let go of the control they had as acute care nurses and instead support the clients without judging the choices they make.

DD GILES

Census

◆ HOW DO I MANAGE DAILY CENSUS FLUCTUATIONS?

Q How can I manage my daily staffing needs during census fluctuation?

A The issue of staffing during census fluctuations is one that many nurse managers are grappling with today. Before exploring several approaches that have been used to deal with this problem, it would be worth your while to determine if you are experiencing fluctuations in both directions or if, like many hospitals, you have instead reached a new "floor" in your census. If you have, you may need to deal with your overall staffing resources, in addition to whatever fluctuations you are experiencing. Regarding the fluctuations, the following may be useful strategies to employ alone or in combination.

To prepare for decreasing census ("flex down"):

◆ Combine units whose census is generally low and cross-train the staff to work with any of the patient types who would be admitted to the combined units. The patients may be segregated

C

by type (e.g., orthopedic surgery patients in specific room numbers and rehabilitation patients in specific room numbers), but the areas are kept in close proximity to each other. Create a staffing pattern that is reasonable for the combined units and, if possible, keep a staff "expert" scheduled in the staffing mix for each type of patient.

♦ Create "sister" units by cross-training staff and rotate the staff between the sister units. Try to make the matches as natural as possible (e.g., ICU and CCU, medical and surgical) and see to it that the expectations for the "flex" staff are clearly delineated and that they are not asked to do anything for which they have not been prepared or trained. Establishing specific competencies for the units is helpful as a basis for coordinating training and/or assignments.

♦ Create a competency checklist for "float" personnel and be sure that any person who floats can perform all required skills. This establishes a minimal expectation for anyone who floats and for the unit to which they float. Units whose expectations or needs exceed the generic competencies (e.g., labor and delivery) need to establish a modified checklist and then only persons who can perform the entire set of competencies would be floated to those units. This strategy assumes that you have either a float policy or a float pool. It is always helpful to identify those staff who like to move around and determine what circumstances make it comfortable for them to continue to do so and to let the other staff—particularly those who need float staff occasionally—know what they can do to make their unit or area a desirable one to float to.

♦ If you have the resources to do so, you can "flex" staff on to projects that need to be done for the organization, such as preparing for JCAHO, thus eliminating the need for anyone to lose pay. If you do not or cannot put people to work on projects, you may have to establish a rotating "flex" schedule for staff either to float, if you need that, or to take time off.

To prepare for increasing census ("flex up"):

♦ Establish an internal "pool" of people who wish to work on a part-time basis. This can be tough to do if you are not able to guarantee a minimum number of hours. You may be able to establish some flexibility with your regular part-time people who would agree to be in a pool for a limited number of hours per month in addition to their regular part-time hours.

♦ Make use of the local external agency that can provide part-time help. Again, this is easier to do if you use this service on a regular basis. Depending on how tightly you have budgeted your staffing hours, this may be a valuable resource to include to some degree in any budget.

A final note on staffing for census changes. Nursing staff generally select the number of hours they work for a reason. The full-time person needs or wants full-time work; the part-time person probably *does not* want to work full time. The worst situation is one of uncertainty. Many staff can and will adjust their time commitments when they understand the circumstances and the situation is made as predictable as possible. The more information you can give the staff and the more they can be involved in the development of the system you choose, the better.

M MURPHY

♦ **HOW CAN I HANDLE VARIABLE STAFFING NEEDS WITH A FIXED STAFFING LEVEL?**

Q What do I do on a unit where I have variable staffing needs but only a fixed staffing level?

A The problem with fluctuations in census has always existed on nursing units such as labor and delivery, postpartum, and emergency departments. However, in recent years of cost efficiency the mandate to not have excess staff has become more important. The flip side of this situation is ensuring quality of care when the patient care needs exceed the capacity of the staff available to deliver care. The issue raised in the question also implies the additional dimension of involving the staff in decision making. The problem can be addressed from both short-term and long-term perspectives, but in all decisions staff need to assist in selecting the solution so they will respond more favorably to the outcomes.

In the short term, traditional solutions can be used to manage downtime for staff (periods of low census), which include tasks such as updating policies and procedures, in-service programs for reviewing old and establishing new treatment protocols, and conducting quality-improvement activities. However, for prolonged or frequent periods of low census, other strategies are needed such as the scheduling of PRN personnel who call in a few hours before their shift to see if they are needed, sending personnel home after they have begun a shift to take annual leave time, and/or scheduling staff using flextime or partial shifts. These latter methods of dealing with low census can cause discontentment among the staff unless they were involved in setting up the program and also determining which nurses use which staffing patterns. Flextime and partial shifts should also be used to handle periods of peak census in that the PRN staff would report to work, partial shift staff would be asked to work additional time (without the need for overtime), and no staff would be sent home.

Longer term solutions may be possible if the institution is organized according to product lines, or grouping of similar services. In this situation, staff can be cross-trained and "pulled" to similar units to smooth the peaks and valleys in census across the product lines. Thus, for example, in periods of census fluctuations, a nurse is prepared to deliver quality patient care in any critical care unit. This program would require the time for orientation and training, as well as changes in appropriate staffing policies to define the units on which a staff member would be qualified to work. Again, staff should be involved, given information when hired that cross-training is a job requirement, and given some choice as to which units they might prefer.

JW ALEXANDER

♦ **WHAT RESOURCES CAN HELP ME PLAN FOR STAFFING ADJUSTMENTS WHEN I HAVE WIDE-RANGING CENSUS CHANGES?**

Q What information do I need to help me plan to adjust my staff when my census needs vary?

A This problem is a very real one and seems to have been a part of nurse staffing concerns almost since the beginning of hospitals. During the past 15 years much has been written about nurse staffing and scheduling. Much of our effort has been directed at creating flexibility and wider options for the nurse practitioner.

Today many hospitals face economic crises, and their alternatives are innovation or closure. Contributing to economic crises is labor, a major component of the health care industry, which itself is now up against economic and staffing crises. When faced with an economic crisis and the need for innovation, one must plan, analyze financial resources, implement, and evaluate. Scheduling nursing resources in a manner that (1) incorporates flexibility toward fluctuations in census and acuity, (2) satisfies nurses, and (3) fulfills patients' needs is a vital challenge in managing the health care work load.

Much work has gone into developing models for predicting census fluctuations and thereby staffing needs. By utilizing historical data and understanding any extenuating or unusual variables, you should be able to forecast census fluctuations with a reasonable degree of accuracy.

Your organization's management engineers will be able to assist you in reviewing historical trends and developing a utilization predictor model, which incorporates variables unique to your unit, physicians utilizing the unit, and your community. The advent of managed care has altered many of the traditional utilization patterns. Further, if your organization, as eventually all will, has a large population of patients insured through HMOs, careful attention must be given to change in utilization and medical practice behavior encouraged by managed care.

To learn how one organization improved its scheduling flexibility by focusing on fluctuations in census during predictable time periods, I suggest you read "Staffing According to Episodic Census Variations" (Capuano, Fox, & Gresh, 1992).

GA ADAMS

Certification

♦ **SHOULD CERTIFICATION AND ACADEMIC PREPARATION BE WEIGHED EQUALLY?**

Q Should certification and academic preparation be given equal weight for determining economic advancement in practice?

C

A While the nursing profession debates the comparable worth of certifications and academic degrees, these credentials are used interchangeably and with varying weights for economic advancement at many institutions. Both certifications and degrees are formal vehicles for communicating to the consumer that a nurse has sufficient knowledge and competency to ensure safe and superior care. Whether this care is any better or is worth more money than that provided by another licensed nurse who lacks these credentials is an issue that must be continually negotiated by nurses with health care agencies and consumers.

Either credential can be acquired by nurses in several ways: academic degrees can be obtained through traditionally structured programs, mail-order degrees, and credits by waiver or examination, whereas certifications are granted through professional organizations, government agencies, and health care institutions. Although an academic degree often costs more time and money than a certification, this is not always the case, and the expense is relative to the person; some nurses are simply not in a position to invest in a degree beyond their basic program.

The nursing profession appears to be taking direction from other professions by requiring academic degrees as a prerequisite to some certifications, like medical subspecialty boards. In this case, both certification and advanced academic preparation are used as incremental, not interchangeable, measures for economic advancement (such as nursing certifications requiring an academic degree as a prerequisite for the certification examination).

Criteria for establishing policy in this areas should address the following:

1. Who are the most appropriate people to decide the issue in your institution in light of the present composition of the professional group?
2. How relevant is the content of each credential to specific jobs?
3. What credentials are required now and will be required in the future by outside regulatory agencies? professional organizations? your institution?
4. How great is the burden of certification renewal versus the one-time investment in a degree relative to the job?
5. Which credentials do you wish to promote in your future group?

In the end, compensation for these credentials will reflect trends in the profession as well as the market.

RG HESS

◆ WHY SHOULD I GET CERTIFIED?

Q What are the benefits of obtaining CNA or CNAA certification?

A Certification is a method often used by professional bodies to ensure that a defined level of excellence or competence has been verified. Certification itself does not guarantee good performance, but it does indicate that a standard of measure has been applied to the knowledge and work of an individual.

The "certified in nursing administration" (CNA) and "certified in nursing administration, advanced" (CNAA) credentials are recognitions applied by the American Nurse's Credentialling Center for competency in nursing management. Certain prerequisites for education and role permit an interested candidate to apply for a certifying examination that tests the knowledge of the candidate regarding a variety of issues that affect the roles of the nurse manager and executive. The advanced certification (CNAA) has usually required the addition of a master's degree and an executive-level role in nursing and the completion of 50 additional examination questions on the certifying examination.

Certification is essentially an acknowledgement that certain requisites have been met and a level of understanding has been obtained. It ostensibly validates the competence and value of the individual to her peers, the patients she serves, and the organization within which she works. It simply extends recognition. More organizations are looking at certification as evidence of understanding and having achieved a specified level of competence in their leadership staff. Some institutions have begun to reward certification through increased pay or benefits. In addition, certification may have an impact on the sense of credibility peers have regarding preparation for and competence in the role to which it refers. Many career advancement programs have certification as a component of the requisites necessary to advance toward new roles with increased responsibility or higher levels of reward.

T PORTER-O'GRADY

◆ IS IT VALID FOR NURSES TO EXPECT THEIR HOSPITAL TO PAY THE EXPENSES FOR THEIR CERTIFICATION?

Q I really believe in the certification process advocated by our national professional organizations. Although the staff seems to like the idea also, they feel that it is the hospital's obligation to finance the process. Of course, there are no budgeted funds to support this process. How do I motivate the staff to become certified and renew their credentials through recertification?

A It is unfortunate that, although nursing has claimed professional status for some time, a glaring difference between nurses and other professionals such as lawyers and physicians is the idea that someone else is responsible for financing nurses' continued development. Some of this is a result of wages that, until recently, have been substandard compared with those of other professional groups. As salaries have increased during this time of change in the health care industry, nursing is offered an opportunity to broaden its definition of professional practitioner as one who takes accountability and responsibility for her own continued professional development.

As staff nurses and advanced practice nurses are brought closer into the budgeting process of hospitals that are facing reduced payments from governmental and third-party payors, the financial constraints on the industry may become apparent to them. It is essential for the nurse manager to share such information with staff, so they can accurately understand the financial status of the organization and the industry.

As the technology and science of health care continue to explode, nurses are increasingly aware of their need for continuing education to maintain competency in their work. How does the organization reward these individuals who rise above the "average" standard of practice? Do promotions and salary increases go to all nurses, irrespective of competency? If so, this reinforces the perceived need for the organization to pay for the difference in the form of a tuition payment for their certification.

How is an advanced contribution celebrated and recognized by the nursing practice? Are certified nurses marketed to the other nurses in the organization, other departments, and the public? Publications and pictures that promote certification of nurses and the work they do is another way to assist nurses with a redefinition of who is responsible for their professional advancement. If we want nurses to assume more responsibility for advanced practice, we must put organizational information systems and reward and marketing structures in place that will make certified nurses an inspiration to all other nurses in the system.

J KOERNER

◆ WHAT IS THE DIFFERENCE BETWEEN CERTIFICATION AND VALIDATION?

Q I get very tired of staff having to be certified in all kinds of clinical procedures. Is that what we really want to accomplish with certification? Can we just validate specific performance and not identify it as certification? What does certification mean in these circumstances?

A The credentialling process simply ensures that there is evidence that each staff nurse is competent to practice in her area and is knowledgeable regarding the equipment being used. Whether you choose to call that certification or validation is probably not important. Most managers consider the certification to be the license, the American Nurses Association (ANA) credential (CCRN, CEN, CORN, RNC, etc.), or any diploma or certificate declared evidence of proficiency. Validation, on the other hand, is a process by which the person demonstrates by testing or by performance that she is competent to execute procedures.

JCAHO requires that each member of the nursing staff be assigned clinical and/or managerial responsibilities based on educational preparation, applicable licensing laws and regulations, and an assessment of current competence. At Saint Joseph's Hospital of Atlanta, we have set up skills labs by division to validate and revalidate at 3 months (for new hires), 1 year, and biannually the staff in each of the clinical areas (depending on the frequency requirement of the standard). Each area has its own trainers, and the participation has been excellent. The staff clearly understand that it is not their manager's problem; it is

C

theirs. In order to receive their annual evaluation, they must have completed skills validations as well as updates of institutional requirements and an annual physical.

MA SORENSEN

♦ **DOES CERTIFICATION REALLY GUARANTEE COMPETENCE?**

Q Is national certification truly a good measure of competence?

A National certification provides evidence of a general level of knowledge within a clinical specialty. However within health care institutions, national certification does not replace competency assessment for hands-on clinical skills and performance. This assessment should be conducted within the clinical setting based on institutional policy and procedures. However, national certification can and should be utilized as a baseline qualification for employment or advancement within a particular specialty area.

C BRADLEY

♦ **HOW DO I ENCOURAGE STAFF TO BECOME CERTIFIED?**

Q I have recently assumed a nurse manager position in a critical care unit. I am the only one who has the CCRN credential. I would like the staff to attain this advanced certification, but when encouraged to do so, they respond, "Why should we? We don't get any more money for it." How do I respond to them?

A People tend to be motivated by their own needs. The nurses must realize the value of certification to their career on a personal basis. As a manager, you must determine the value of the certification of nurses to the unit and to the organization. Once the value has been defined, logical approaches may be considered. What impact does certification have on quality of patient care or on marketing the qualifications of the nursing staff for the unit?

Options include:
1. Mandate certification as a requirement to work on the unit.
2. Provide monetary recognition for certification.
3. Incorporate certification requirements into a clinical or career ladder program.
4. Continue to encourage nurses to enumerate the advantages of obtaining certification.

SH SMITH

♦ **HOW DO I PREPARE FOR THE CNA EXAM?**

Q How should I prepare for the CNA(A) examination?

A There is generally no "official" way to prepare for certification. Applying for it implies that a level of competence has been achieved; certification simply validates its presence. However, there are consistent areas of performance that are assessed in the nursing administration certification examination. It is also assumed that the educational and role prerequisites have been met before applying. That is a baccalaureate degree and manager role for the certification in nursing administration and a master's degree and an executive role for the certification in nursing administration, advanced. Application must be made to the American Nurse's Credentialling Center, Suite 100 West, 600 Maryland Avenue, S.W., Washington, D.C. 20024-2571; phone (202)554-4444.

There are a number of preparation programs that are offered periodically at different places around the country. They are usually privately sponsored, so quality and content may vary. The credentialling center cannot recommend specific programs without compromising its independence in examining and certifying. Often universities or medical centers will offer a review course if enough nurses are interested in certification.

I have always recommended that the candidate for either examination be familiar with hospital and health care operations, including staffing, labor law, finance and budgeting, standards of care, and professional standards related to the employment of nurses and the practice of nursing. The advanced examination also requires a basic knowledge of health policy, national policy issues, reimbursement, and social issues. Both examinations will have a substantial number of questions on current leadership strategies and roles.

Review of current information and concepts and a grounding in fundamental principles in these areas should be adequate as a foundation for the examination. A further review of multiple choice test taking will be helpful in preparing for the multiple choice format of the test. Most helpful is a relaxed and positive attitude toward the test. The proctors of the examination provide more than enough time to complete the exam without having to rush through the questions. The rewards in accomplishment, advancement, and personal satisfaction are certainly worth the effort.

T PORTER-O'GRADY

Chain of Command

◆ HOW DO I GET NURSES TO FOLLOW A CHAIN OF COMMAND?

Q How do I get the nurses I work with to follow the chain of command when a situation occurs with medical management of a patient that will lead to detrimental results?

A In order to get nurses to follow the chain of command in this situation, an environment of trust must be present and the nurses must be adequately educated in the process. To feel comfortable in dealing with the situation or even reporting it, the nurses must know and feel that a positive outcome will occur because of their intervention. This involves trust between all levels. The manager must empower the staff to proceed according to established policy and procedure. And the staff must trust that the situation will be taken care of once they notify the appropriate individuals.

Before all of this can happen, the nurses must be educated as to the proper procedure and chain of command. They must know who the available resources are and how to contact them. These resources can include risk management personnel, nurse managers, or off-shift supervisors. An ethics round table as well as a professional consultative service should also be available to assist the nurses through the process. The resource role is to facilitate the problem solving process so that a positive outcome can occur.

Education about the process can occur during orientation at the division level as well as at the unit level. The information should also be reinforced whenever needed. Case studies and patient care conferences could be used as methods to educate staff and management. Role modeling by management and staff utilizing the correct chain of command with positive outcomes is a methodology that can be used. Follow-up sessions with the staff are also important to ensure understanding.

Proper education, an environment of trust, and effective communication throughout the process are essential to ensure that nurses follow the correct chain of command. It is with these key elements that positive patient outcomes in this type of situation can occur.

K KERFOOT

◆ WHAT CAN I DO WHEN STAFF GO OVER MY HEAD TO MY SUPERVISOR WITH PROBLEMS I SHOULD HANDLE?

Q Several of the staff feel strongly about some staffing issues and recently have begun to bypass me, talking directly with the director, to whom I report, about their views. This is undermining my credibility and making it very difficult to solve problems in a collaborative way. How can I handle this situation?

A The staff's actions may mean many things. Among other things they may indicate that staff do not think you are taking the issues to the director; staff may feel you disagree with them and are not representing their views; they may feel you are not

C

listening to them; or they may think they are helping you to get your message across to the director.

Sit down with your staff and tell them how you feel. Try saying the following:

I feel undermined when you go to the director to talk about unit issues and do not include me. I expect that if you feel the director needs to be involved in unit matters that you first discuss this with me and that we negotiate our strategy. There are times when it might be more helpful for me to ask one of you to come with me to talk with the director. You have a unique perspective on staffing that I do not have. However, we need to agree on who will present what and how we will support each other's positions. We also need to be clear on points we disagree on in advance and not use our meeting time to 'get' each other. Let's review what your concerns are and what mine are. Then let's identify who will go with me to meet with the director. The two of us will meet to plan our presentation. After the meeting the two of us will meet with the entire staff and share the outcome of the meeting.

By doing this you show respect for their opinion, but you clearly demonstrate that you are a part of this unit and will be included in the process. By stating that you and the staff representative will meet with the rest of the staff after the meeting, you also are showing respect for the staff's need to know about the decisions resulting from the meeting.

It is important for you to recognize that there will be times when the staff should be free to meet with the director without your being present. However, you should help them understand that if you are made aware of their concerns you will be better able to support their efforts if others question you about them. In a decentralized model, people should be free to work with whoever is able to resolve the situation.

As the nurse manager, you should also examine whether you have been forceful and convincing enough in presentations to the director. It may be that you will have to take a stronger (and riskier) position if in fact serious staffing issues are present. You should also examine how well you have given feedback to the staff. It may be that you are communicating well with the director but are not "closing the loop" with the staff in giving them information about the outcomes of your meetings with the director.

JE JENKINS

Change

♦ HOW CAN I KEEP FROM BEING OVERWHELMED BY CONTINUOUS CHANGES?

Q Change is the norm in our current environment. How can I avoid being overwhelmed by the pace of change?

A A nurse in one hospital I visited told me about a bulletin board in a nursing station on which was posted a diaper with this sign: "Only Babies Like a Change!" Fyodor Dostoyevski wrote that "Change is what people fear most." My belief is that people don't always fear the content of the change, but rather fear that the transition to the new state will be painfully mismanaged.

Think of change as having two components:
1. Content—What will be different?
2. Process—How will this affect my job?

The underlying concerns therefore are, Am I capable? and What are the rewards or losses to me and the people I care about? An astute manager will work hard to address these underlying concerns as completely as possible *before* the change, and then to build in ways to stay responsive *after* the change.

The way the transition is managed makes a lot of difference. Some classic hints are:
1. Clarify your authority bases and others' expectations of you and the staff.
2. Build on already existing strengths.
3. Be clear and honest on "before and after" behaviors you will expect.
4. Don't promise the world. Be realistic!
5. Involve the right people.
6. Inform and educate more than you think is necessary.
7. Make sure you as a manager are comfortable with the change first.
8. Build a structure for evaluation before you begin.
9. Don't ever count on 100% agreement or satisfaction with the change.
10. Remember that change is never linear (one thing at a time).

In the complex institutions providing health care, change that really matters is usually complex too. Consider how many people are affected by just changing the Kardex location or introducing new forms or a new piece of equipment. One thing in all of this is clear to me: if the nurse manager doesn't want or like the change, it will never actually occur. Your staff are watching like hawks for your true feelings and values. So when minor or major change is in the offing, look to yourself first and do your own homework to become comfortable with the change.

K ZANDER

♦ HOW CAN I HELP STAFF COPE WITH CHANGE?

Q The uncertainty and change occurring in the health care field is very unsettling. Sometimes I doubt my ability to lead others through this time. What management skills are most valuable in helping me and my staff thrive through all this chaos?

A Rapid and continuous change is now a permanent part of every manager's life. Today not only management skills are important but, in addition, leadership skills are essential. The successful manager must be able to lead change with well-developed skills in the area of facilitation, development, communication, vision, and coordination.

The manager must be able to assist staff in understanding and accepting the change while at the same time giving support so that they may verbalize their fears and concerns. The staff should be provided with an explanation of why the change is necessary and be helped to explore the impact it will have on them. Help the staff to identify the positives and negatives of the impact. If possible, include the staff in the change process so that they have some opportunity for involvement. The more involvement they have, the more ownership they will feel and the less conflict will arise. Expect conflict to be a part of the implementation. As the manager, you should feel comfortable with conflict and view it as a positive and necessary step. However, you will need to develop the change process. Staff skill development

may be necessary to smooth the change transition. In addition, you will need to provide vision and encouragement. Cheerlead the process but also assess the pace and make adjustments as needed. For every change, whether imposed or self-stimulated, a process for implementation should be initiated. The employees involved should be part of the implementation plan development. Minimally the plan should include:

1. Description and reason for change
2. Impact
3. Barriers and strategies to barriers
4. Responsibilities and accountabilities assigned
5. Steps in the implementation process
6. Resource requirements (time, expertise, etc.)
7. Education needs
8. Structure and system changes
9. Expectations and role changes
10. Time lines

SF SMITH

♦ HOW CAN I PROMOTE REVAMPING OF OUTDATED HOSPITAL NURSING PRACTICES?

Q Do you have any strategies to redirect nurse managers, administrators, and physicians to change the antiquated structure of nursing found in most hospitals?

A It seems some of us are holding solidly to antiquated ways in hopes of reducing our stress in these times of change and uncertainty. I would like to describe a method used to develop new nursing practice strategies as well as to facilitate communication among nursing staff, administrators, and physicians. This method may be effective in redirecting all involved because it offers support for each player while encouraging new, yet meaningful ways to organize and work. Revisiting the values and purposes for our work, and sharing these, can be reassuring. Remembering these values and purposes can free us to explore new structures for nursing.

1. Nurses can begin by examining the real purposes of nursing. What is the unique focus of nursing?

C

What nursing and related knowledge is essential for nursing practice? What is the focus of nursing in the hospital as you see it practiced and as you think it should be practiced? What are similarities and differences?

2. It may be useful to examine purposes and processes of other professions, especially of medicine. Since we can often more clearly define nursing by describing what it is not, it may be useful to describe the purposes and functions of medicine as non-nursing. This can also help us explore the purposes and processes shared by nursing and medicine.

3. Move on to use this approach in examining administrative structures that support nursing, including relations with administrators and physicians.

In one situation, values held by nurses led to selection of nursing theories that viewed the person as whole and unique and recognized the importance of nurses at the bedside as well as involvement of the family. Innovative practice strategies based on these nursing values included assurance that practice decisions were made as close to the bedside as possible by individual nurses and that the role of administration was clearly to facilitate nursing at the bedside by management of resources to support nursing. Nurses were more self-assured and satisfied with their nursing when they could articulate the focus of their practice. They seemed to share increased respect among themselves, and relationships with physicians were generally more comfortable. Some nursing decisions to change practice, such as means of reporting and recording, were challenged by physicians. The comfort and confidence of nursing staff assisted communication and negotiation so that changes provided opportunities for growth for physicians as well as for nurses.

ME PARKER

◆ HOW CAN I INVOLVE STAFF IN CHANGES TO BE MADE?

Q How can I help the staff I manage "see" their role in an expanded context so we can better plan changes in care together?

A Teamwork should be the guiding principle for all health care managers in this time of health care reform. In particular, nurse managers have a critical role to play in the future health care system. Nurses need to understand that day-to-day activities add up to the overall effectiveness of the organization. Involve the staff in planning and make sure they are aware of the broader political and financial issues that have an impact on their practice and the institutions they work in.

Today, nursing exists in a rapidly changing environment in which even the most seemingly inconsequential decisions can have enormous ramifications in the future. Provide leadership for staff and encourage them to keep abreast of health care reform efforts along with the goals of your institution.

P MARALDO

◆ HOW DO I COMBAT RESISTANCE TO CHANGE?

Q How do I deal with staff who have always worked at the same hospital in the same arena and believe there is only one way to do things? I am frustrated by their resistance and am getting worn out trying to cope. I need support.

A Individual behavior styles and corporate cultures of organizations are powerful components. By carefully planning for change and relating the needed change to the mission and strategic plan of the organization, you will gain support for your decision to initiate change. The proposed change should be communicated to administration and when appropriate to the nursing staff to ensure their understanding of the change and to gain their support.

The staff affected should be involved in the change process at the earliest stage possible. The staff input will be valuable to avoid serious oversights during the implementation process. Be aware that normal emotions accompany change. Some people are fearful that they will not be able to adapt to the required change, others feel the change will only cause more confusion and interfere with rather than improve care, and still others take personal offense since they were instrumental in developing the current process.

When initiating change, the following points should be considered:

1. Be sensitive to the reasons people resist change.
2. Seek input and feedback from those affected by the change.
3. Listen to the objections; some may be valid.
4. Plan for change.
5. Allow time for the change process when possible.
6. Seek out the informal leaders and gain their support for the change.
7. Accept that some people may not be able to adjust to the change and will resort to the fight, flight, or apathetic coping mechanisms.

SH SMITH

♦ HOW DO I STIMULATE CREATIVITY?

Q How do I motivate and stimulate creativity in staff who have a history of longevity and a marked resistance to change?

A When resistance is manifest in a staff, its cause must be identified. It is unfortunate that in too many traditional systems conformity to one norm has been standard practice, with organizational policy and reward structures based on cybernetic principles. A response–feedback loop has been in place that rewards compliance with one way of being and one standard outcome. Suddenly systems are beginning to require creativity and innovation. This invitation is extended to individuals who have spent their entire career in a system seeking and rewarding conformity.

If a more spontaneous performance is desired of employees, second generation cybernetics must be introduced. In this case diversity, rather than conformity, is the goal. People are rewarded for their unique and varying contributions rather than conformity to a standard norm. Just as we encourage a small child to walk, so the manager must encourage and celebrate any small efforts that deviate from the norm but are clearly focused on a shared vision and outcome goal.

A second resistance to change is fear. If it is a fear of punishment, the manager must make clear the level of autonomy, authority, and accountability being given the staff for innovation. If it is a fear of failure, a working definition of failure must be made explicit (failure is not having tried) so that all know the standard of expectation for themselves and others. If it is a fear of appearing foolish, strong educational and support systems must be in place for those willing to risk as they learn new ways of being. These are the challenges and opportunities for managers trying to establish a new culture for innovation.

J KOERNER

♦ HOW DO I DEAL WITH STAFF WHO RESIST CHANGE?

Q How do I deal with senior, experienced nurses who resist change and are looked up to by other staff?

A This is not an uncommon situation, given the diversity of our workplace today. What is first and foremost in importance is to avoid giving in to your own feelings of frustration and labeling these senior nurses as resistant. The key question here is "what is getting in the way of these individuals' accepting change?" None of us likes change, particularly drastic change. By creating a climate that encourages dialogue and disagreement, you may be able to help these nurses to discover their own blocks to accepting the change. Sometimes senior nurses are the designated spokespersons for individuals who are less comfortable with expressing their real concerns. You may want to strengthen the work group commitment to the change by stating that there seems to be disagreement and by engaging them in an exploration of the change.

The nominal group technique is a process that could be very helpful in this situation. This tool allows you to define any issues and problems that need more discussion and will engage the group in the definition of areas of disagreement. After using this approach, you need to work to resolve prioritized problems related to the change. This approach emphasizes the equal and mutual concerns of each person about the impending change and prevents one or

C

two people from dominating the work group. The nominal group technique also places the accountability for problem solving with each individual. You might want to ask an outside facilitator to lead the discussion, depending on the intensity of the issues.

In using the nominal group technique, follow these steps:

1. *Generate Issues, Ideas, and Concerns.* You must help the group come to agreement about the perceived problems with the change. Using free-flowing discussion, engage the group in generating a list about the issues needing discussion. Write the list on the blackboard or a flip chart so that everyone can see it. Then ask each member to silently review the list and to jot down any corrections or additional ideas.

2. *Share Ideas and Concerns.* Open up the discussion once again, and add ideas to the list. Continue the process of open discussion and silent thought until no more ideas are generated. *Require that each person contribute one idea, until everyone has participated in the discussion.* There is no evaluation of the ideas presented at this point— they are simply added to the written list. The group will need regular reminders not to evaluate responses. If evaluation of ideas does occur, it will reduce the openness of the group and how comprehensive the problem list becomes.

3. *Discuss and Clarify.* This is the stage in which the discussion is opened to clarify perceptions of the issues identified thus far. The group is encouraged to ask questions about the meaning of anything on the list, as well as the context in which it was discussed. Avoid arguments about meanings and seek clarification instead. Prevent the group from engaging in evaluation. The outcome of this stage is to achieve agreement on the meaning of each idea.

4. *Prioritize Issues and Plan for Resolution.* Ask each person to silently review the list and to assign a priority to each item. Limit the selection of issues to the five with the highest priority. Ask each member to state her priorities from 1 to 5, with 5 being the highest priority. Tally the priorities for items selected. The five items with the highest tallies are the most important to the group. Once priorities are determined, move the group into problem solving for each issue.

After the work group has committed to resolving issues within the change, the senior nurses may still remain negative. At this point, individual confrontation by the manager is needed. This work may be made easier by the fact that the work group's involvement in an open discussion and problem solving process will generate peer pressure when certain members of the group refuse to participate in being part of the solution.

CK WILSON

♦ **WHAT CAN I DO TO BLOCK STAFF'S SABOTAGE OF INNOVATIONS?**

Q Sabotage of innovation by colleagues is a reality where I work. Are there any early warning signs that can help me?

A Innovation happens on the spur of the moment. There's no way to predict who will curtail it or, for that matter, who will fuel it. But *who* doesn't matter. Your ability to move the organization forward with innovation depends on *what* is done, not by whom. Evaluate your planning strategy for innovation. Don't turn this process into a witch hunt. Identify your goals, give people a chance to help you achieve those goals, and fearlessly move forward. There is no substitute for trial and error.

P MARALDO

♦ **WHAT IS THE BEST WAY TO DEAL WITH OBSTRUCTIVE PERSONNEL?**

Q I have been instructed by the nursing director to implement a new approach to patient care. Most nurses on my unit are older than I am, have worked in the area for many years, and know the doctors very well. Some say they are not going to change and that I will probably be the one to leave. How can I help encourage change to a new model without being driven out?

A To transform resistance into a sense of joint accountability and excitement for the change, the manager must possess the skills of a diplomat, the self-confidence of a tightrope walker, and the caring and adaptability of a nurse. However, successful implementation of these roles requires the active mentoring of the nursing director.

To promote this mentoring relationship, you should meet with the nursing director and ask the following questions regarding the change:

1. What is the rationale?
2. What are the specific promoting and opposing factors?
3. What is the timetable?
4. What are the available resources?
5. What approach would she recommend? (You should come to the meeting ready to suggest an approach.)

During the change process, you should meet regularly with the director to inform and brainstorm. Before these meetings, send the director written progress reports. Also, prepare possible strategies to deal with the issues you plan to discuss at these meetings.

A suggested framework for promoting shared responsibility is the "Treasure hunt change model." This model involves the following steps:

1. *Define the "treasure" and why it should be sought.* Clearly explain the change, and stress that it is vital to implementing the vision of the organization. Explain this to all who will be affected (e.g., staff, physicians, other disciplines). Also, identify how implementing this change will benefit the individuals being asked to make it. Do this in practical terms. An example might be that research has shown that the new delivery system improves staff and patient satisfaction. Another example might be that it will improve the financial status of the organization and therefore provide enhanced job security.
2. *Draw the map to get to the treasure.* Assign a task force to outline the steps to achieve the change. This group must have the autonomy to decide the best path to take. Members should include yourself, risk takers, "nay sayers," and informal leaders. In addition to the nursing team members, invite representatives from other disciplines who will be affected by the change. Provide specific objectives, a timetable, and resources.
3. *Decide how the value of the treasure will be determined.* The task force should develop evaluation tools to monitor the change for its efficiency and effectiveness. This will avoid squandering valuable resources.
4. *Send out a scouting party to follow the map.* Implement a pilot project to evaluate the planned change and make revisions to the plan as needed.
5. *Train the treasure hunters.* Success of a change is directly related to how well the participants are prepared to deal with it and to implement it. Ill-equipped treasure hunters are set up for frustration and failure.

MC HANSEN

♦ HOW CAN I HELP STAFF PREPARE TO ACCEPT ADDITIONAL RESPONSIBILITIES?

Q Our organization has experienced tremendous change in role expectations of the nursing leaders at the unit level. We have gone from "head nurses" to "nurse managers" with increased responsibilities. Our staff, predominantly prepared at the diploma or associate level, are having difficulty understanding and accepting the difference. How do we go about helping them to help us make this a successful endeavor for everyone concerned?

A When organizations go through significant change, people often exhibit a natural tendency to resist, to want things to stabilize (i.e., return to "normal," as it was) regardless of their educational background or positions. It is important to help the people who are less than enthusiastic appreciate what has *not* changed, because it has worked, as well as the benefits of the change. Ultimately, everyone needs to experience the change in a positive way. In the beginning, you may need to explicitly point out the benefits so that they will be noticed.

There are often some staff who do appreciate the change. You need to support those people and encourage them to share their perspective with others. Finally, it is a good idea to *listen* to the comments of those who voice some dissatisfaction or concern. They may have something valuable to add to the situation that you, in your enthusiasm, had not considered. Keep in mind that you do not have to have an instant answer for every challenge. It is perfectly okay, and sometimes even desirable, to back off and take time to think and then come back to the issue after you've had a chance to reflect on it and consider

C

the other's point of view before responding. Change is always difficult; be patient and persistent, and give it time.

M MURPHY

♦ **HOW CAN I SUCCESSFULLY MANAGE CHANGE WHEN MY BOSS IS NOT SUPPORTIVE?**

Q My organization is in the midst of a major delivery system change. I have learned that my boss is not actually supportive; she is providing only lip service. As a manager responsible for the program's success on my unit, what should I do?

A You are in a difficult, but common, situation. You will want to do your best to successfully implement the new system in a win–win manner. There are several ways to help you act effectively:
1. Realistically assess your boss' style and needs as best you can. Does she need a great deal of support and information? Does she prefer you to proceed independently unless you have problems? Match your reporting style to her needs. Make it your business to clarify expectations and communication to the best of your ability. Do this while making sure your boss does not lose face in any way, privately or publicly, in the process.
2. Be alert to information needs your boss has. Be as realistically positive about the new delivery system as you can, without being overenthusiastic. Endless positiveness can alienate your boss, further contributing to a closed mind. Be aware of benefits and payoffs for your unit, the patients, and your boss.

   It may be that your boss needs a chance to get used to the idea and to estimate its effects. It may be that she is uncomfortable because she herself doesn't thoroughly understand the concepts and applications. Use opportunities that come up to casually give her newly published articles and other information. As you continue to learn, you are sharing your new knowledge with her, with the emphasis on *sharing*, rather than on *teaching*.
3. Find a constructive support system for yourself. This *does not* mean that you find others to com-

miserate with or complain to. It *does* mean that you find a trustworthy, objective, nonjudgmental person who understands the system well enough to offer meaningful support on a regular basis. Ask whether this person is willing to offer this support. This gives you someone to bounce ideas off of, role-play with, and use as a reality check. Good luck in implementing this new delivery system. Remember that change is hard for people at all levels, and sometimes hardest for those in management positions. The *known* can be very hard to give up.

J HIXON

♦ **AS A NEW MANAGER, HOW CAN I CHANGE OLD ATTITUDES?**

Q I recently accepted a head nurse position with a larger scope of responsibility. In my first 3 months, I recognized that there were several employees on the off shifts with very unprofessional behaviors. However, no one has ever dealt with them. As I learn more about this organization, it seems that there is a real reluctance to "make waves" with the staff or to engage in activities that produce conflict of any kind. Yet I believe that the patient care is suffering. What should I do?

A You evidently spent the first few months evaluating your organization and your staff—now you are beginning to evaluate your role and how to make it more effective. At the same time, your supervisor and your staff have been evaluating you. It is now time for some action. You need to concentrate on changing the culture. Begin by asking everyone on your staff to individually meet with you. Have a sign-up sheet and request that everyone allocate 30 minutes to discuss unit concerns. During these meetings take the opportunity to get to know your staff members. Ask questions like "What's great about this department?" and "What do you think should be the first thing we focus on together?" While you exchange ideas, be sure you indicate to each individual that you intend to address her concerns. Then tell each person about some ways that this can be accomplished. For example, you may want to establish some unit-based committees to look at nursing practice. Check this out during these meetings to see if your idea would be supported. Staff members are generally very aware of problems affecting patient care; by establishing a committee, you can raise these concerns in a group and no one person would have to feel responsible for "making waves."

Since you've identified several employees on the off shifts as having unprofessional behaviors, pay particular attention to their interactions. Sometimes these behaviors continue because supervision has been lacking, so spend regularly scheduled time on the off shifts. If you have an assistant or a resource nurse on these shifts, communicate your requirements to her as well and give her the responsibility of addressing any inappropriate behaviors she observes.

Other opportunities to change the culture and increase levels of professionalism might include:

- Getting the staff involved in making presentations. These could be brief case reviews at staff meetings or reports from conferences they may have attended.
- Involving them at multidisciplinary rounds. This not only would provide them with good information on their patients but would allow them to contribute to the plan of care as well.
- Asking them to represent their unit on a hospital-wide committee.

Any of these related activities would work in your favor in reinforcing the need to change how things currently are. Of course you should always role model behaviors and coach your staff along. Of primary importance is how you now regard and treat staff who are making progress with you versus those who are not. If you have been clear with your expectations and are fair in your interactions with the staff, they will grow to respect your judgment and will want to work with you toward further improvement. Remember that this process takes time. Don't get discouraged by individuals who continue to test you. Be firm and consistent with your requirements, recognize and reward your good employees, and remind yourself often that ultimately, the patients will gain from all your efforts.

One final comment on making waves—be sure to keep your supervisor informed of all of your actions; that way, if conflict should arise, you will have the support of your boss.

V MANCINI

Clinical Nurse Specialists

C

◆ HOW SHOULD THE CLINICAL NURSE SPECIALIST'S ROLE BE VIEWED?

Q How do clinical nurse specialists align in an organization most effectively? Are they consultants (conventionally reporting to the chief nurse executive or the nurse manager)? What is the most effective way to utilize the clinical nurse specialist?

A The clinical nurse specialist (CNS) role varies in each organization I have worked with, and may even vary within departments in an organization. The role will evolve with the development of the staff the CNS works with. Let me try to deal with your questions one at a time.

First, the alignment of the CNS in the organization will depend on the structure and maturity of the organization (I am speaking of maturity in terms of the organization's use of advanced practitioners and of the education and experience of employees) and on the role designed for the CNS. I have worked with CNSs who were focused on staff education, others who specialized in managing complex patients, and others who worked mainly on case managing and discharge planning. Each is a slightly different role. The focus of a CNS will be narrower if staff nurses are relatively inexperienced with their patient population. The role can broaden as the staff are able to support the patients and their own educational needs. When staff are inexperienced, they will need more educational and consultative support for specific patient needs. As the staff members mature and gain experience, they begin to support new staff themselves and are experienced enough to manage most patient problems. With this experienced staff, the CNS can focus on advanced clinical issues for a broader population both on and off the home unit.

When a CNS is first introduced to a facility, it is probably appropriate to have her report to the nurse executive. However, I find that the reporting relationships can become divisive for managers and CNSs. The CNS needs to work in very close con-

C

cert with the manager of the department, supporting the patient population that the CNS works with. The level of maturity of the managers in the development of their role will also help define to whom the CNS should report. Whom the CNS reports to is probably less significant than the presence (or absence) of collegial relations between the CNS, manager, and staff. Reporting will also depend on the number of direct reports an individual can manage. If the nurse executive has a large work load, the CNS will likely have better support from a director or manager.

Further, in aligning themselves in the organization, it is important for CNSs to define their role and to share their role and expectations with clinical staff so that the CNS can be used effectively as a resource. If a CNS is to be involved in research, her work and results needs to be shared so that others understand the contribution of the CNS.

In response to the second question: I see the CNS role as a combination case manager and educator. I believe that advanced practice nurses must not only practice to support patients, but also to support their colleagues. We need role models and teachers in order to become more skilled in patient care delivery and professional practice. I do not see CNSs as "in the education department" per se; they need to be more available than that to support nursing staff and patient and family care and education. I think they are most effective when assigned to a patient population or patient care area. Utilization of CNSs will vary with facility and patient population. My preference is that nurses who function in many capacities provide patient support and education, patient assessment and intervention, staff education and development, role modeling, and clinical research. All are services we need in order to manage the patients we care for. No CNS can take on all of these roles at once, but she may focus on different aspects at different times in her own career development and that of the organization and population she serves.

I would suggest that the role of the clinical nurse specialist be defined with input from nursing staff, nurse managers, administration, and medical staff. The goal is to identify a role that will be useful to the patients and organization. Input from the individuals who are expected to use the CNS for support encourage the success of the role.

M PECK

◆ HOW CAN I JUSTIFY USE OF CLINICAL SPECIALISTS?

Q We have used clinical specialists in our hospital for a number of years; however, our chief operating officer has no appreciation for their contributions and is continually asking us to consider eliminating those positions. We have valued them a great deal but it is difficult to translate that into numbers. We are very concerned. What can we do?

A In order to justify this type of position, the role needs to be evident in relation to patient care. Whether the clinical nurse specialist directly provides patient care, provides staff development to improve patient care, or enhances systems or standards to improve care, this must be made clear. The clinical nurse specialist's role should be evaluated by staff nurses, patients, and nursing managers (depending on whom the role serves). Those people can best explain the value of the role to the organization. Each role in today's organization must contribute to cost effectiveness and quality of patient care as defined in the hospital and nursing department strategic plan, or the position faces possible elimination. These roles are very important and, if well performed, will meet individual organizations' needs. Clarify and articulate your needs and describe how the clinical nurse specialist meets them.

D SHERIDAN

Coaching

◆ HOW CAN I HELP MY STAFF FIND ANSWERS TO THEIR PROBLEMS?

Q How do I ask the right questions to assist in encouraging my staff to find their own answers?

A New organizational models, quality improvement initiatives, self-directed work teams, and professional practice models in nursing all require the nurse manager to actively engage in staff development. To do this, you must be prepared to act as a coach and to be skillful in the application of key facilitation skills. Coaching is a purposeful relationship between the manager and employees. It may involve problem solving over a performance issue or how to negotiate organizational politics, or it may involve teaching new technical skills. Regardless of the nature of the problems, the coaching is entered into by the employees. Your role as the manager and coach is to facilitate the exploration of the issue so that the employees are successfully guided through their own thinking and problem solving. Together, you will develop insight or information (in the case of teaching); this should help the staff plan strategies for problem resolution.

Facilitation skills and experience in applying adult education principles are necessary for effective coaching. There are four basic facilitation skills applied to the coaching process:

1. *Active Listening:* Showing you are paying attention, being fully present in mind and body.
2. *Clarifying:* Restating in your own words what you are hearing to enhance and validate understanding.
3. *Summarizing:* Pausing in the conversation periodically, so that what has been identified or decided is verified and understood.
4. *Using Open-Ended Questions:* Purposefully asking questions that require thought and dialogue rather than "yes" or "no" answers.

There are other skills that can also help you increase your effectiveness as a coach. You may find that you could benefit from more training in facilitation skills. Contact clinical nurse specialists prepared in behavioral health, in your organization or your community, in order to locate training opportunities.

As a manager you probably feel pressed to provide the answers. Remember that coaching fails when the coach is much more focused on getting the "right" answer than on allowing an employee to struggle through finding the answer.

For example, an employee may be struggling with understanding the value of a new program. We are tempted to label this behavior as resistance. Instead, the manager-as-coach will ask the question: "What is getting in the way of this person's comprehending the value of the program and participating in it? By creating a climate that permits open discussion, expression of doubts, and even disagreement, the manager creates opportunities for the employee to become involved in exploring the reasons for not participating in the program. Together, the coach and the nurse may identify serious misinformation, fears about being unable to develop the skills needed for participation, or personal problems interfering with the need to accept change at work.

One word about dealing with personal problems. The coach works with the *whole person.* If a personal problem is the source of work problems, it is appropriate to identify that and refer the person to the appropriate resources. Too many times we shy away from this difficult situation, but it may be the core of the issue.

In order for a manager to help employees to find their own answers, a coaching role should be assumed. This means replacing controlling and directing of employees with coaching and facilitation and mutual collaboration. Remember: people can never be forced to find their own answers, but they can be stimulated to use their energy in the development of problem-solving expertise and self-confidence.

CK WILSON

◆ HOW CAN I BRIDGE THE GAP BETWEEN STAFF WHO ARE ACTIVELY INVOLVED IN MANAGEMENT AND THOSE WHO ARE NOT?

Q All managers have some staff nurses who are active and participate and others who choose not to participate. How can I, as a manager, encourage peer support of those who choose to become actively involved? It appears, at times, that there are too many nurses out there who don't care to get involved, resent the higher expectations, and look at their colleagues' involvement as dumping more of a clinical work load on them. How can I help both groups bridge their gap more successfully?

A A nurse manager's role would be far less complex and stressful if nurses entered the profession with a sense of belonging and moved from mutuality and acceptance of one another up the hierarchy of needs to professional self-esteem and ultimately to professional self-actualization. However, in reality there are many professional nurses who choose to remain at the lower levels of the professional hierarchy (survival and security) and never advance beyond that point for multiple and varied reasons.

Both of your questions can be answered by identifying accountability for professional practice and consequences for lack of that accountability. Nurse administrators and managers have, until the relatively recent past, rewarded task-oriented, standardized procedures and processes based on manual dexterity and precision while also supporting a clear division of work. Rewarding such thinking and behaviors denied professionals' need for interdependence, shared commitment, and affiliation. What nurse managers have learned over time is that there are many roads to their goals. Motivation, self-esteem, and trust come both from within the individual nurse and from the professionalism fostered on the individual unit. Some professional nurses will refuse to contribute to their unit and profession beyond basic expectations and will express feelings of powerlessness and victimization if they are requested to move beyond those basic expectations. Some nurses will always have a selective perception, be that high or low, regarding the criteria for professional accountability. Such variations add to the challenge of the nurse manager's job in orchestrating staff harmony and coordination.

Three helpful hints for the nurse manager in these areas are:

1. Be very clear on what makes up satisfactory professional behavior and competence on the unit. These behaviors and competencies need to be identified in outcome-oriented results, including the perspectives of quality, quantity, time, and cost. Responsibilities need to be realistic and progressive, with progress measured at regular intervals, beyond and outside of the annual appraisal process.

2. Offer varied options for demonstration of those behaviors and competencies. Some nurses will chose to demonstrate them at the survival and security level of task-oriented and technical care and advocacy, whereas others will demonstrate those competencies at a higher level of professional participation and self-actualization. What is important to emphasize here is that any of the defined options, once agreed upon, are acceptable, and if they are not met, the nurse manager will confront the issue and predetermined unit-based or personal consequences will be activated. Nurse managers have often been inconsistent in the past either by not defining the acceptable expectations clearly or by identifying, but not implementing, the consequences when lack of staff nurse accountability was apparent.

3. Evaluate your unit for role confusion, current trust level, degree of threatened self-interest or fear of failure, knowledge or communication deficits, false assumptions, inaccurate perceptions of intended changes, diversity of perceptions, unrealistic expectations, and basic differences in interests or goals. As with most management models, it is better to deal with weaknesses or issues inherent in the unit structure before beginning to address professional motivation, mutuality, acceptance, and self-actualization issues. After the nurse manager is assured the unit is functioning at a high level of professional performance, then the less motivated individual staff nurses can be asked what they are doing to improve their personal level of practice, how they have contributed to the unit and the profession, and in what specific ways they are going to improve practice and reconfirm their professional commitments.

BV TEBBITT

◆ HOW CAN I HELP STAFF DEVELOP ORGANIZATIONAL SKILLS?

Q How can I assist the less experienced staff on my unit in developing organizational skills in managing a group of patients? They need coaching in problem solving, prioritizing, and organizing.

A Staff can develop organizational skills for managing multiple patients by (1) using appropriate staff as role models; (2) practicing time-management techniques; (3) acquiring proficiency in clinical skills, particularly those that are usually time consuming for the novice; and (4) gaining varied experiences.

1. Lengthy orientations and formal preceptor programs are effective but self-limiting and expensive. When these resources run out, arrange for a balanced distribution of experienced and less experienced staff when assigning patient care. Foster an atmosphere of collegial support and consulta-

tion, not criticism and competition, and encourage team spirit.

2. Teach time-management techniques to new staff, including
    ♦ Planning the shift in advance by separating activities into categories of "must do" and "nice to do."
    ♦ Delegating appropriate activities to ancillary staff.
    ♦ Accomplishing multiple tasks at one time when entering a patient's room.
    ♦ Collaborating with other staff to save time and learning how and when to say no to those who unnecessarily waste staff's time.

3. Provide early practice opportunities necessary for staff to become proficient in tasks such as inserting IVs and NG tubes, and in more complex skills, such as documentation. These activities tend to dominate a new nurse's time and inhibit further organizational development. A mutual assessment by you and new staff nurses should easily generate an appropriate list of problem skills.

4. Provide increasingly complex, but controlled, challenges in patient assignments for less experienced staff. Staff are generally more willing to tackle complex problems if they perceive that support is easily available. Take advantage of patient rounds to help nurses prioritize their work. Frequent scheduled opportunities, designed explicitly to evaluate their management of patients, are helpful, particularly if the sessions are expected and nonthreatening.

RG HESS

♦ WHAT DO I DO ABOUT STAFF WHO ACCUMULATE EXCESSIVE OVERTIME?

Q How do I approach a staff member whose skills and work performance are excellent but who accumulates excessive overtime?

A It is common for nurses to assume that clinical practice issues supersede all other performance factors. For this reason overtime and other behavioral problems such as excessive absences are often left unaddressed. This is unfortunate, since such issues affect the overall level of unit function and may lead to morale problems with the rest of the staff.

The question implies that this is your first counseling session with the employee. Factors you will want to consider in developing an approach are how long standing the problem is, what actions, if any, have been taken by previous managers, and how any other overtime problems on the unit have been handled.

Set aside uninterrupted time and meet with the employee. As basic as it seems, you should clearly define what constitutes excessive overtime. Staff's perception of *excessive* may differ significantly from that of the manager, who is accountable for managing the unit resources. In the first session get the practitioner's view of why this problem is occurring and what might be helpful regarding its management. If the problem is of relatively recent onset, has anything occurred in the staff member's work or personal life that lends itself to a particular solution?

Present your perspective of the situation from a management point of view, focusing on how this problem extends beyond the caregiver and affects the work environment on the unit. At the end of the meeting, a clear direction should be set.

1. Establish specific goals and outcomes related to the use of overtime. These should be clear, measurable, and not open to negotiation.
2. Set time frames for regular evaluation, using the established goals as a guide.
3. Define next steps if outcomes are not met. Be sure to familiarize yourself with personnel policies in regard to progressive discipline to ensure consistency should initiation of the policy become necessary.
4. Write an account of the session to be signed by both you and the employee so that expectations are clear and not subject to misinterpretation of what was said.

Follow up meticulously. Receiving the message that handling this issue is important is part of the learning process for the employee.

B FOSTER

♦ HOW CAN I DISCOURAGE A VACATIONING NURSE FROM CHECKING UP ON HER UNIT?

Q One nurse on our unit always calls in numerous times during her vacation to see how things are and if she is needed. She has even visited the unit at

C

times when she was on vacation. Is this appropriate? If not, how should I respond?

A This nurse is demonstrating a need for affiliation with the work group. In addition, depending on her job description (does the nurse have any management or overall long-term responsibilities for the operation of the unit?), the nurse may have a need for control or she may feel unable to let go of aspects of the job for which there she bears ultimate accountability. If the situation is the former, then the behavior is not appropriate; however, if the situation is the latter, in the short run the behavior *may* be appropriate.

In either situation, a counselling session is needed. Before the counselling session, you should gather more information as to how great a problem this behavior is to the operation of the unit (i.e., is the behavior negatively affecting the productivity of the scheduled staff? do the remaining staff find the behavior bothersome?). This information will assist you in conducting your counselling session. Follow the principles of good counselling by letting the staff member know of your concerns and requirements while allowing her to talk, but do not allow the discussion to become one of blaming and offering defensive excuses.

In the session, suggest other ways to meet affiliation needs, such as religious groups, professional organizations, and family. Emphasize the importance of the use of vacation time to rest, relax, and rejuvenate, even if vacation activities involve just "a change of pace." This change should be complete and thus should not include frequent checking in to the work environment. Small exceptions may occur in periods of change on the unit, and the nurse may call in to be informed so that on return she is emotionally and psychologically prepared to deal with the changed situation. Of course, the nurse could be encouraged to obtain this information in a more *social* manner, by talking to a trusted staff member when she is off duty.

If the behavior is motivated by the nurse's sense of control over some aspect of the work responsibilities and the inability to let go, then the counselling session also needs to address ways in which the nurse can delegate these responsibilities during periods of absence. If other staff truly are not prepared to assume these responsibilities, then your job is to help

develop their abilities, as well as to serve as a "safety net" and resource during the nurse's absence.

JW ALEXANDER

◆ **SHOULD I HELP STAFF SOLVE PERSONAL PROBLEMS?**

Q A nurse whom I supervise complains constantly about her personal life to anyone who will listen. What can I do?

A In this situation the best approach is the direct approach. The manager should counsel the employee regarding professional behavior and professional boundaries. It may be necessary to help the employee understand the inappropriateness of personal information in the work environment where the public or other professionals may overhear. The employee may require very specific examples of what behavior is appropriate and where it is appropriate. The manager should not be pulled into actually counselling the employee regarding her personal problems. If the employee asks for help, she should be told to seek outside counselling or outside resources.

The manager should clearly articulate the expected behavior and the expectation that if it continues, the disciplinary process will be initiated.

SF SMITH

◆ **HOW SHOULD I DEAL WITH A NURSE WHO IS A HABITUAL COMPLAINER?**

Q What is the best way of dealing with a worker who constantly complains?

A The worker who constantly complains can be highly disruptive and distracting to the rest of the staff. This is a type of behavior that may go unaddressed because the employee manages direct patient care at an acceptable level. Relationships among members of the work group are often not addressed as a part of practice, thus allowing dysfunctional behavior to continue.

As the manager, you need to meet with the employee and directly address the behaviors. If this is a long-standing issue, you need to be prepared for resistance to acknowledging the behavior as a legitimate problem. Be concise and focused on the behavior, and avoid being distracted by side issues the staff member may try to introduce.

1. Indicate clearly why this behavior is a problem, to the extent that ownership exists.
2. Set the expectation that the employee will bring solutions and approaches to issues that help resolve them. Simply complaining will no longer be acceptable.
3. Structure follow-up counselling at relatively short intervals since this is an ongoing frequent concern. Consider engaging the staff member in work related to an issue he or she has indicated needs change as a part of the follow-up. Exposure to the larger considerations of the problem can broaden the employee's view of the situation.

The staff's level of maturity in not confronting negative behavior indicates the need for education and practice in managing conflict and other negative behaviors. Your management of the problem can serve as a model to staff.

B FOSTER

♦ WHAT SHOULD I DO ABOUT AN EMPLOYEE WHO MAKES TOO MANY PERSONAL PHONE CALLS?

Q One of our nurses has a girlfriend whom he is always calling during his work time. They do not talk long, but he does call frequently even though we have a policy against the use of work time for personal calls. He is a great nurse and is well liked by both staff and patients. How should I handle this?

A Your staff nurse may not be aware of the policy and needs to be reminded of it. He may also be aware of the policy but hopes it will not be applied. If he is a good nurse and has engaged in no other behavior that offers any reason for concern, this should be fairly simple to address. Ask him if you can speak to him privately and describe what you have

observed and the policy that addresses it. Let him know that you have always applied policies fairly and consistently and that this behavior is unacceptable. He must know that you expect him to fully comply. If he is open to your dialogue, he should be able to accept the parameters you suggest.

Sometimes there are extenuating circumstances that warrant exceptions. If there are some short-term concerns that require frequent conversation and this does not threaten his work effectiveness, some dialogue and accommodation may be necessary. There are sometimes unusual or extenuating situations that demand moderation and management judgment. Whatever the situation, the rules should be fairness and consistency, sensitive moderation where necessary, and just resolution of inappropriate behavior as quickly as possible.

T PORTER-O'GRADY

♦ SHOULD I INTERVENE IN PATIENT–STAFF RELATIONSHIP?

Q One of the nurses on the unit has been spending an increasing portion of her time with one of the male patients on the floor. It appears to me they are attracted to each other. When I spoke with the nurse, she accused me of making a big deal out of nothing and of being suspicious. I am concerned; how should I handle patient–staff "special" relationships?

A This challenging situation highlights the importance of maintaining the highest standards of professional conduct in our patient interactions and the difficulties that may be encountered when these standards are not self-imposed. First, you are dealing with making a judgment call about whether something inappropriate is going on. Given that there is clearly disagreement among at least two professionals (you and the involved nurse), I would ask for the assistance of a neutral third party, such as your supervisor, in validating the legitimacy of your concern. Discuss the specific behaviors you are observing, how they differ from this nurse's interactions with other patients, and the conclusions you have drawn.

C

It is essential that as health care providers we recognize the vulnerable and often dependent position patients are placed in. At times, their lives are literally in our hands. We must safeguard against anything other than strictly professional interactions and recognize that there is a risk of confusion about the nature of relationships in an environment characterized by dependence, warmth, caring, and genuine concern.

It is somewhat disconcerting that the nurse in this situation doesn't demonstrate alarm at even the *appearance* of impropriety. One would expect a zealous effort to eliminate even the slightest hint of concern immediately. If your supervisor concurs with your assessment, enlist her assistance in addressing this concern with the nurse and taking whatever steps are necessary to ensure a strictly professional relationship.

JE BEGLINGER

♦ HOW SHOULD I APPROACH A NURSE ON MY UNIT WHO HER COLLEAGUES FEEL IS NOT DOING HER JOB?

Q There is a level II nurse on our unit. One year of training has been invested in her. It appears to her colleagues that it has failed. Her nursing care is questionable at times; however, there is simply nothing tangible to prove that. Our staffing is tight. What should I do with her?

A The first thing to do is go talk to her. Find out what she is feeling and what she thinks is going on. Ask her about her own assessment of her nursing skills and knowledge base. Find out if there are areas where additional training could increase her proficiency. Maybe she needs further skills development or maybe she feels she is doing very well and has no insight into the apparent problem. No nurse is ever going to be proficient in every aspect of her practice. We all have special talents and gifts that are displayed in different ways. There are, however, minimal performance requirements to which all nurses must conform. As her nurse manager you should do the following:

1. Talk to her as outlined above. Validate her assessment if she thinks there is a problem.
2. With that information and the feedback from her colleagues, you will need to determine as best you can what the problem is, if any exists. Is it incompetency or immaturity? Is she overwhelmed by the pace or complexity? Is she feeling unsupported? Is there a relationship conflict?
3. Once you've determined what you think the real problem is, plan a course of action to resolve it. Some obvious action alternatives may include more training and educational support or a mentor relationship with one of your more experienced nurses. In some cases, a transfer within your hospital system to an area that better matches her skills and strengths may be appropriate but should not be pursued as an early strategy. Unless you find serious incompetency problems or attitudinal issues, I would not recommend discharge at this early stage.
4. Meet with her again and share with her your perspectives and your plans. Gain her input and support for the action plan. Make sure she understands your expectations of her. During the implementation of the plan, give frequent feedback and reassurances.

As a nurse manager you can expect to find all types of people who develop at different rates and some who may never live up to the norm or standard that evolves within a group of nurses who work closely together. Your challenge is to motivate all your staff, encourage them, and find ways to capitalize on their strengths. If all your efforts fail and no progress is evident after 3 months of concerted effort, then you should move forward more intensely with transfer plans or with a more formal disciplinary process.

CCC LEVENS

♦ WHAT CAN I DO ABOUT A MANAGER WHOSE STAFF RESENTS HER?

Q We have a manager who is very popular with her peers in management. She also has done a great job of managing the budget and keeping her unit operating efficiently, and she has met all the goals set for her by nursing administration. She is considered quite a "golden girl" by her fellow managers. Her staff, however are very unhappy with her. She frequently shines at their expense. She manipulates and rigidly controls behavior and does not tolerate objection or assertiveness. What can we do?

A This is a very unfortunate and challenging set of circumstances. However, it is not as uncommon as you might think. This "queen bee" behavior permits an individual to shine at the expense of others and in her own exclusive best interest. Breaking through this pattern is difficult, but there are some things that can be done:

1. Make sure that the feelings regarding this manager are generally shared by the nursing staff. Define together specifically what issues they share in common with each other about this manager's behavior.
2. If you have not collectively confronted this manager in the past, it is time to do that now. On the outside chance that she is not aware of her behavior, she needs a chance to become aware that such a behavior exists. If she has given evidence of punishing those who confront her, you may need to carefully consider whether this step needs to be modified, through the presence of a third party who can mediate the dialogue.
3. If necessary, request that her supervisor be present during the combined discussions about the discomforts of the staff with her inconsistent and apparently destructive behavior. Stick to the issues and provide examples of the behavior so there is a context for enumerating the difficulties the staff is having with her.
4. Clearly present the staff's needs for communication and role expectations for discussion and negotiation. Allow for response and indication of corrective action or an indication that the manager is willing to explore her behaviors and adjust them to the realities of the time and the unit.
5. State clearly the behavior change desired or other formative activities that the manager can identify with in order to give form to the expectation you have for changing her behaviors in her performance as manager in the organization.

Visibility of the negative behaviors is an essential ingredient for addressing these activities. After having exhausted all your resources as a staff member, you will need to partner with others who recognize what is truly happening and can assist you in addressing these aberrant and negative behaviors.

Also, examine your motives and those of your colleagues to be sure that you are not just reacting to something that you simply don't like. If you are clear about your motives and the behavior of the manager is not seen by those who can assist you in making change, you are on your own. Through staff partnering, it is possible to address these issues directly and to work together to change them. It is important to know that such corrective actions are very difficult and rife with political implications, so care and caution and consideration of the risks must be clear to the staff. Seeking a mentor or trusted advisor can also help the staff discern the appropriate response and to take positive action in resolving this difficult situation.

T PORTER-O'GRADY

◆ HOW SHOULD I CURB A STAFF MEMBER'S MANIPULATIVE ACTIONS?

Q An employee of ours is manipulative. She demonstrates manipulative behavior with regards to scheduling, patient assignments, and with other staff members. What suggestions do you have for interacting with a very manipulative nurse?

A Cooperation and a spirit of camaraderie are essential to the success of a group that must function as a team to accomplish its purposes. These are certainly essential characteristics of the caregiving team. Effective behavioral management begins with a clear understanding and consensus by team members of the desired and essential behavioral characteristics and is ensured by assuming shared responsibility for monitoring and addressing individual and group behaviors.

In a professional work group it is inappropriate for the manager to assume the role of mother or policewoman as it relates to staff behaviors. It is appropriate, however, for the manager to model, coach, and facilitate the staff's identification of the behaviors they believe are appropriate in the practice environment and to effectively address situations in which behaviors are inconsistent with the standard that has been set.

One very effective approach is to incorporate the behavioral expectations of the caregivers into a unit

C

mission statement. A mission statement articulates the purpose and ideals of the group, and its development can serve as an excellent stimulus to get people really thinking about what they believe and value. Examples taken from a mission statement of a medical–surgical unit serving oncology and geriatric patients follow:

We recognize the importance of effective communication skills to maximize positive outcomes.

We are committed to provide competent, caring, and personalized service to patients and their families, utilizing the latest technology and professional skill and knowledge available.

We are committed to providing an environment that strives for well-being of body, mind, and spirit.

We are committed to each other as people, as family, and as staff to optimize therapy and return patients to their normal environment.

Clearly established behavioral norms for the unit provide the basis for dialogue when unacceptable behaviors are observed.

A manager's time is well spent engaging the staff in discussions about how adult professionals relate to one another. Dealing openly with the discomfort that normally is experienced by anyone when constructively addressing a behavioral concern is a part of the developmental process. Practice sessions may be indicated and useful. One unit director I know has been actively working with her staff on their inability to communicate effectively with one another. At a recent staff meeting she had them each offer a compliment as well as a constructive suggestion to someone in the room. This proved a very painful exercise, and her "grapevine" feedback suggested the staff didn't feel very positive about the experience. This affirms the challenge of developing effective communication skills and the need for the manager to assess where her staff are and stick to a plan focused on their developmental needs.

This approach lays the foundation for dealing with manipulative or any other unacceptable behaviors. Early in the staff's development you will assume a greater role in modeling the constructive confrontation of behaviors that are inconsistent with expectations, thereby stressing the impact these behaviors have on the group's ability to work together. At the same time, you must continue to coach those who are affected by inappropriate behaviors to constructively deal with situations as they occur. All behaviors

are encouraged, enabled, or tolerated. For someone to successfully manipulate, someone else has to allow the manipulation.

JE BEGLINGER

♦ **HOW CAN I IMPLEMENT PROGRESSIVE CORRECTION WITH AN OBSTINATE EMPLOYEE?**

Q What are the best ways to implement progressive correction with a staff member whose attitude and behavior cause disruption among the other staff and who creates an obstacle to change?

A Implementing progressive action requires careful planning. The process requires patience, objectivity, and flexibility if informal attempts to improve the staff member's performance have not been successful.

As the nurse manager, you should design a plan of performance expectations with time frames for implementation. You and the staff member should meet to discuss the plan and to assess the individual's ability and commitment to use the plan to improve role performance. During the meeting, you should elicit feedback from the staff member to refine the strategies developed to enable the nurse to meet role expectations and contribute to the overall performance of the team.

Focus discussion on the following:
1. Role performance
2. Participation as a team member
3. Professional development
4. Evaluation of progress

During the meeting, offer the staff member an opportunity to question the plan or process. It is important to assure the staff member that the information discussed will remain confidential and will not be shared with other staff members unless they are in leadership positions. At the end of the meeting, summarize the key points of discussion, schedule your next meeting, and ask the individual to describe her understanding of the next steps.

Remember that a staff member who requires corrective action may not understand how to initiate behavioral change. Therefore it is helpful to clearly identify undesirable behaviors and actions, delineate specific corrective strategies, and discuss the effect that these actions will have on the individual, other staff, and patient outcomes. If the staff member is unwilling or unable to make a commitment to the plan, you should outline the next steps, including dismissal.

Although implementation of progressive correction is not a pleasant task, it offers you and the employee an opportunity to work together on improving performance and understanding role expectations. It is important that you not assume responsibility for the success or failure of the staff member, but serve as a facilitator for professional development.

AMT BROOKS

◆ HOW CAN I KEEP PERFORMANCE EVALUATION FOCUSED?

Q Whenever I counsel an employee regarding her performance, she immediately refocuses the conversation to my performance, which puts me on the defensive. How should I refocus the discussion and respond to this critiquing of my performance?

A One of the least pleasant aspects of the work place is dishing out criticism. It's hard to receive, hard to give, and especially hard to give well. Yet criticism and praise are both essential tools for improving the performance of the people for whom you are the leader.

Remember that it is your responsibility to make sure that you and your staff work to the best of your abilities. If the person your are counseling makes you think twice about correcting him or her, then that person is stopping you from doing your job. Holding on to that thought should help eliminate any reluctance you might have about confronting the situation.

Remain focused. Concentrate on doing what you are supposed to be doing—analyzing and correcting her work. Be consistent, don't stray, and don't let your employee's reaction sidetrack you. A consistent focus on work-related issues is your best strategy.

As much as possible, it is best to deliver praise and criticism at different times. That way your employee will really hear the praise when you compliment her and, of course, your criticism will be heard clearly, too.

LG VONFROLIO

Collaboration

C

◆ HOW DOES AN ORGANIZATION SUPPORT NURSING AT THE SAME TIME IT SUPPORTS A MULTIDISCIPLINARY PATIENT CARE APPROACH?

Q How can an organization support the discipline of nursing if it also supports the emerging models of a multidisciplinary approach to patient care?

A Historically our organizations have functioned based on newtonian physics; each division is a separate and distinct unit: autonomous, independent, and with little if any relevance to other units. We are now viewing organizations through the lens of quantum physics, which describes units in terms of their *relationship* to each other. No longer do we view ourselves as distinct, autonomous, independent units or departments but rather as an important part of a whole. We can achieve our goals and mission only in relationship with other departments or units.

To support nursing, we must clearly define the role of nurses within the organization and how they work with other disciplines to achieve the institution's mission and goals. Our main focus as health care providers must be on the patient and community as external customers and other departments as internal customers. Each discipline brings a unique art or skill to meeting or exceeding customer needs and expectations. Process management can help delineate roles because it identifies who (discipline) owns which process (task) and therefore has the responsibility and accountability for its implementation, quality, and outcome. Organizational processes are no longer structured according to organizational box or department but by who manages the specific part of the process. Admitting a patient, for example, is not the sole responsibility of the admitting department because several departments own parts of the admitting process, so the responsibility belongs to all of them.

Flowcharting multidisciplinary processes can also help define each discipline's specific contribution to the anticipated and planned result. Flowcharting visually identifies the overall importance of the discipline for a successful outcome. In flowcharting most

C

hospital processes, nursing's contribution becomes extremely clear.

Nursing can be more strongly supported in an organization when it is viewed as a team player whose only goals are quality outcomes than when it is viewed as an autonomous unit vested with self-interest. When you break down the barriers between the departments, you strengthen nursing's position as a team role model. For example, change of shift report is traditionally a nursing task. In becoming truly customer focused, include all the disciplines that treated the patients that day: PT, RT, dietary, and even housekeeping, who may have heard some valuable information from the family. With practice, these reports need take no more time than when nursing does them alone, but the new method improves continuity for patients, shares understanding of roles between disciplines, opens communication between departments, develops a heightened level of mutual respect, and positively affects the outcome.

RM HADDON

◆ HOW DO I BEGIN TO CREATE A PARTNERSHIP WITH PHYSICIANS?

Q How do I create an openness to start collaborative partnerships with physician chiefs of service for visioning and planning change?

A Nurses bring incredible strength to the table as competent, consistent, caring, and compassionate members of the team. We need to use all these behaviors to influence new behaviors and relationships with other colleagues.

Initiate open, frank discussions regarding nonvolatile issues that yield more areas of agreement than disagreement. The art of negotiation is a skill that would be worth reviewing. Generally speaking, "core values" that deal with expected patient outcomes are a safe agenda item. Early identification of values allows all the stakeholders the opportunity to define areas of compatibility and areas that may become problematic.

Do your homework and recognize the precious commodity of time; tolerance for endless and pointless meetings is minimal. Be honest, use restraint, and choose your battles carefully. Identify champions of particular systems, approaches, and processes. Steer

clear of the "people issues"; retain "care values" as the achievable outcome goal and the point of departure.

Partnership generally implies each partner shares equally in the risk and benefits of the relationship. This is a higher order relationship than collaboration, in which parties share information and may determine a common path toward a desired outcome. I would separate the two and clearly define the preferred relationship.

The partnership relationship rooted in a clearly articulated value system of patient care delivery systems and outcomes seems only natural and provides common ground to foster further development of patient-centered integrated delivery systems.

LM JOHNSON

◆ HOW CAN I HELP STAFF DEVELOP AN INTERDISCIPLINARY APPROACH?

Q How can the nurse manager assist staff to develop a better organizational perspective and interdisciplinary approach to patient care?

A As health care organizations put their quality improvement systems into place, this reorientation to a broader, interdisciplinary focus by nursing staff will become easier for the nurse manager to facilitate. In quality improvement the customer path is followed throughout the organization with the emphasis away from individuals and onto systems. Expectations are more clearly defined regarding the responsibility for quality improvement and interdisciplinary efforts by *all* staff. As the nurse manager, you can also begin to discuss how customers are defining quality and their expectations for nursing care outside of the nursing unit. Building on existing and currently effective organizational and communication structures and relationships with other disciplines helps address both paranoia and apathy. Don't involve other departments or disciplines for the sake of involvement alone, or to meet only nursing's needs. Ask for their involvement when their participation is needed, timely, and mutually meaningful. Identify clear expectations, and limit the time commitments expected of others. Integrate nursing's activities and clinical outcomes with those of other departments and disciplines by suggesting methods for application of those outcomes in their individual settings, particularly those that may enhance cooperation from others, such as more efficient support services or improved turnaround time and more satisfied customers, both internal and external to the unit and organization.

BV TEBBITT

◆ HOW CAN I GET OTHER DEPARTMENTS TO COOPERATE?

Q We need to form clinical partnerships in our managed care approach. We are having difficulty helping other departments understand what this means to them. How should I handle this?

A Nursing is not the only department affected by a change to managed care. Acknowledging the fact that other departments are having difficulties is a start. The nurse manager needs to establish ongoing verbal communication with the managers of other departments in order to identify issues and to attain resolution together, through collaboration. Managers in all departments in our institution are held accountable as a group for meeting the financial goals of our facility. No department can operate in isolation in a managed care environment and have the institution survive.

DD GILES

◆ HOW CAN I IMPROVE COOPERATION BETWEEN NURSING AND OTHER DEPARTMENTS?

Q Nursing has been having considerable problems getting the pharmacy to work effectively with us. The nursing staff is very angry about late arrival of medications, incomplete order filling, and a lack of flexibility on the part of the pharmacy staff. How can we get them to work *with* us?

A This is an excellent example of a complex interdepartmental problem that is all too common in health care today. The concepts of continuous quality improvement (CQI) help us to look at such situations in a way that focuses on the processes

of how we do work and helps us avoid focusing on blaming individuals. As a manager of this nursing unit, you can set the tone for collaborative problem solving with the manager of the pharmacy. To do this, you must acknowledge to the pharmacy that the system of administering medications to patients requires the pharmacy and nursing staff to work together. This really means that nursing owns part of this problem and pharmacy owns part of this problem, and that the solution must be found by working together. Understanding that you share a common goal to meet the patients' health care needs is the first step. Next, see if you can get the pharmacy manager to agree to form a small task force made up of one or two of her staff, one or two staff nurses from your unit, and any other key players in this system, like messengers, clerical staff, or supervisors. Once this group is gathered, explain that you are interested in improving patient care and you need their help to make sure that patients get their medications in a timely fashion. To begin, have the group make a step-by-step description of how a medication gets from point A (the physician's order) to point Z (patient ingesting and absorbing the medication). What you will find if your organization is typical of most is an incredibly long, protracted, and complex process consisting of many steps. These steps will probably involve at least five or more people and often include repetitive work (also known as rework). If you have charted each step on a chart pad where the group can see the procedural steps outlined, the group members will probably be able to identify several areas in the process that are common causes of inefficiency:

1. Too many steps in the process.
2. Too many hand-off points where one person's work depends on another person's work.
3. Places where rework is done.

Fixing the flaws in such systems is one of the best ways for quality improvement to occur and to get interdependent work groups to see the benefits of collaboration toward a common goal. If you have a training session available in your area or organization on CQI techniques and tools, sign up. As our organizations grow more complex, the ability to facilitate multidisciplinary work groups to solve common problems by redesigning and improving the work systems becomes a critical management skill of the future.

MC ALDERMAN

C

Collective Bargaining

◆ HOW WILL CHANGES IN THE WORK WORLD AFFECT UNIONS AND COLLECTIVE BARGAINING?

Q The whole world of work is changing. How will that affect unions and the collective bargaining process?

A Yes, the whole work world is truly changing, but in the area of labor–management relations, hospital administrators, managers, and supervisors will continue to be confronted with human relations problems. Employees have rights, especially if they are discriminated against, unfairly treated, or inadequately paid. Good managers also have responsibilities, which include protecting employees. We have a difficult balance to maintain in health care today—we have a *primary* responsibility to protect our patients. Those hospitals that are organized will continue representing their employees. Managers will continue to sit at the bargaining table. All supervisors should be well informed and involved in the negotiation processes.

JG O'LEARY

◆ IF EMPLOYEES ASK HOW TO GET RID OF THE UNION, WHAT SHOULD I DO?

Q The nursing staff is organized under a collective bargaining agreement. Several staff members have come to me and asked what they could do to get rid of the union. As management, what can I say?

A This could be a very sensitive situation that must be handled carefully. Remember that if you persuade them or unintentionally influence your staff members to eliminate the union and they are still unhappy about their work situation, you would probably be the one to take the blame. By all means listen to them; let them ventilate. They are probably

seeking your advice because they respect you. Most important, be aware that discouragement of union activity by hospital management is considered an unfair labor practice. Thus it is important that you maintain a very objective position with these staff members. Establish from the beginning of each conversation with your staff members that you are maintaining an impartial position.

Remember that the staff *is* the union. An organization (in this case, the union), after all, is composed of individuals. If it is not representative of their needs, whose fault is that? Do they provide input to their bargaining unit representatives? If they do not like the union, you can explore whether they are actively involved with its operation. Allow them to describe those situations that have made them dissatisfied with their union. Is their discontent because the union is placing unrealistic demands on a stressed hospital situation? Are they unhappy with the delegates that represent them? You may suggest that they speak to the union representative and get involved with decision-making committees within the collective bargaining unit.

LG VONFROLIO

◆ HOW SHOULD I DEAL WITH HARASSMENT FROM UNION MEMBERS?

Q We're at a serious point in our contract negotiations. There are several militant union members in our organization. They have been pressuring, harassing, and intimidating some of the nursing staff who are not as rigorous about the contract issues. As a nurse manager, what responsibilities do I have to deal with this issue and how do I approach it?

A You are in a most difficult situation. Seek help from nursing administration and your director of services. They should provide support and the needed information regarding what you as a manager can and cannot do with your staff. You also should have the professional advice of hospital counsel because there are many rules and regulations regarding your employees' rights and your responsibilities as a manager. There are many booklets published listing what you can do as a manager, and what you cannot do. You cannot coerce or threaten your staff. You can and should maintain open communications with your employees. Continue with your staff meetings and encourage these militant members to voice their concerns, and always attempt to provide them with honest answers. Do not avoid these individuals; they may be identifying serious problems.

JG O'LEARY

Committees

◆ WHICH COMMITTEES ARE REALLY NECESSARY FOR NURSING SERVICE?

Q It seems that in nursing we are burdened by a huge number of committees that really have no meaningful outcomes. Just what committees should exist in the nursing service and how do we avoid having useless committees?

A Over the past 10 years, hospital implementation sites for shared governance models have had an opportunity to start from scratch and redesign their committee structures. While these structures are often customized for the environment, four basic standing committees consistently emerge to address the ongoing concerns of the nursing department.

Standing committees and their areas of concern usually include:
1. *Nursing practice committee*—nursing care and practice standards, nursing conceptual frameworks, and delivery of care.
2. *Management committee*—budgeting and planning, fiscal management including human resources, systems, and operations.
3. *Quality assurance committee*—risk management, standards compliance, and mechanisms for data collection, analysis, evaluation, and recommendations.
4. *Education committee*—assessment and enhancement of the educational and professional needs of the nursing staff and supporting groups and the conduction of research and its publication.

From these committees, *ad hoc* committees can be formed to address specific projects and tasks, and then be disbanded after they have achieved their goals.

The easiest way to guard against too many committees is to be very specific, in writing, about their purposes and activities. There should be a coordinating committee that decreases duplication by reviewing minutes and making sure that these committees are communicating with one another.

RG HESS

◆ WHAT CAN I DO ABOUT A DYSFUNCTIONAL CLIQUE ON A COMMITTEE?

Q What do I do if there appears to be a powerful dysfunctional clique on a given hospital committee, which maintains the status quo?

A The direction you choose to take depends on whether you are a long-time member of the committee or a new member. Let's assume you are a new member and have noticed the situation you describe.

Nominal group technique would be a safe way for all members to speak up and share their perceptions. The following steps can be undertaken:
1. Members define the mission of the particular committee.
2. Members describe how they can contribute to achieving the mission.
3. Members describe obstacles to achieving the mission.
4. Members describe strategies of how to overcome the obstacles.

Chances are that the clique's behavior is a group reaction to the mission. This may surface during the brainstorming sessions as well as individual member motivation to accomplish the mission.

Ideally, there is a nursing administration facilitator assigned to the committee with whom you can meet and describe your desire to pursue this exercise. She can then facilitate the process and help move it along.

JM McMAHON

◆ WHAT DO I NEED TO LEARN TO BE A GOOD COMMITTEE LEADER?

Q I am a new committee chairperson and unfamiliar with leadership process in managing my committee. What specific skills should I be developing in order to provide successful committee leadership?

A Organizations in today's health care environment should focus on leader behaviors that promote employee autonomy, foster creativity, and encourage employee involvement. Current leaders should strive to create a culture of caring professionals, encouraging all nurses to function at their full potential.

As a committee chairperson you should be prepared to effectively utilize the collective energy, time, and resources to achieve a predetermined outcome, usually through consensus building, and rarely by majority vote.

According to Crosby (1990), effective group leaders are "willing to learn, ethical, available, determined, energetic, reliable, sensible, humble, intense, pleasant."

The "force of the positive," expecting the best, is one of the most powerful and least thought about weapons you can bring to a meeting. Think positively and speak positively. Use this approach to make yourself someone people admire and emulate when they want something accomplished (Bennis, 1989a).

Bennis (1989b) believes that leadership can be felt throughout an organization. It gives pace and energy to the work and thus helps to empower the work force. Empowerment is the collective effect of leadership. According to Bennis (1989b), in organizations with effective leaders, empowerment is most evident in four themes:

- *People feel significant.* Everyone feels that he or she makes a difference to the success of the organization.
- *Learning and competence matter.* Leaders value learning and mastery, and so do people who work for leaders.
- *People are part of a community.* Where there is leadership, there is a team, a family, a unity.
- *Work is exciting.* Where there are leaders, work is stimulating, challenging, fascinating, and fun.

Leaders have the ability to identify opportunities to help those with whom they work to improve their abilities and skills. The greater the improvement among members of the group, the better group members will perform their jobs and ultimately the entire organization improves.

J TROFINO

◆ HOW CAN I IMPROVE COMMITTEE MEMBERS' PARTICIPATION?

Q There is one member on the committee that I chair who never speaks, even though she has much to contribute to the meeting. On the other hand, there is another who is constantly talking and has little to contribute. How do I change the focus of these two members?

A As a committee chair, it is essential that you clearly understand the purposes of the committee and the positions and responsibilities of the chair and members on the committee. It is helpful to periodically review this information with the committee and encourage dialogue about expectations held by each person on the committee. The chair should be willing to, with genuine honesty, share her guiding philosophy. For example, is it expected that the chair will set the agenda and make assignments or will the chair serve as facilitator to assist the group to determine goals and means of working? With this sharing as an example, the chair may invite members to move toward similar sharing of individual beliefs and expectations. It is useful to recognize and respect the unique talents, interests, experiences, and individual concerns of each person and encourage use of this information in determining goals and tasks to be accomplished.

With this information and these processes as a backdrop, it is easier for the chair, or for a member, to engage in dialogue about observations and concerns in the group. The chair can also approach each of the members in question with individual observations of behavior. The most effective opening is to seek information to help in understanding an issue or problem. The chair could say "You seem hesitant to talk in the committee and I'm especially concerned because I know you have a lot to offer the group. Can you help me understand why you talk so little and how I can help us all to benefit from what you know?"

It is important that people be respected for their interests, talents, experiences, and requests for growth opportunities when committee assignments are made. The literature of nursing and organizations describes use of the Myers-Briggs Type Indicator (MBTI) as a safe and helpful tool for providing information to individuals about their interests, ways of seeking information, communicating, relating, and problem solving. This tool can help bring to awareness increased knowing of the self and appreciation of the preferences of others. You may contact Consulting Psychologists Press, 577 College Avenue, Palo Alto, CA 94306 for a list of publications and general information about the MBTI.

ME PARKER

Communication

◆ WHAT IS GOOD FEEDBACK?

Q What is considered good and ongoing feedback?

A A definition of feedback includes data that are reflected back to the employee. Good feedback entails providing data for the purpose of promoting growth and self-esteem. The primary purpose of feedback as used by a nurse manager would be to reveal to your staff member your perception of her performance or behavior. This involves not only describing the staff member's behavior but also evaluating it and telling her how you feel about the behavior. Feedback helps other people learn how they appear to others and what interpersonal impact they have. It is essential to personal growth and development.

Feedback is usually offered to (1) clarify, (2) reinforce, (3) educate, or (4) reprimand actions. Some examples of the semantics of feedback are as follows:
- ◆ "Is this what I heard you say? . . . " to help clarify the intended meaning.
- ◆ "What you asked Mary if she needed any help, I felt good" or "My reaction to that is . . . " could be feedback that is useful for instruction.

It is important to be aware that feedback can help or harm a person's self-esteem, and it must be utilized sensitively. One of the best resources that I would recommend is the video "One Minute Manager" by Paul Hersey. It is an excellent video covering a number of issues, including feedback. It is not only helpful but also humorous, and you may want to share it with your staff. A useful tool to help you obtain feedback from your staff regarding the effectiveness of your leadership style is the leadership effectiveness style "Lead Others" (Hersey & Duldt, 1989).

SR. M FINNICK

◆ HOW CAN I IMPROVE MY COMMUNICATION SKILLS?

Q Sometimes it seems that my superiors do not really understand what is happening in the delivery of everyday nursing care. How can I do a better job of explaining what my staff does and what resources they need to perform well?

A Just as managers feel that corporate administrators do not understand their work and what they need, administrators often feel that managers do not understand the constraints of the corporate reality of limited resources. It may be a sign that communication and systems perspectives need to be adjusted on both sides.

It is essential for the nurse manager to fully understand all staff activity so that appropriate information, human, material, and financial resources are made available to them to complete their work. At the corporate level, it is equally essential that administrators know of the overall needs of the corporation, community, and the industry while keeping their financial situation balanced to develop and maintain a healthy organization. Both management levels share one common goal: a commitment to quality care. This is the unifying principle around which both groups operate.

An environment based on mutual respect for the expertise of each management level, coupled with a trust in the judgment and accuracy of information shared between the two, is more essential than fully knowing in detail the scope of responsibility of each. A nurse manager may never be able to acquire all the resources needed to do an optimal job because that level of resource simply does not exist for the institution. Thus she must work with all other managers to ensure that the resources that exist are fairly allocated. Further, the manager must assist staff in understanding corporate reality through providing accu-

C

rate and clear information. This may be an invitation to reexamine rituals and practice patterns to identify new and innovative ways to stretch existing resources further, keeping a focus on the essentials for quality care.

J KOERNER

♦ HOW DO I DEAL WITH A DIFFICULT ADMINISTRATOR?

Q I report to a new nursing administrator. Although we are not having conflict, I am having difficulty getting my point across and having my unit's needs met when I meet with her on a regular basis. What are some strategies to enable me to deal with my administrator more effectively?

A A new nursing administrator has a great deal to learn about the job, the role, and the organization. Her ability to fit into that role is undoubtedly her first priority. The success of the nursing administrator is often based first on how she is able to build her relationships with stakeholders in the organization. These stakeholders include physicians, peers, boss, and directly reporting employees. It often takes a year for a new nursing administrator to feel comfortable knowing the "politics" of the organization. It is important for those reporting to her to be sensitive to this and to support their new boss during this time. The manager needs to take a leadership role in helping the nursing administrator acclimate to the new role effectively. It is important to find out from her what her needs are to help ease her transition into the role. The nursing administrator has many constituents to please and respond to during this time. Seeking ways to support this transition will pay dividends once the role is firmly in place.

How does she like to receive information? Is it in written form such as a formal memo or notes? Does she prefer it to be verbal? Face-to-face or over the phone? Find out what works best for her and design your relationship and reporting of information around this. What are her expectations of you? Does she want you to function autonomously or does she want to be informed regularly of your activities? How often does she want to meet, and how does she want to structure the time together? It is critical to clearly understand and appreciate her expectations and the best way to meet them. Find out from her how to help her be successful. What does she want to know more about? The most critical factor, when beginning a working relationship, is to clearly understand each other's goals and expectations. Take time to get to know her. We sometimes get so caught up in doing the job that we lose sight of knowing the person and what that person's values, beliefs, and goals are. The manager needs to determine the congruency of thinking and recognize differences and openly discuss them. Let her know you want to develop a strong collaborative, collegial relationship that enables her to meet her organizational goals and, at the same time, utilizes the strengths you bring to the organization. She needs to know where you see your strengths and your opportunities for growth as well as how you would like her help to achieve your goals.

When preparing to meet with her, I recommend you prepare for the meeting in this way. First, prepare an agenda. List issues on which you need her help or advice, as well as these that require information about your area. This portion of the meeting focuses on the manager's issues. The second part of the meeting should focus on providing information the nurse administrator has requested and increasing her knowledge about the organization. It is important to negotiate an agreement on the structure of the meeting. Once you have agreed on the format of the meeting, then assume responsibility for ensuring you are prepared for the meeting. The agenda items should be well prepared, clear, and easy to get through. Responding to her questions, concerns, or thoughts is an opportunity for you to learn new insights from a different vantage point—the nursing administrator's.

It's crucial to remember, from all of this, that the organization's success depends on support and collaboration from all levels of the organization.

J TORNABENI

♦ HOW CAN I CORRECT MISCONCEPTIONS?

Q I have very strong convictions and commitment to my profession, but when I express those as a manager I'm often accused by the staff of being opinionated, rigid, and narrow. That is not what I want to project. How do I deal with these perceptions?

A As a leader, you can project an image of confidence that can be intimidating to staff, particularly if you are their department manager or administrator. It is important to be sensitive to this when you speak or express your opinions. You may limit the input you receive by expressing your own views too quickly and too adamantly. It is hard to listen if you are more concerned with communicating your own views. I would suggest that you attempt to always solicit employees' opinions first in any discussion and then compare and contrast these to others before offering your own opinion.

The terms "rigid" and "narrow" may indicate that staff do not feel that you can accept other views and opinions as being useful or valuable. Acknowledging differences in views and seeking clarification are important listening behaviors to learn. Commitment and convictions are terrific as long as they do not infringe on others' rights to hold other, equally valued opinions.

C BRADLEY

◆ HOW CAN I MAKE SURE ALL STAFF ARE INFORMED ABOUT POLICY CHANGES AND STRATEGIES?

Q Some of the staff members on my unit never seem to be aware of changes and policies. What strategies should I utilize?

A Problems with communication are very common in nursing units whether large or small. Because the nursing unit operates 24 hours a day, so much goes on within the unit and throughout the hospital that it is often difficult to keep everyone informed. Since many departments constantly interact with each other, the policy or news in one department may directly affect another. Employees may view changes in policy or structure as threats instead of challenges if they begin to fear that information is being kept from them or if misleading or incorrect information is released. Managers should not get frustrated by having to repeat the same information and must experiment with different types of communication methods to decide which ones are best for each particular unit.

There are several steps that can be taken to facilitate communication:

1. Informal notes can be written by hand or typed on the personal computer daily or as often as needed to relay necessary information. Messages and reminders can be posted to emphasize important changes, make corrective adjustments, or praise staff for jobs well done.

2. Everyone's time should be used judiciously. Representatives from the nursing unit need to adequately and appropriately report information from nursing committees or multidisciplinary task forces. The representative should take notes to stimulate her memory when reporting back to the nursing unit. This will eliminate the standard reply of "nothing much" when she is asked about what happened at the meeting. It should be remembered that old news to one nurse might be new information to someone else.

3. Communication books are often helpful. The manager's communiqués are signed and dated when they are placed in the book. Employees are responsible for reading and initialing the book appropriately before their shift begins. Responsibility for keeping current should be shared between the staff and the manager. Employees cannot expect to be personally notified about decisions, and they should not be excused for *not* knowing if the opportunity for obtaining the knowledge was given.

4. Monthly staff meetings are essential. The staff meetings should be repeated, and adequate coverage should be provided so that all staff have the opportunity to attend. Agendas need to be preset so that all important points are covered. Staff members who work full-time should be required to attend at least 75% of these meetings. Minutes of the meetings should be available.

5. Informal staff or shift meetings are helpful on a weekly basis. The more that staff have the opportunity to interact with the manager, the more secure and interested the staff will be in obtaining the information about a change in policy or structure.

BH DUGGER

◆ CAN I HELP MY STAFF IMPROVE COMMUNICATION SKILLS?

Q As a nurse manager, how do I facilitate the development of communication skills among the

C

nursing staff and by the staff with patients and other departments?

A Communication skills, although of utmost importance, usually receive little attention. We concentrate our efforts on developing technical skills because they are easily defined and measured. Perhaps the best way to facilitate the development of your staff in this area is to look at your own abilities. How do you role model effective communication for your staff? What is your style when speaking with other nurses, physicians, or patients? For example, when addressing a colleague, you probably pay attention to the following:

♦ You speak directly with your peers, you avoid talking about them in the cafeteria or the conference room, and you discuss issues openly and honestly but always privately.

♦ You avoid putting colleagues down and, whenever possible, you openly compliment what they've done.

♦ You respect their privacy and protect them by not contributing to gossip.

♦ You support their efforts by attending programs they may be offering or by attending and participating at meetings they have called.

♦ You nominate them for task forces as a compliment to their skills.

Similarly, when communicating with physicians, you do so respectfully—even when the issue is a difficult one. When there is disagreement, you listen to the opposing view with consideration. You acknowledge your differences. If you role model this way, you will be reinforcing positive behaviors.

You may also want to consider sending your staff to workshops designed to enhance communication skills. Or perhaps your organization offers such workshops. If not, at least think about conducting some role playing during which you describe a situation and then have members of your staff play it out. Observers can then comment on how the communication came across. Help your staff to recognize nonverbal messages in their body language and facial expressions. Be candid with them, especially if there are obvious areas needing improvement. Tell your staff that you will commit to observing their communication patterns more carefully and that you will provide them with feedback. Then follow through with your commitment and be sure to recognize and applaud each positive behavior.

V MANCINI

♦ **HOW CAN COMMUNICATION BETWEEN SHIFTS BE IMPROVED?**

Q What methods are good for improving communication between shifts?

A This sounds like the D-E-N (day-evening-night) syndrome. This is a common malady found in many hospitals today. Basically, the signs and symptoms of this syndrome are the following:

1. The night staff reports off to the day staff and the day staff is not happy with how the unit was left, but they do not inform the night staff of their dislike.

2. At the beginning of report for the evening shift the day staff informs the evening staff that they would like them to inform the night staff not to leave the unit in the same condition that they did the morning before. The evening staff reluctantly accepts this responsibility.

3. When the night staff arrives, they are informed that the day staff was not happy with the way the unit looked the morning before. This is not the best way to start your shift, so the night staff simmers on this situation all night and by the time the day staff arrives the next morning the night staff is not in a friendly mood. Moreover, if the day shift thought the unit was a mess yesterday—just wait! Report is tense and they do not talk about the problem.

We frequently communicate in this fashion because we are not skilled in direct and open communication. Because ineffective communication skills are learned behaviors, they can be unlearned and replaced with more effective methods. To begin with, the staff must recognize that what they are currently doing is not effective. Then, and only then, are staff able to be receptive to changing their behavior. The basic principles of communication that I call the "Five Rights of Communication" are:

1. *The Right person.* Always communicate with the right person. In the D-E-N syndrome, the evening staff should have encouraged the day staff to speak directly with the night staff. Stepping forward to solve someone else's problem creates a dependency relationship and encourages passive-aggressive behavior.

2. *The Right time.* When things are tense and uncomfortable, it is usually not the appropriate time to speak to someone about a problem. People often

need time to cool off and process the meaning of the interaction. However, you can make an appointment with the other person(s) to resolve the conflict. At that time, speak calmly and specifically about what behaviors you find conflictual.

3. *The Right way.* Choosing the appropriate channel for communicating is very important. A general rule is to always give bad news in person, and good news can come through most channels.

4. *The Right language.* Words must be carefully chosen. Selecting direct, simple words is a good rule of thumb.

5. *The Right of the receiver to give feedback.* Just telling someone something is not communicating with them. You must seek feedback so that you know, without a doubt, that you have been heard.

Communicating effectively is as much an art as a science. Practice with effective communication techniques can improve your ability to communicate with colleagues, facilitate collegial relationships, and improve patient care. The manager must continually monitor staff interactions to assess how communication patterns affect the workplace and patient care. Providing education and feedback will enhance staff's ability to communicate effectively.

GL CROW

◆ HOW CAN I ENCOURAGE MORE HONEST AND DIRECT COMMUNICATION?

Q In the process of building a team within my operating room, I am trying to foster more open communication. I find that this is difficult to get started. The mostly female staff are much more comfortable with messages imbedded in humorous statements or comments spread secondhand. What can I do to help them learn to communicate more honestly and directly?

A Schedule some brainstorming sessions about communication. Ask the group to describe what "open communication" means and looks like to them, how it is handled, what are examples, and most important—what they see as the benefits of open communication. Next have them select two or three models that they most prefer using, such as direct expression of feelings through "I" statements, focusing on goals and tasks rather than behaviors, or using

a facilitator at all meetings who will process group communication and dynamics. Once these models are selected, ask the group to decide how they wish to handle group members who communicate outside the new boundaries, such as those who continue to use secondhand messages.

The key is to have the group own the communication process they wish to use to achieve certain goals. During your brainstorming sessions, have them role-play to get used to each other and this new style of communicating.

Next, teach the group the art of asking questions. When done properly, asking questions is nonthreatening and immediately moves a person from a child or parent state to the adult state as described in transactional analysis, a very powerful communication methodology. If the questions focus on goals and tasks, you can decrease the amount of emotion and "old baggage" that come into play.

Finally, have the group practice active listening skills: listen both for what someone is saying and for the hidden nonverbal messages. Sometimes listening is more important and effective for opening honest communication than constantly verbalizing.

Communication is an art that can be learned. It takes repetition, practice, and time. Keep at it. Let the group select the structure and boundaries, and you can act as facilitator and role model.

RM HADDON

◆ HOW CAN I GET STAFF TO SHARE INFORMATION BETWEEN SHIFTS ACCURATELY?

Q The shifts on my unit do not share information effectively. What can I do to improve the situation?

A Jones et al. (1990) indicate that "frank and open communications can minimize suspicions, correct misunderstandings, and build teamwork."

Nursing research has demonstrated that communication between the nurse leader and staff nurses can affect staff morale, productivity, and job satisfaction. Furthermore, it is essential that all nursing staff receive the same message, thus creating a more seamless transition between the shifts and ensuring consistent high-quality patient care outcomes (Kennedy et al., 1990).

Selective considerations in establishing a strong communication network between shifts should include the following points:

- Provide sufficient time for discussion in an atmosphere conducive to communication.
- Present simple, clear, well-defined facts. Simplicity will enhance universal understanding.
- Summarize presentations and reclarify at the end of the presentation.

Each individual and her contribution to the unit should be valued and acknowledged. A team-building philosophy that supports the concept of service excellence should prevail and be clearly evident in both words and actions toward patients and colleagues (Redland, 1992; Brown, 1991; McConnell, 1989).

Communication mechanisms to enhance intershift communications should be developed by staff, in an atmosphere that is open and receptive to all suggestions and concerns. Active listening should be encouraged; educate staff to listen with one ear for *meaning* and one ear for *hearing*. Management should be listening to staff and staff should be listening to one another (Raudsepp, 1990).

Leaders should always maintain direct eye contact when communicating with staff. Keep lines of communication flowing by informing staff of all organizational changes. Make time for staff to listen to issues and present positive suggestions so that communication breakdown may be minimized.

Maintain a highly visible, approachable posture with each shift, visiting with staff regularly during their shifts. Use humor when interacting with staff to help put members at ease and allow greater group participation. Praise and acknowledgement of staff by managers and fellow staff members should be encouraged and openly practiced (Redland, 1992). The development of open, positive communication among staff and between shifts is an ongoing process requiring constant nurturing and support to maintain at high levels.

J TROFINO

◆ HOW CAN I WORK WELL WITH A SUPERVISOR WHO IS A POOR COMMUNICATOR?

Q How does one work with a superior who does not communicate clear expectations?

A This can certainly be a challenge when a person is working with unclear expectations. If the supervisor is not clear, it becomes incumbent upon the nurse to ask questions and seek clarification to a greater degree than if expectations were made clear. In other words, in a very nonthreatening way, ask your supervisor what it is that she would like for you to do and what outcomes she would like to see for you to be successful. Ask questions in a general sense and then very specifically so that you can get a clear idea of what your supervisor expects from you. If this ambiguity continues, you may also want to assertively ask your supervisor to set clear expectations that she believes will help make all of you a better team with improved outcomes.

KJ McDONAGH

◆ WHAT STEPS SHOULD I TAKE TO RESOLVE COMMUNICATION PROBLEMS WITH MY STAFF AND OTHERS?

Q I recently received a phone call from the director of another department informing me that one of my staff had been "very rude" to one of her staff during a transaction. I value my relationship with the director but I know that the behavior mentioned is not characteristic of my staff member. What would be the first steps in resolving this situation?

A Even the most conscientious employee can have a bad day, so you might begin by initiating a conversation with the employee relating to her how the interaction had been perceived by the other involved employee. Convey your surprise at the feedback and that the described behavior seems inconsistent with this employee's usual approach to her job. At this point you might elicit the employee's perception of the incident and ask whether there is anything particular going on with her that is influencing her ability to perform her responsibilities in the manner you expect. Her response will dictate your next action. If she acknowledges inappropriate behavior, assist her in determining if any follow-up would clear the air. If she perceives the situation completely differently, you and she may want to sit down with the other involved employee and director and try to determine where communication broke down.

This is a critical communication exchange for a number of reasons. Ideally, feedback from employee to employee should not flow via directors. The objective of the managers in this situation is to model constructive resolution of conflict to eliminate the need for them to run interference in the future as much as to bring some closure to an incident that may leave residual negative feelings and jeopardize otherwise good working relationships. Utilize the following to guide your discussion:

- Convey your confidence in both people and their positive intent.
- Focus on really hearing both perspectives.
- Elicit the employees' thoughts on preventing recurrence and how the two directors may be of assistance.
- Demonstrate the commitment the directors have to the departments' working constructively together.
- Acknowledge anything that perhaps should have been done differently.
- Above all, utilize this opportunity for learning and growth, not punishment.

JE BEGLINGER

Competency

♦ HOW DO I ENSURE COMPETENCY?

Q How does the nurse manager ensure competency?

A Even before making a job offer, be sure that your hiring practices mandate that prospective employees are competent. Once the individual is hired, your orientation process should be discussed and understood fully by the new employee in terms of time lines and expected outcomes.

Performance-oriented behavioral objectives should be discussed in relation to your organization's practice standards. Be sure that these competency statements are clear, behaviorally stated, and measurable. These statements should indicate that competency exists or that it can be demonstrated. Once your new employee has successfully completed the orientation process, it should be clear what specific competencies will be mandated on an annual basis, such as fire and safety regulations and the right to know laws. Many nursing organizations enlist the help of the nursing education department to conduct classes and maintain these records. Lists can be generated from that office that will call your attention to employees whose mandatory competency requirements are coming up for renewal. It is recommended that you post this list for your staff so that the responsibility of renewal rests squarely with them.

You can formalize this further by having a policy stating that if an individual is not up to date on the mandatory requirements, the salary increase associated with the performance review will be held until the requirements are met.

An additional step that would help you to ensure competency would be to implement mid-year performance reviews. Stay in touch with off-shift supervisors or preceptors and resource nurses regarding the performance of the individual coming up for review so that you can give that nurse specific feedback. Take this opportunity to reinforce the areas needing improvement so that the issue will have been resolved by the time of the annual review.

Last, provide as many educational opportunities as possible for your staff to remain competent. Support their attendance at nursing grand rounds or workshops, encourage certification in their field, and make VCRs and educational videos available to them on the unit so that they can view them during break times.

In summary, if you hire competent employees, orient them fully, establish processes for mandatory requirements, provide learning opportunities for them, and review their performance regularly, you will have done your part in ensuring competency.

V MANCINI

♦ HOW CAN I ENSURE THAT COMPETENCY REMAINS THE FOCUS OF PERFORMANCE EVALUATIONS?

Q I have worked hard to develop staff involvement in performance evaluation. I want to keep staff focused on competency and performance outcomes. What elements do I need to include in order to ensure that competency remains the focus of performance evaluations?

A Once you have developed competency statements for the job categories being evaluated, it is important to use those statements to guide the actual evaluation. Competency statements describe the performance expectations of persons holding specific jobs. To retain the emphasis on *performance* rather than *personalities,* the evaluation should include *behavioral* evidence (observed) of the employee's ability to demonstrate the competency. In addition, any feedback or correction plans should also be behavioral and specific, so the employee can know when she has met the expectation or specifically what she must do in the future to demonstrate the expected competency.

M MURPHY

◆ WHAT SHOULD I DO IF ONE OF MY EMPLOYEES CAN'T READ?

Q I have an employee who I think can't read. What should I do?

A The first concern always is patient safety and ensuring the quality of nursing care of individual patients. If nursing care is not threatened, your focus can be on the welfare and growth of the employee.

In a genuinely open, honest, and caring way, describe the experiences or situations you have observed that have led you to believe the employee cannot read. Tell the person your concerns. Ask the employee to help you understand ways you can be helpful. There are a host of reading learning programs in your community you can suggest to help your employee learn to read.

ME PARKER

Computerization

◆ WILL COMPUTERS CHANGE NURSING PRACTICE?

Q How will computers change the future of nursing practice?

A As Naisbett (1982) noted in his book *Megatrends,* we are now an information society.

Health care is clearly at the heart of this technology explosion. So much information is being generated about patients each day that it is often difficult to convert these enormous data bases into useful information. Computerized monitoring, computerized testing, telecommunications technology, teleconferencing, electronic storage and retrieval of information, centralized computer systems to track supply ordering, admissions, staffing, patient bills, laboratory data, and hundreds of other information sources are all commonplace in health care today. As a result, nurses will have many critical roles to play in the information age; some are extensions of their current roles and some are totally new roles.

Nurses of the future will need to be computer literate. More important, nurses will need to serve as a bridge for patients between the high-tech world of health care and the personal and high-touch needs of humans with health care problems. In addition, integrated systems of the future, capable of instantly communicating patient information around the world, will require nurses to be constantly vigilant in safeguarding the confidentiality of patient data. Finally, the huge, rapid electronic collection of continuously generated data will require nurses to see the overall, "big picture" view of patients.

A critical skill to develop will be the ability to translate large volumes of data into meaningful trends and patterns of information reflecting the whole person. The ability to step back from intense and detailed technical reports and to see the significance of the human being and his or her place in the context in which he or she lives will be a key normalizing and essential role of nursing. As a nurse manager you will need to help your staff become computer literate while maintaining and enhancing their human relations skills. As a nurse leader you will have to role model technologic adaptation and the need to be a skilled data manager dedicated to the integrity of the patient's holistic nature. This means learning new skills and using new technology while acting as a change agent for those who might be intimidated by the computer age.

MC ALDERMAN

◆ WILL COMPUTERS MAKE MY JOB EASIER?

Q What can computers do to make my job easier?

A Computers can be of great assistance to you in four areas: access to information, decision making, your own learning, and communication.

1. *Access to information*—Have you ever been in a situation in which the administrator has asked you to quickly investigate a patient fall complaint? Would having the most recent patient satisfaction data and the patient fall statistics for this month at your fingertips be helpful to you in your investigation and response? Of course it would. In the same vein, wouldn't it be great if the patient information was up to the minute, rather than several hours old? Unfortunately, the situation in many organizations is that information about patient falls and the "real time" status of the patient is often difficult and time consuming for a manager to retrieve. The person who collects the fall information is not available, the nurse caring for the patient is tied up with another patient and has not charted yet, the x-ray has been read but the report has not been sent to the floor—and the list goes on.

Access to an integrated clinical, quality, and financial information network would eliminate the time you spend chasing down information. By simply turning on the personal computer in your office, you could retrieve the information you need to complete an effective investigation and to initiate corrective actions.

2. *Decision making*—You may have some experience with automated patient classification systems, which have been used to make decisions about resource management. The trend is moving away from the traditional, quantitative systems, to systems that emphasize patient standards, as well as previously underemphasized nursing assessment and outcome evaluation (Finnegan, 1993).

The wealth of software programs available to the small business owner today is incredible. Many contemporary software programs can be utilized by managers to make decisions about budget planning and monitoring, salary program management, regulatory record-keeping, and project management.

3. *Learning*—One of the most difficult accomplishments for managers is the pursuit of their own learning. Finding the time to get way for conferences, go to school, or simply keep up with journals is sometimes impossible. Many business journals and newspapers, such as the *Wall Street Journal,* are available on-line to subscribers. Look for more and more nursing publications to move in that direction.

There are also many tutorials available to you. For example, the American Organization for Nurse Executives, in collaboration with Medi-Sim, Inc., produces a software program teaching financial management to nurse managers. The journal *Computers in Nursing* publishes an annual software directory and is a good resource to locate computer-assisted education software.

4. *Communication*—Have you ever had to manually send the same information to several different departments at one time? Have you missed an important meeting because a memo was lost in the mail? Do you spend a significant amount of time playing "telephone tag"? The answer is yes, unless your organization provides you with electronic mailboxes. In these systems, you can send and receive information via computer and not rely on the mail or be tied to the phone. If you are in a meeting when the other party responds to your request or vice versa, the information can still be communicated and stored until you can retrieve it. As health care organizations expand into large networks, electronic mail will become a necessity.

It is important to remember that automation by itself is not the answer. Beware of organizational initiatives that may be flawed, resulting in fiscally draining outcomes. Flawed initiatives do not adequately take into account the viewpoint of the bedside practitioner in the design and implementation of information systems. Some projects attempt to replicate an inadequate paper process, rather than taking advantage of new technology. The goals of the project may be fraught with disagreement among managers, vendors, and professionals about the dimension of the system. Finally, beware of initiatives that do not have the strong input of nurses with nursing informatics background.

CK WILSON

◆ HOW DO I KNOW WHICH COMPUTER PROGRAMS TO BUY?

Q There are many computer staffing and scheduling programs on the market. What is the best way to select one that will meet my needs?

*A*Points to consider when selecting a staffing and scheduling program are numerous. One factor that seems to cause great difficulty, if not adequately addressed before purchasing a system, surrounds the question of system function. Regardless of the size of your hospital, or the sophistication of a software package, in the final analysis the functions of the system must match the needs of the organization. Therefore the selection must not be a decision made by a few individuals, but rather one that incorporates the thinking of all levels of management. Begin by documenting, as specifically as possible, the functions that will be required, and outline them in a written request for information (RFI) from several vendors. Some general functions from which you might develop your detailed specifications include recording, maintaining, and printing information related to

- Available employees by category, skill level, qualifications, and status.
- Preferences, expertise, and recent assignments of float personnel.
- Staff use of overtime, sick time, holidays, LOA, education time.
- Schedule preferences of each staff person, and the unit's cyclical schedule.
- Organization-wide staffing work sheet.
- Master staffing plans based on budgeted units of service and standard for hours of care.
- Position control documents, including filled and vacant positions.
- Turnover reports, number of hires, transfers, and terminations, with reasons.
- Staff productivity data and analysis.
- Employee history profiles relating hire date, license number and expiration, and education record.
- Variances in actual and required staffing.
- Staffing needs by skill level based on individual care requirements (acuity).
- Scheduling guidelines for each unit and employee.
- Nursing costs per hour, per patient day, and per unit of service.
- Trends and graphs of nursing resource use.

In preparing the RFI, include information about your organization's size and number of employees that the system will need to manage. Request that the vendors specify how their product handles the functions identified, and the time frame required for implementation. Finally, give the vendor a deadline date

by which you need to receive the information. Although outlining functions is merely the first step in the selection process, it is a most important step in ensuring satisfaction with the purchase.

SA FINNIGAN

♦ **HOW DO I LEARN ABOUT COMPUTERS?**

*Q*How do I obtain Automated Data Processing (ADP) support when I don't know what I need and don't have time to teach myself about what I need, and the organization will not hire a consultant for me?

*A*Computer literacy is rapidly becoming a required skill to function effectively in the health care environment. Institutional strategic planning objectives frequently identify the incorporation of "informatics" as a critical element in the system of integrated care.

You will be well advised to reallocate your time and avail yourself of the learning opportunities that are commonplace in most settings. Specialized educational courses for beginning users are provided by major vendors of automated systems, academic settings provide classes for various levels of interest from novice to advanced, retail stores with major product lines of computer services provide entry-level learning opportunities, and some vendors eager to sell their products will come on site with their equipment and walk you step-by-step through your objectives and show you what the automated system can provide.

Major educational settings are providing courses in informatics as part of the routine curriculum. Obtain permission to audit such courses. Business schools offer short-term courses, generally tailored to give a basic foundation.

Networking with facilities in other hospitals that have implemented a management information system is yet another option; many of these options can be conveniently planned to accommodate the working individual and are not financially prohibitive.

Finally, an institutional direction with time lines for introducing integrated management of patient data at all levels would be an initial step. This would provide a clear definition of your needs and the systems and applications to support this global strategy, thus avoiding a fragmented approach to patient data management.

LM JOHNSON

♦ WILL COMPUTERS REDUCE DOCUMENTATION TIME?

Q What can we expect from computers that will reduce documentation time?

A Groups of people are working to achieve an open, standard-based computer system to allow greater communication regarding patient information than that provided by the present closed, proprietary systems currently in use. Standardization of communication would mean that all health care providers would use similar words to describe health care problems and interventions. This demonstrates the need to solidify a common language among nurses and ultimately among health care providers. One major influence to standardizing nursing terminology has been the work of the North American Nursing Diagnoses Association (NANDA). There is an urgent need for nurses to be part of the development of the interdisciplinary language rather than having it externally imposed. This would facilitate entering patient data in one area only and having these data available when needed for that patient, thus eliminating the frequent duplication that currently exists, requiring numerous entries in patient charts.

Clinical information systems presently automatically acquire, display, and report crucial information where and when it is needed. The transition to computerized documentation requires an initial investment of time, energy, and money. Time and energy are needed to thoroughly assess the elements that are useful for inclusion in patient documentation. Time and energy are also incurred in the start-up phase of learning and adapting the system. Remember that learning a computer system can be likened to learning a second language in that it is evolutionary and perfected through practice. Cost is obviously a factor

in purchasing an information system. In addition, allocation of funds to facilitate the education of nursing staff cannot be overlooked. Once an integrated system is in place and patient information can be entered from the multitude of treating providers (e.g., via insurance forms, doctor's office forms) who can then interact with one another, documentation time will certainly be reduced. Hewlett-Packard's excellent booklet, "Choosing a Clinical Information System" (1990), and Roy Simpson's (1992) *Technology: Nursing the System* are recommended for additional information in this area.

SR. M FINNICK

♦ ARE THERE POCKET COMPUTERS THAT REDUCE DOCUMENTATION TIME?

Q Are there pocket computers that can be downloaded into main computers to reduce time spent documenting?

A Computer technology and its application to nursing documentation are rapidly making their way to the point of care delivery. Currently, two types of hand-held computers are available for use at the bedside. One type requires downloading at the end of a shift, and the other works off of a radio frequency and functions like a personal computer without the need to download. Limitations of these computers are due primarily to their size and in the case of the radio frequency type, their limited range (Health Care Expert Systems, 1993; Hendrickson & Kovner, 1990). Technology is changing rapidly, and new models will probably be on the market soon.

Applications that would result in significant time savings for nurses include daily charting, nursing assessment, and discharge instructions. However, this would require free text ability and a keyboard, which the hand sets are too small to accommodate. Finally, the time in waiting for hand sets to download can become an inconvenience; in addition, misplaced or missing hand-held sets can contribute to computer downtime and nurse frustration (Health Care Expert Systems, 1993).

The introduction of newer concepts like voice-activated computers for nursing documentation may

C

respond to nursing needs with greater efficiency and fewer disadvantages (Trofino, 1993).

J TROFINO

Confidentiality

♦ WHAT DOES CONFIDENTIALITY MEAN?

Q What does confidentiality mean? We have to share patient information to properly care for the patient. Is confidentiality really a myth?

A Confidentiality can be defined as the condition and the resulting obligation that certain information about a patient will not be shared with any personnel other than those directly involved with the aspect of care that requires such knowledge. Most institutions have confidentiality policies stating that case discussion, consultation, examination, and treatment are confidential and will be conducted discreetly. Patient's rights include the promise of confidentiality. Most computer systems have code access, but confidentiality is of concern when so many have access to records all over the hospital. There are mechanisms that can be instituted to check which persons enter the computer access of each patient. Some hospitals have taken disciplinary actions against personnel for accessing information on patients for which they have no professional responsibility.

Ways to avoid breaks in confidentiality are:
1. Never discuss patients or patient information in public areas such as elevators, public corridors, cafeterias, and open rooms.
2. Ask yourself if the information you are passing along is necessary for patient care or outcome. Report pertinent clinical information and refrain from the tendency to gossip about family or other situations.
3. Screen persons asking for patient information for correct identification and intent.
4. Follow the "golden rule," and talk about others only as you would want someone to talk about you.

5. Encourage others to use these rules, and remind them to lower their voices or step into another room to discuss detailed patient information.

BH DUGGER

♦ HOW CAN I EXPLAIN WHY I FIRED SOMEONE WITHOUT BREAKING CONFIDENTIALITY RULES?

Q Several nurses in our facility feel that a recent decision to terminate a nurse was unfair. How can I explain to them that she was terminated with just cause, without breaking rules of confidentiality?

A This is one of the most difficult situations a nurse manager may ever face. Having to deal with all the issues surrounding a decision to terminate someone is difficult enough without having to defend your decision to others. Clearly, you can't disclose any information regarding the confidential employee situation. This being the case, you have no choice but to let your past credibility as a reasonable and fair manager speak for you. In some instances the institution's reputation as a reasonable and equitable employer will offer a complement to your credibility. In the very best of cases, you can say to your nurses that you are not in a position to disclose confidential information related to any employee. Validate with them that you understand their need to feel that everyone is treated fairly and that you are committed to that also. Ask them to trust in your reputation and the institution's reputation for acting fairly and equitably over the years. Use their confidence levels in you and the system to give them the reassurance they need. If the trust levels are sufficient, this should satisfy their concerns about the fairness of the situation. You may still have to provide them an outlet to deal with the changes this may bring about on the unit from a social perspective, but the question of trusting that a fair decision was made is at least put to rest.

Unfortunately, some managers don't have the luxury of having developed that level of trust between them and their nurses. It may be because they are new managers or it could be that their past history has been less than exemplary in this area. If you are a new manager and don't have a history within this institution, you can share with your nurses what your past experiences have been regarding terminations and even your philosophy on how one should go about making such difficult decisions. Be careful not to talk about specifics, but rather attempt to communicate a healthy respect for the concept that everyone deserves a fair deal from their employer, while at the same time acknowledging that that is a two-way street. Ultimately, if they pursue specifics, you will have to ask them to trust you and they will choose whether to do so based on their perception of your trustworthiness.

If you have a clouded history of inconsistent decisions regarding termination or if the institution somehow has created suspicion over the fairness of recent decisions, you have a very difficult task. Easing their concerns may be impossible. Over time and with visible consistent and fair treatment of everyone by management, the trust level should change. All you can do in these situations is attempt to develop rapport and trust with your staff and ask them to support you in doing your job, just as you attempt to do for them. In order to avoid this problem in the future, nurse managers need to concentrate their efforts on developing a trusting relationship with their staff by keeping them involved and informed, as well as being open, fair, and honest toward all.

CCC LEVENS

Conflict

♦ HOW DO I RESOLVE CONFLICT AMONG STAFF?

Q How do I go about facilitating the resolution of ongoing conflict between and among various staff members?

A It is important for them to be reminded of what parameters or boundaries exist for their behavior. Clearly the conflict must not interfere with safe, competent, and caring patient care. Second, it must not introduce legal risk to patients, staff, or the organization. Third, it must not lead to severe morale

issues on the unit. When one or more of these conditions are likely, the manager must take action.

Sit down with the individuals involved and reiterate your expectations (and when yours have been articulated, those of the staff). Be specific. For example,

Each person is responsible for her own interpersonal relationships and you are therefore expected to resolve your conflict directly with the person with whom you are in conflict. You may come to me for advice and I will help you find ways to resolve the conflict with each other. I will not solve conflicts for you because I believe you are able to and should do this yourselves. I expect that you will resolve this conflict within 3 days. If you are unable or unwilling to do this, I expect to hear from you within those 3 days.

Work with them. They may not be successful the first time. Help them to think through options and to try again. Praise their efforts and successes. Be supportive if they are not successful, but insist on their resolving their own interpersonal problems. Don't be trapped into being a parent and solving conflicts for them.

JE JENKINS

♦ HOW DO I CLEAR A QUARRELSOME ATMOSPHERE BETWEEN TWO CAPABLE WORKERS?

Q Two staff members in my department are having a great deal of conflict over any issue that comes up. I have talked with them both, but they don't seem to be able to control themselves when a conflict arises. They are both capable and I don't want to lose either of them. How should I resolve this situation?

A This situation needs to be resolved as soon as possible. One could interpret that there is strong competition between these two staff members. This usually arises from feelings of inferiority. Their individual strengths need to be identified and competencies acknowledged. Keeping this in mind, it would seem apparent that you have discussed the conflict with the two of them. Have you discussed it with them together? If not, that may be a good place to start. An open discussion between the two of them

C

and facilitated by you or a psychiatric CNS nurse, if available, may assist the two of them to better understand the underlying reasons for their conflict. Two capable people ought to be able to recognize the destructiveness of their interactions when a conflict arises.

An assessment of this situation may also need to be made as to its impact on the staff working in this area. Sometimes the environment is such that this problem is perpetuated, and others encourage the continuation of the conflict interactions of the two staff members to give fuel to their conversations. Again, this needs to be addressed with the group of staff members. If all possible solutions have been tried, then you may need to recommend that one or both of the employees move to another unit. Ignoring the situation is not a solution. The facilitation needs to have a goal, based on your style, of whether the encounter is one of confrontation and conflict resolution, or one of establishing effective communication between the two staff members.

SR. M FINNICK

◆ WHAT CAN I DO TO HELP PEOPLE WHO MUST WORK TOGETHER BUT CONTINUALLY ARGUE?

Q How do I assist a unit educator and nurse manager who work together but have frequent conflicts?

A It is assumed from this question that the persons involved are peers or at least that no line relationship is involved. The answers will generally fall into establishing common goals and negotiating conflicting issues. The problems often fall into one of the following areas. The nurse educator is disruptive of the manager's authority on the unit; the educator is intent on fulfilling goals on the unit that do not match or tie into those of the unit. There is a personality problem; the manager does not support educational programs and feels educators should do patient care. As a person interested in solving this conflict, the first thing for you to remember is that it is not appropriate to judge the validity of each person's complaints, only to recognize that conflict exists. The primary issue is that both persons are paid to reach the goals of the organization, and by their work, have a positive impact on patient outcomes. When each person complains about the other in your presence, listen carefully, state that you understand the complainant's feelings, and ask the complainant to identify where she thinks the other person is coming from with her actions. Are they related to the same goals and values as those of the complainant but with different priorities? Where are the similarities in beliefs and values? Over a period of time, you can help each person to notice the similarities rather than concentrate on the differences. When appropriate, perhaps a meeting over coffee could help them understand each other's goals and how their methods to achieve those goals are causing unnecessary friction. The discussion could then lead into how to build on each other's strengths for a unified goal of quality care and personal and professional goal achievement.

If the conflict is occurring from an open personality conflict, the approach, although the same, would differ slightly in the initial steps. After listening in a nonjudgmental way to one person complain about the other in subjective, emotional ways, you may need to point out that both of the persons involved are role models and that their feelings may be getting in the way of achieving goals. The challenge for all people in leadership roles is to move past personal likes and dislikes and look for those positive attributes that exist in all and to be able to work as a team to reach goals. Nonjudgmental listening with the continual response of moving each person back to her primary purpose should be your role. Mutual goal setting, respect for each other's roles, consideration for staff who become involved in the conflict, and above all, their responsibility to quality patient care, should be stressed.

S LENKMAN

◆ HOW DO I RESOLVE QUARRELS BETWEEN RNs AND LVNs OVER DUTIES?

Q How do I clarify the constant conflicts between registered nurses and licensed vocational nurses regarding their roles and accountabilities?

A To achieve the most cost-effective skill mix while maintaining quality care, the level of skill required of each care provider needs to be clearly understood. This level of care is defined in state laws, and every nurse manager is responsible for understanding it. The state law privileges by licensure and limitations then need to be reflected in hospital job descriptions. These job descriptions actually serve as the hospital's policy regarding who can do what.

Cost effectiveness is enhanced by permitting each provider to work to her highest skill level. For example, a licensed vocational nurse may be able to start IVs in some states, but in others certification may be required. To maximize use of a licensed vocational nurse, a hospital should then be sure its licensed vocational nurses are certified and competent at starting IVs.

The registered nurses on each unit then need to decide on a care delivery model and with the licensed vocational nurses decide how they will work together to deliver care. Excessive role overlap creates increased role confusion and usually results from inappropriate skill mix when hiring. For example, if a registered nurse needs a partner to help with routine ADLs but needs little help with medications, perhaps a nursing assistant would be a more appropriate partner than a licensed vocational nurse.

In order to achieve the appropriate skill mix on a unit, explore each of the following steps with your staff:

1. Review the patient population of the unit and tasks to be performed for these patients.
2. Delineate the tasks by level of provider skill required.
3. Decide on a care delivery model—how will care be divided and delivered—usually some modification of primary, team, partnership, and total patient care.
4. Hire the skill mix needed for your patient population.
5. Discuss as a team who does what and how to achieve maximal quality and efficiency.

D SHERIDAN

♦ HOW CAN I CONTINUE TO WORK FOR A BOSS I DISLIKE?

Q I don't like my boss. There is nothing about her style or approach that I can tolerate. These past 2 years have been very difficult for me. What can I do about how I feel?

A One of the vagaries of management is the possibility that you won't like or get along with some key players in the organization. It is not possible to like everyone and sometimes the conflict is as fundamental as individual behavior and personality. If you can confront your own feelings and sort out specifically what you have trouble with, you can clarify some of the issues with your boss. In any relationship, it is generally not true that only one of the parties has all of the problems. Some self-assessment should be helpful as well.

If there is a real problem with her behavior and she is open to discussing your differences of opinion with her, you should do so, and soon. Some people are willing to confront perceptual conflicts without the need to penalize those who identify such issues. However, often this is not true, and individual confrontation may be risky. It is sometimes advisable to seek out a neutral third person and ask for guidance with regard to appropriate approaches. New insights regarding how you might pursue your differences may result.

If after consideration and self-assessment, you still feel unable to cope with the differences and finding some common ground appears impossible, some change is necessary. If the work you do is hampered or you are unhappy with circumstances you can't change, you have to make some decisions. Whether you stay in the role will depend on what you think may change in your relationship, and what you can handle with regard to what you can't change. When person and position don't fit together, it is always wise to move to a more satisfying role. This is a final option and a serious one; it should be carefully considered when you can no longer tolerate nor change your situation.

T PORTER-O'GRADY

♦ WHAT DO I SAY TO A STAFF MEMBER I BELIEVE IS TRYING TO UNDERMINE MY AUTHORITY?

Q A nurse on my unit is constantly undermining my authority and creating problems among the staff, causing great dissension within the ranks. I believe her motivation is to get me fired so she can take over my job. How can I confront her with this issue?

C

A There are two possible responses to this scenario. If the person is salvageable and capable of contributing to the unit, you should develop a strategy to gain her support. The challenge is for you to effectively channel this individual's energy toward productive and supportive behaviors. If the person is not salvageable, you must recognize this and develop a plan for how you will either convince her to leave or document her out of the system.

Is the person salvageable or not? Either way, you need to let the nurse know her behavior is noticed. You should first meet with the nurse to find out from her how she feels things are going and if there are any concerns or suggestions she has about the unit. You should then ask her if there is anything she would recommend you do differently to make the unit function better. After carefully listening to all of this and assuming the nurse would have little constructive criticism, you need to share with her what has been observed, heard, or experienced. It must be clearly stated that it cannot continue and must stop at once. In all likelihood the nurse will deny there is any truth to your comments. Then, depending on your assessment of the nurse's long-term contribution to the unit, the plan should unfold.

If you believe the nurse should stay because of her potential to contribute to the success of the unit, you should share with the nurse your desire for her to be successful. You should share with the nurse thoughts about how she could contribute to the success of the unit and reaffirm your willingness to work for that success.

You need to have a well thought out strategy and plan of action that moves the nurse from undermining and sabotaging to supporting and participating in the changes within the unit. It is important to get the nurse's commitment to be proactively and positively involved. You must also share with the nurse what behavior and performance expectations are necessary for her to succeed.

Another strategy would be to give the nurse a project in which she clearly understands the goals and expectations of the project and is empowered to accomplish the project the way in which she feels it needs to be done. Weekly meetings should be held to monitor progress and to ensure behavior and performance changes are recognized and reinforced. Likewise, if problems or old behaviors resurface, they need to be addressed immediately.

You could help her find and attend management training classes or encourage her to go back to school. Often, it is through this kind of conflict that the strongest relationships and support are built. Conflict can be, and often is, very healthy. It is important to encourage people to talk openly and freely about their ideas, disagreement, or opinions. This needs to be done face to face and openly, not behind closed doors, with physicians, or in an arena in which nothing can be resolved; in these ways environments can be destroyed. Typically, negative energy can be channeled into positive energy with sincere and frequent coaching, firm written behavior expectations, and peer pressure. It is often those individuals who cause managers the most grief that also provide them the most opportunity for managerial growth, if the manager is mature enough and confident enough to deal with the individual in a proactive way.

On the other hand, if you feel the nurse is not salvageable, then you must develop another plan of attack. After talking with her, you should let her know you are aware of her "behind the scenes" activities. You should let the nurse know that you will not tolerate this kind of disruptive behavior on the unit and share with her the behavior and performance expectations necessary for her to succeed. This must be done in writing. You need to clearly articulate and document what is expected through measurable goals. Weekly or bi-weekly meetings should be set up in which the past week's performance is discussed, addressing what went right and what didn't. Each meeting should end with a written summary of what was discussed and be signed by each participant and put in the nurse's file. This should continue until enough documentation has occurred to justify the nurse's termination or until the nurse decides on her own to quit or transfer.

It is important to ensure that the human resource liaison is aware of your employee issue and provides the proper coaching or support if necessary. Taking the time and energy to clearly articulate and document for the nurse your expectations and how she has or has not complied provides the opportunity for the nurse to come to her own conclusion that the job is not right for her. You may also assist the nurse to find a job more suitable for her talents, desires, or personality. As a manager, you are responsible for treating everyone fairly. This often takes an inordinate amount of time, but it contributes significantly to the respect and admiration staff have for you. If staff members see that the manager is willing to take time to help them grow and be successful or even to leave gracefully, then staff will reciprocate. It is the willingness to give that stimulates others to give back and is a key indicator of success for a manager.

J TORNABENI

◆ HOW CAN I GET HONEST FEEDBACK FROM MY STAFF?

Q I frequently hear from my supervisor that my staff has concerns about my management performance. Also, I am told by the assistant managers about conflicts among staff members. How can I promote honest face-to-face communication from staff regarding my management performance and better conflict resolution among staff?

A There are two separate issues being addressed in this scenario. Both of these issues deal with the process of climate creation at the unit level. Climate creation is the operation of addressing the human psyche. It involves both intrapersonal (within yourself) and interpersonal (with others) dimensions.

In order to promote open face-to-face communication and feedback from staff regarding your performance, you must be open to receiving feedback and listen to staff. This is not easy and will take practice if you are not accustomed to it. Feedback is necessary if you expect change to happen; however, it can also be uncomfortable. The use of techniques such as using "I" messages can promote healthy communication of feelings. Techniques like this one can be inserviced to the entire staff with time allotted for practice. There is proven success with many of these interventions.

Self-esteem is directly related to a person's ability to receive feedback and resolve conflict. To the degree that you are secure with your "self," you will be able to support and build esteem in others. In other words, I will be more threatened by your feedback if I lack confidence in myself. It is important to be sensitive to this fact. As a manager, you may decide to seek additional coaching or referrals for those staff members who are threatened within this process.

Conflict resolution is another topic for group inservicing. There are speakers available who specialize in how to approach conflict and appropriate ways to resolve conflict. It is important to move with these issues as a group and to allow for practice. Designing this learning as an expectation for all staff promotes a healthier unit climate.

MT SINNEN

◆ HOW CAN I COPE WITH A PERSON WHO CONTINUALLY PROVOKES ME?

Q There is a staff member on our unit who continually attempts to force me into anger and raising my voice, hoping I will lose control. How do I deal with this person?

A Think about the reasons why this person is constantly pushing you to the brink, and then find the common element that links all these situations together and evaluate the problem. Half of the responsibility rests with you, so identify your role and figure out ways to correct it. There is little you can do to change the way others behave, but there are many ways for you to correct your own behavior.

Look at your interpersonal relationship with this person. What does your body language convey when you are speaking with the person? What feelings does this person conjure up in you when you think of her? Possible reasons for this person's behavior are resentment or envy, or she simply thinks you're doing something wrong. Deal with the person directly. Meet with the person at a time when neither of you is in the heat of an argument or difficult situation. Explain that you expect to avoid future confrontations starting now. Solve the riddle and then proceed head-on to confront the root of the problem, not the individual incidents that provoked the outbursts.

P MARALDO

◆ HOW SHOULD I RESPOND TO A SUPERVISOR WHO CONTINUALLY CRITICIZES NURSING ADMINISTRATORS?

Q I have a weekend supervisor who tends to be nonsupportive and "bad-mouths" decisions made by nursing administration. How can we respond to her when she behaves this way?

C

A It is important to find out why this supervisor is acting in this manner. It might be that this person feels left out of the decision-making process and therefore finds it difficult to be supportive of the decisions being made by nursing administration. Before providing feedback about the behavior of "bad-mouthing," it may be worthwhile to investigate just how and where the role of the weekend supervisor fits within the decision-making process at your institution. Supervisors often have a global view of the organizational issues because of their institution-wide role and therefore have a different perspective that can add a new dimension to decisions. Are they allowed to be heard? Are their concerns, opinions, and suggestions taken into account?

It is essential to provide feedback to this supervisor about the "bad-mouthing" behavior. Allowing this to continue can be detrimental to the climate of the organization. In providing this feedback, take the following into account:

1. Examine the behavior and its effects. Utilize concrete examples within the dialogue.
2. Stress the need for a cohesive, supportive management team.
3. Question her satisfaction within the supervisory role or other reasons for the behavior.
4. Outline and agree on specific interventions that will increase satisfaction and participation and decrease the nonsupportive behaviors.
5. Make it a point to reevaluate the situation.

MT SINNEN

Consultants

◆ HOW DO I EVALUATE CONSULTANTS?

Q What criteria should I use to assess consultants?

A The health care industry is overflowing with consultants, both within and outside the industry, who claim to have the expertise in whatever it is that you need to have done. Consider the number of people currently claiming expertise in quality improvement programs! Your question is a very important one. I hope the following questions can guide you in assessing consultants:

1. *What is the professional background of the individual?* You should examine whether the individual has a recognized background in your particular area of need. Has she published or presented workshops, or can she provide you with a list of clients who have experienced her work relative to your needs? You want to determine if the person truly has expertise in the area you need and is not just marketing a newly developed program in order to increase her client base. If the conversation becomes difficult, it may tip you off that the person is inexperienced.
2. *What are the values of the consultant?* Are they compatible with yours? If you are hiring someone to bring about significant change, you want someone who has the same beliefs about people and nurses and change as you do. What methods of social influence will she use to bring people on board?
3. *Does the consultant have a theoretic framework or model that is logical and psychologically satisfying to you?* Are the processes and instruments grounded in a solid base of information? Some consultants will present a slick "package" of activities that seem to work. Ask pointed questions about the outcomes at each step of the process, and why the processes must proceed in the manner outlined. If it seems fragmented, illogical, or confusing, the program will most likely not produce the desired results.
4. *What is the nature of the consultant's organization?* Are there other members of the organization who may be working with you? What is their level of expertise? When will they be used during the project? Explore the resources available to the consultant that are critical to the project. Statistical analysis may be important, for example. Does the consultant have easy access to this resource? How is the work of associates monitored and evaluated?
5. *How does the consultant assess and diagnose your needs?* Regardless of the model or processes used, the consultant should have a feel for your organization's and staff's strengths and weaknesses. What methods will be used to build a base-

line before the project begins and at key points during the project? This requires a working knowledge of research or evaluation methodology, including interview and observation techniques.

6. *How will the consultant transfer the ownership of the change and close the project or move it to the next stage?* Beware of individuals who promise magical results—or cannot tell you at what point in the project to expect desired behavioral changes.

7. *How will evaluation of the project occur and how will the consultant demonstrate accountability for her work?* This question is aimed at establishing mutual agreement about the definitions of success. The frequency of reporting, the content of the report, and who will receive the report should be discussed. I have found that the criteria for success are rarely described clearly. Both parties may think they have agreement, but often it is more global in nature. *Specific* behavioral changes should be identified, as well as shifts in how work will be done and what quality and cost outcomes to expect.

The way for this to happen is to engage prospective consultants in an *intensive* interview process. A consultant is not worth hiring if she is hesitant about participating or she offers only expansive, evasive, or general answers. Also, if she does not have the information you request, she may lack the requisite skills for the success of your project. This extensive contracting process ensures that both parties are going in the same direction and prevents blaming or the inclination of either party to avoid real change.

CK WILSON

♦ WHAT SHOULD BE INCLUDED IN A CONSULTANT'S CONTRACT?

Q What should be included in a contract with an outside consultant?

A There are perhaps as many types of contracts as there are consultants. However, from the nurse manager's perspective the following should be specified:

1. The overall scope or purpose of the project, including the intended outcomes; this is usually defined in the contract's introductory paragraph.

2. Specific objectives, with the emphasis on *specific.* The more clear you are in identifying what is to be accomplished, the better the odds the project outcomes will be successfully achieved.

3. Time lines both for the individual specific objectives and overall project completion. Be sure to identify what action either you or the consultant will take if time lines are not met as originally defined and agreed on.

4. Methods to be used in project design and completion, whether in needs assessment, questionnaires, sampling plans, surveys, data collection, or analysis.

5. Access to necessary people and data within the organization for the consultant to most effectively design and complete the project.

6. Total and itemized budget costs, specifying what the budget covers, such as development of methods, printing, processing and analysis of data, discussion and meeting time, preparation and presentation of final report, and personal consultant expenses. You need to understand exactly what *is* and what *is not* covered so that there are no assumptions that result in surprises as the project progresses.

7. Nature of the relationship with the consultant, whether as an independent contractor or as an employee. The variance here is in who pays benefits and/or income taxes, for whom, and when.

8. Copyrights, inventions, patents, and technology rights, in the event such may be an outcome of the consultation process. This item has become imperative for nursing as work redesign has been undertaken by health care organizations.

9. Assurance of confidentiality for data, findings, conclusions, and recommendations. This includes who has the exclusive rights to the consultant's final report.

10. Conditions for termination of the contract by the organization or the consultant, and time frames for the same.

11. Schedule of payments, which most consultants require at various times, particularly for extended projects. Often payment is scheduled in

C

parts; for example, a set amount is due on signing of the contract, another on completion of data collection, and the last on delivery of the final report.

12. Authorization to proceed, formalizing the agreement outcomes, time lines, project cost, and payment schedule with the appropriate organizational and consultant signatures.

Concluding advice on consultant contracts is to have the agreement reviewed by the organization's legal counsel, before obtaining signatures, to ensure legal restrictions and/or requirements are addressed and met in the contract.

BV TEBBITT

◆ HOW DO CONSULTANTS CALCULATE FEES?

Q How do consultants calculate their fees? Is there a formula?

A There are probably as many formulas as there are consultants. However, there are some key areas that must be considered when setting fees. The fees must cover the business expenses (salaries, rent, taxes), provide enough incentive that the consultant wants to continue working, and provide sufficient income to the individual consultant to meet expenses and enjoy life.

The rate billed to a client includes the salary to the consultant, a factor for the research and development required to offer the service, overhead expenses (phone/fax, postage, secretarial support, travel, miles accumulated), and benefits (health, life, disability, and unemployment insurance; taxes; vacation; retirement). Then a profit must be considered based on what the competition is doing and charging. Whether the economy is in a recession or is thriving will also affect fees. Consultants must also consider that occasionally a client does not pay for services rendered. To minimize this and not penalize good clients, the consultant will usually require partial payment up front and then regularly during the project. Then if a client does not pay on time, the consultant can decide if she wants to continue working.

Formulas that are used include the following:

1. Rule of Threes:

$\frac{1}{3}$ = Salary of consultant
+ $\frac{1}{3}$ = Overhead plus benefits
+ $\frac{1}{3}$ = Profit
= Total yearly revenues (TYR)

Billing Rate = TYR ÷ Yearly billable hours

2. Modified Rule of Threes:

$\frac{1}{2}$ = Salary of consultant
+ $\frac{1}{4}$ = Overhead plus benefits
+ $\frac{1}{4}$ = Profit
= Total yearly revenues (TYR)

Billing Rate = TYR ÷ Yearly billable hours

3. Exact Costs Method:

Hourly rate = Exact costs
+ Profit requirements
÷ Yearly billable hours

Consultants may charge by the hour or by the day, or for a fixed amount per project. Sometimes a consultant may be paid on retainer to ensure availability, when specific services are required for a fixed period of time, and to ensure a steady income.

JE JENKINS

◆ HOW CAN I GET RID OF AN UNSATISFACTORY CONSULTANT?

Q We made a bad decision in hiring an outside consultant. How do I go about terminating our contract with her?

A Review the contract agreement. Determine the components of the agreement that the consultant is not fulfilling. The process may be more difficult to address if there is not a termination clause in the contract. Discuss the contract and the situation with the people at the hospital who are responsible for contract negotiations and risk management. Depending on the nature of the contract and the situation causing you to want to terminate the contract, legal counsel may be warranted. All contracts should be carefully written to include roles, responsibilities, and expected results.

SH SMITH

Cost Control

♦ WHAT PART OF A FINANCIAL REPORT SHOULD I PAY ATTENTION TO?

Q When I am reviewing a financial report for my area of responsibility, what components should I pay special attention to?

A To review a financial report, develop a system of review for yourself that can be used each time the report is published. The following steps will provide a guide for better understanding of the financial report and your unit's performance within the budget.

1. Initially perform a gross comparison of *actual* expenses and revenues with the *budgeted* expenses and revenues. Identify where there are variances, both positive and negative. Compare the actual units of service (or any other measure of activity used in your organization) with the budgeted units of service. The activity level often will provide an explanation about variances that have occurred. Expenses may be greater than budgeted if the activity level was greater than expected. Generally, expenses can be expected to increase proportionally with the activity level. Flexible budgets create changed budgeted expectations when volume changes occur. To check variances from the budget, calculate the actual and budgeted cost per unit of service and compare. If there are discrepancies, look for explanations based on the variances.

2. Variances are often explained by volume, price or rates, or quantity. Review each category that is in variance and determine the cause for the variance. *Volume variances* are caused when the volume is less than or greater than expected. Checking for the cost and/or revenue per unit of service will give information about the volume variance. Greater volume will often result in a larger gross revenue, but the type of volume may reflect a different case mix requiring more resources for care. As an example, if the increase in volume consisted of higher acuity patients, staffing levels may exceed what would be expected for that level of volume. This type of variance is called a *quantity variance,* which occurs when more resources than expected were used for a given workload. Quantity variance occurs not only with staffing expenses, but also with supplies, equipment rental, telephone expenses, and any other expense resulting from direct patient care. Negative quantity variances should be investigated, since they may also reflect productivity problems. Further analysis would include a review of productivity reports and a comparison of budgeted and worked full-time equivalents (FTEs). *Price or rate variances* occur when the expense for supplies, rentals, or salaries is higher than expected. The use of registry nurses, an increase in the use of overtime, or any other arrangements for nurses who receive a higher rate of pay than expected will cause a rate variance. *Price variances* will occur when supplies or any other expense category costs more than was expected or projected during the budgeting cycle.

3. Once actual and budgeted expenses and revenues are compared, review the revenue section of the financial trend report for the case mix information. Determine the types of patients that were seen for the time period such as the percentage of publicly assisted patients, commercial insurance patients, and contract patients. These types of payor categories will give you an indication of the types of reimbursement that will be received for services. Many financial reports will specify the deduction amount and provide a total for net revenue. Compare the actual net revenue with budgeted net revenue to determine any variance. Variances could be caused by a change in case mix resulting in more or fewer deductions, a decrease or increase in volume, or a rate increase or decrease. Compare net revenues with gross revenues for the percentage of deductions or discounts.

   Look for the net income line, which is the amount of money left after expenses are subtracted from net revenue. This number should be a positive. If it is not, expenses will need to be investigated.

4. Further financial analysis will include a review of direct and indirect costs. Direct costs refer to the cost of resources used for the direct care of patients and may include salaries for caregivers and

C

expenses for supplies and equipment. Indirect costs reflect expenses that are charged to the unit but are not directly used in providing patient care. Salaries of managers, clinical nurse specialists, and others not directly providing patient care are included in this category. Because hospitals differ in how they define these categories, investigate what constitutes direct and indirect costs for your unit. As an example, some hospitals include ward clerks as direct costs but others do not.

5. Financial information is meant to be compared and reviewed for trends. Compare budget with actual; this month with previous months; this year with previous years; your hospital with other hospitals. Compare one number with another by developing your own ratios to review trends. Hospitals differ in what kinds of financial reports are shared with specific levels of managers. Other financial reports that may be used are income statements, balance sheets, and cash flow statements. These reports are used for more global analysis of the financial solvency, use of cash, and investments made by the hospital.

JF STICHLER

ity outcomes will capture and retain market share. Reducing the cost of production will become the manager's primary contribution to the bottom line.

Managing day-to-day operations in the current environment is increasingly challenging. The importance of involving the staff in monitoring and controlling expenditures is critical. Maintaining active involvement in changes in clinical practice that affect budgetary constraints is also essential. The challenge to be innovative and creative in providing patient care is vital; thus the involvement of all direct care providers in these activities is necessary. By maintaining staff involvement and a close scrutiny of changes in clinical practices in a prospective and timely manner, day-to-day operational issues can be managed more effectively and efficiently. Staff needs to receive consistent and frequent information concerning budgetary considerations to be able to make worthwhile contributions. A collaborative working relationship with physicians also enables staff to be innovative and provide creative alternatives. The challenge to be fiscally responsible while providing quality patient care with optimal patient outcomes should be the vision.

J O'MALLEY

◆ WHY IS REVENUE GENERATION NOT AS IMPORTANT AS COST CONTAINMENT?

Q Why is revenue generation not as critical to the bottom line as cost containment? How do I manage my day-to-day operations in this environment of shrinking reimbursement and pressure on the health care system?

A In today's fiscal environment, inpatient services are typically reimbursed in some form of capitated, or fixed, fee arrangement. Furthermore, hospitals in the future may be contracting with managed care companies to provide a "lifetime of care," from birth to death, in which they are paid a flat fee to provide for the complete health needs of an insured. In this scenario, successful organizations will be those who are most efficient and can become low-cost providers. Low-cost providers who achieve qual-

◆ HOW DO I EDUCATE STAFF TO UNDERSTAND THEIR RELEVANCE TO THE BUDGET?

Q I need help in assisting my staff to understand that most dollars on the unit are spent by them in providing service. How can I increase their awareness of their involvement in expenditures?

A Health care is a labor-intensive field, which means the majority of expenses are involved with salaries and fringe benefits. Thus your staff, by providing care to patients, are involved with the largest expenditure. Education is the best tool to increase staff awareness. Many staff nurses have little idea of how much supplies cost and much less of an idea how much of the total budget is consumed by fringe benefits.

The approach to this education can take many forms. One is to involve the staff in the annual budgeting process. Depending on the policies of your institution and the current financial management knowledge levels of your staff, information can be disseminated at staff meetings or you could establish a task force to work with you in preparing the budget. This approach will make them aware of all the expenditures for your unit and how they are distributed. It will also provide insight into where cost savings may be incurred, and into how to prioritize for capital expenditures based on what they feel is needed to improve efficiency and effectiveness of patient care. This approach can be continued throughout the year by involving them in the review of periodic financial reports and the evaluation of the variances.

Another approach is to have some variation of a game such as "The Price is Right." The price of expenditures on your unit can be the "game" items and the staff would guess their amount. This approach can be either in a traditional game format or carried out over a period of time as a silent auction. As a follow-up to this activity, the staff can then be asked to develop scenarios to show how they used supplies, equipment, and time differently because they were aware of the expenditures that they have control over. A contest can be held to determine the "best" scenario.

JW ALEXANDER

♦ HOW CAN I ENCOURAGE STAFF TO DECREASE COST AND INCREASE QUALITY?

Q My corporation is in a "decrease cost and increase quality" mode. Needless to say, this is a challenge. How do I enlist all personnel on the unit in this effort?

A The challenge to increase quality while decreasing cost seems to be the byline of today's health care reform. It is essential to involve staff at all levels in these efforts. Begin by having a staff meeting and explaining what the vision is from the corporate standpoint. Use overheads or handouts that clearly and succinctly point out concepts that your organi-

zation is trying to implement. Then take those concepts from a global level to a more specific unit-based level. Ask for ideas and input. Form sub-groups that can come up with creative ideas on how to do things right. Without using gimmicks, yet with lots of spark and creativity, develop the program so that it is fun and employees feel the reward of doing things more effectively and efficiently.

KJ McDONAGH

♦ HOW DO I EVALUATE PATIENTS' CARE NEEDS AND SELECT THE RIGHT DELIVERY MODEL?

Q I have been asked to reduce costs on my unit. Staffing is as tight as I know how to make it with our current care model. What tools and methodologies are available to assist me in evaluating the care needs of our patient population and in selecting the most appropriate care delivery model?

A A methodology used to guide the process of restructuring the nursing care delivery on a unit level is job redesign. In this approach, roles are designed that meet patient care requirements, maximize productivity, and support professional nursing practice.

There are a number of process models that can be utilized in approaching work redesign, all of which begin with the identification of desired outcomes. These outcomes can include categories such as cost, staff mix, and standards of quality. Next a comprehensive assessment must be made of the current status of these desired outcomes on the nursing unit. The assessment includes a review of staff mix, clarification of the roles and responsibilities of each employee type, and quality and financial measures. This information can be enhanced further by analyzing the actual tasks of the staff.

After reviewing the literature a method of care delivery can be selected and adapted to the institutional needs based on the goals and assessment results. At the time of selection, the evaluation measures should be developed based on the stated objectives.

J O'MALLEY

◆ WHAT SHOULD I DO WHEN ASKED TO MAKE BUDGET CUTS THAT MAY AFFECT PATIENTS' SAFETY?

Q It seems that we are always asked to "cut back" and be more cost effective in our staffing. What can I do when I'm asked to cut my budget to a level where I feel that I can't meet regulatory requirements or patient safety needs? Administrators don't seem to understand these issues.

A It is difficult being a manager in this era of focus on cost reduction. The impact of the United States' spending 14% of our gross national product on health care and not receiving the benefits that the public believes should come from spending this amount of money is directly felt by every nursing manager across the country. In other words, this is not just an institutional issue, but an issue that has finally been recognized at a broader level and that will require very detailed nursing department–specific strategies. However, nursing managers should not be put in a situation in which they feel budgetary cuts are causing regulatory violations or possible problems with patient safety.

In addition, regulatory requirements are typically designed to meet a minimal level of standards of care, not optimal or maximal levels. Therefore it is incumbent on the nursing manager to discuss these issues clearly and discretely with the appropriate hospital administrator. To begin with, meeting to discuss the issues verbally is usually the best method. If you do not feel that you have been listened to, a letter following up your conversation to your administrator would be the next appropriate step. If you still do not feel your concerns are being heard, you should let your immediate supervisor know that you feel obligated to follow the chain of command and go to her immediate superior.

You should also have your rationale for why you believe patient safety or regulatory requirements are being jeopardized. You must have data and facts assembled, not just a "gut feeling" that this is harming patient safety. Good sense and laws require nurses to follow through appropriately with the administrative authorities when clinical issues such as these arise. After all, a fundamental role for all nurses, whether in a clinical area or in management, is to be strong advocates for our patients and their safety.

KJ McDONAGH

◆ WHAT ARE SOME ELEMENTS OF RESOURCE-BASED RELATIVE VALUE SCALES?

Q I have recently heard of resource-based relative value scales as applied to physicians' incomes. I am not sure that I understand what this is and means. What are the basic elements of this process?

A In 1989, Congress passed the Omnibus Budget Reconciliation Act of 1989, which was designed to regulate Medicare reimbursement fees. The government arm that administrates this legislation is the Health Care Financing Administration (HCFA). To implement this process, HCFA consulted with researchers at Harvard University and the Physician Payment Review Commission to develop a new fee schedule. Thus the resource-based relative value scale (RBRVS) was born.

The two major goals of the RBRVS are to reduce Medicare spending and to distribute Medicare payments more equitably among physicians. HCFA designed the RBRVS with a complicated formula. The formula is the basis of reimbursement and is designed to capture a more accurate picture of the "physician work." The fee schedule includes all payments for services including tests, radiology, anesthesia, nuclear medicine therapy, and physician payment.

The implementation date for physician service reimbursement was January 1, 1992. At that time, physicians could no longer charge Medicare a "reasonable or customary" prevailing charge for their services but were required to accept the new fee schedule. The fee schedule applies nationally.

The relative value of each service covers:
◆ Estimate of average physician time and effort (work).
◆ Practice expense (overhead).
◆ Malpractice insurance.

This scheduling fee is over a 5-year transition, with approximately a third of the U.S. physician services presently paid on the RBRVS fee schedule. The other services will move gradually into the new system until 1996, when full RBRVS rates will apply to all services. New physicians will be paid on the RBRVS scale immediately.

Under the old Medicare fee schedules, procedures and specialty services received greater reimbursement. In RBRVS, reimbursement is higher in those specialties that spend more time with the patients. Thus the winners in RBRVS are those physicians who practice general, family, or internal medicine, whereas the losers are those in surgery, anesthesia, and cardiology. It is clear that physician income will be affected. According to the AMA, it is estimated that Medicare payment to physicians could be reduced by as much as 16%.

In addition, it is probably not realistic that the RBRVS will stop with Medicare reimbursement. Blue Shield apparently has plans to adopt the same system at a future date. Therefore it is imperative that physicians and their staff become aware of these charges and incorporate them into their billing system correctly and efficiently.

Some issues and concerns that may be seen by hospitals and physicians are as follows:

- ♦ Hospitals and physicians could face long-lasting effects on their financial arrangements and medical staff relations.
- ♦ Changes in physician practice styles and business arrangements may occur in response to reimbursement pressures.
- ♦ RBRVS will redistribute Medicare dollars and will limit aggregate outlays to some physicians.
- ♦ Physicians may increase business ventures.
- ♦ Physicians may look to the hospital to ease reduced incomes.
- ♦ Physicians could change contractual relationships.
- ♦ Interest in control over both professional fee and facility charges may increase.
- ♦ Physicians may respond by moving services in institutional settings to independent sites.

J O'MALLEY

Cost Effectiveness

♦ **HOW CAN I KEEP MY STAFF FROM THINKING THAT I AM CONCERNED ONLY ABOUT MONEY MATTERS?**

Q How do I stay current with fiscal issues, keeping them relevant to staff's day-to-day needs, without always sounding money conscious?

A As is so often the case, information sharing and education are the fundamental ingredients to balancing the cost/quality equation. The process of budget development and management is typically very foreign to the clinical staff, which is a sad irony since they are major managers of the resources utilized in the provision of patient care. Begin by assisting your staff in understanding how the fiscal management relates to the overall mission and strategy of the hospital. Changing perceptions from managers as penny pinchers to managers as stewards of the resources can be facilitated by assisting your staff in achieving a broader understanding of the relationship of financial concerns to the ability of the hospital to achieve its mission.

The mission, strategic plan, and service priorities of the hospital lay the foundation for a discussion at the unit level of how each unit fits into the whole and what needs to be accomplished at that level to contribute to goal attainment. The fiscal realities must be well understood by everyone involved in the provision of care. This is accomplished through discussion of health care reform initiatives, your changing local health care environment, discussion of changing patient demographics, acuity, length of stay, and any other observable changes that have an impact on your ability to deliver care effectively. The staff should be involved in the budget process along with you, developing an understanding of how predictions about future volumes are made (and contributing to that process), determining the necessary human and material resources needed to care for the anticipated patients, identifying strategic opportunities, and considering opportunities to rethink standard approaches to care delivery.

One very effective strategy for assisting staff in taking a more active role in evaluating the effectiveness of their approach to patient care is the utilization of site visits to units that deliver similar services to a similar population. The opportunity to converse with colleagues about how they address challenging issues and to compare staffing strategies and any other areas of interest has proven very effective in focusing staff on how they might become active stewards of the available resources. One nurse who was a member of a unit staunchly committed to their way of doing things participated with other nurses in a number of site visits to see how other facilities were functioning. She recently described her unit's transformation this way, "I think we stopped trying not to change and started focusing on which changes will be best."

JE BEGLINGER

◆ HOW CAN MY UNIT IMPROVE OUTCOMES WITHOUT INCREASING COSTS?

Q I believe my staff is highly cost effective. What are some tools that we can use to compute the value of various clinical and unit activities undertaken at the same dollars, and improve outcomes?

A There are many tools that have been developed to "cost out" nursing care at the aggregate level. These tools in some way calculate the number of units of service provided (hours of patient care or number of clinic visits) and divide the units of service by the total cost to determine a cost per unit of service. A variation of this method can be done to look at specific activities, such as preoperative teaching or discharge planning. At this level of analysis, it may be difficult to separate all details of the activity from other activities and likewise to separate the costs. But since your ultimate goal is to improve outcomes at the lowest cost, the inclusion of extra aspects of care and costs shouldn't matter.

Once you have determined which unit activities you want to analyze, you can determine the costs associated with those activities. Items that need to be included in the determination of the cost of the activity (or unit of service) are direct and administrative personnel expenses (both hourly rate and fringe benefits), supply costs, and a portion of indirect costs such as utilities or maintenance. With some effort, the indirect costs should be obtainable from your financial office, and with simple division you can calculate the proportion related to the activity of concern.

Now that you have an idea of what makes up the clinical or unit activity and its component costs, you will need a measure of outcome. Outcome measures can be drawn from a variety of sources to include your quality improvement activities, patient comments or more formal surveys, and length of stay or infection control data.

You are now in a position to vary components of the activity, monitor the subsequent costs, and deter-

mine the effect on outcomes. Through these activities you will be able to justify your sense of cost effectiveness and discover areas where further improvements can be made. In addition, if this methodology is used with other units within your institution, you will now have a common denominator for comparison.

JW ALEXANDER

◆ HOW CAN I EVALUATE EFFECTIVENESS OF NONPRODUCTIVE TIME?

Q What methodologies are available to evaluate the effectiveness of nonproductive time such as time spent on education, orientation, or quality improvement teams? Please answer this in the context of decreased cost and increased quality of patient care.

A The concept of "nonproductive" time has long plagued nursing; the title itself suggests that it is of marginal value and must be justified in a manner that differs from "productive" time. Terminology that more accurately reflects this essential component of the professional nurse's work is "indirect time," that is, time spent on the work of nursing other than the direct caregiving activities. The evaluation of time spent in this area is of key importance to the nurse manager who finds herself managing in an environment of increasingly constrained resources. The need to make wise investments and realize a maximum payback from those investments exists as never before in health care.

The most important first step in evaluating the effectiveness of any undertaking is to have a very clear understanding of what the objective was in choosing a particular strategy or course of action. The actual outcomes achieved are then measured against the intended objective.

Educational support of staff poses a unique challenge as we move into an era of having to differentiate what we need to know from what we may like to know. Identifying the educational needs of staff may be accomplished in a number of ways. Needs assessments are a common method used to define areas of practice in which the nurses perceive their greatest learning needs. Quality improvement activities are another frequent source of information about staff learning needs. Once the educational priorities have been determined, you can establish clear objectives for learning. The extent to which learning objectives are met through the educational offering determines the effectiveness of the strategy.

Orientation experiences should be specifically tailored to the expertise and experience of the practitioner. The essential competencies for safe practice in the clinical area that has been selected should be clearly defined. The first step of the orientation experience should be validation of those competencies already mastered by the orientee and identification of unmet learning needs. Learning experiences should be structured to meet learning needs in a style that is most compatible with the orientee's learning style preferences. This will ensure assimilation of new knowledge rapidly and comfortably. Demonstrating competence in the chosen area of clinical practice without being required to needlessly "relearn" areas of practice in which competency has already been achieved is evidence of effective use of time.

Continuous quality improvement activities offer an objectively measurable investment in indirect time. Through these activities, a team of individuals analyzes a particular process that is a component of the work they do. The objective is to improve the process. The first step of the team's work is generally to create a flow chart of the process as it currently exists. As they work through the steps of the process, they identify areas for improvement. A great deal of data collection is undertaken to facilitate a full understanding of problems and opportunities. The improvements in newly designed processes can easily be quantified in the form of decreased time, fewer steps, fewer errors, and increased patient satisfaction.

JE BEGLINGER

◆ HOW CAN I ENCOURAGE MORE COST-EFFECTIVE USE OF RESOURCES?

Q As a nurse manager, how can I influence the organization to use resources on the unit in an efficient and cost-effective manner when the heads of these departments are part of the "good old boy"

network and exclude nurses from the information cycle?

A Of all the tools you have at your disposal, those used for total quality management/continuous quality improvement (TQM/CQI) are probably the strongest. If you identify a better way to use resources and document how it is better and then demonstrate your method with data, you will be listened to. The quality improvement methodology requires that you focus on the patients and their needs and expectations. If you show with a flow chart or otherwise illustrate the current process and then illustrate a more effective method along with a proposal for trial and evaluation, your administration is very likely to support you with a trial. You need to do your homework first. You need to know about state and federal regulations that may apply, the political concerns that your proposal raises, and the other departments involved (talk to them before turning in the proposal). Also talk to your supervisor so she can support you with administration.

The "good old boy (or girl) network" is alive and well in most places. One way to deal with it is to be objective and to provide data. Objective data, demonstrating how something does (or does not) work better, will do more to sell your proposal to the established group of leaders than any amount of complaining about the existing network.

M PECK

◆ HOW CAN I CONVINCE STAFF THAT CLINICAL DECISIONS HAVE FINANCIAL IMPACT?

Q How can I assist the staff to understand the financial implications of their clinical decisions?

A There are a number of ways to do this. I work with one manager who reviews financial summaries with her staff every month. By hearing how much they have spent and what it was used for, they have a better understanding of what they are able to affect. We are just beginning to implement a computer program that enables staff to see how their staffing decisions affect cost per day for the unit. This needs to be balanced with discussion of clinical priorities, but it helps to see how staff decisions affect costs.

C

We find that once educated to financial issues, staff will make cost-effective decisions. The education is important. We spend time in nursing orientation to discuss the political and economic realities that we are dealing with in our facilities so that nurses know what is happening with federal, state, and private reimbursement.

We are also learning to include staff at budget time, to help us prioritize how we distribute the resources we have. For instance, a number of units with patient populations with high dependency needs decided to increase the number of care providers by using certified nurse assistants (CNAs). While this decision meant fewer RNs, there are now CNAs assigned along with the RNs to patients. Patients see more staff and are able to get help with ambulation and activities of daily living in a timely manner. There are other patient care areas in which assistive personnel would not support optimal patient care. In these areas the staff are trying other approaches like the evaluation of in-line IV filters to reduce costs.

We instituted a case management system in 1989 and began tracking some of our practice patterns and the financial effects. This was helpful to us, particularly in identifying and eliminating those practices that had no apparent clinical effect, but cost money (such as admission the night before surgery for some surgical patients and weekend stay-overs just because no one was around on Saturday mornings to facilitate discharge with home care).

Staff and patients resent a focus that is on money and cost savings only. They are, however, aware of their personal financial limits and can relate those to patient concerns about the cost of care. We have found that educating staff and sharing information openly help staff to understand their role in our financial viability.

M PECK

Costing Care

◆ WHO SHOULD BE INCLUDED WHEN COST OF NURSING IS CALCULATED?

Q In our community we are beginning to have more managed contracts; therefore our nursing administrator wants to identify the cost of nursing. Should the unit managers, clinical specialists, and unit clerks be included even though they don't provide direct patient care?

A The answer to this question rests with a clear understanding of the purpose of the information being gathered. The negotiators for various third-party payors in the managed care arena are going to be looking to the hospital to provide services at a discounted rate because of the large volume of potential patients on whose behalf they are negotiating. It is essential to your hospital's financial health that any discounts from charges that are negotiated still provide enough revenue to cover the cost of caring for the patients who will be covered by the contract and a sufficient profit margin to allow for expenses such as acquisition of state-of-the-art equipment. All individuals involved in the provision of care, whether direct or indirect, must be accounted for in the total cost of nursing care. You may find it useful to think in terms of whose salary and benefit costs must be covered in nursing by the reimbursement for patient care.

JE BEGLINGER

◆ CAN NURSING COSTS BE TIED TO DRGs?

Q I am anxious to develop a way of determining nursing's contribution to the DRGs that we serve at the unit level. How can I begin to directly tie my nursing costs to the DRGs so that I can determine what percent of those dollars is driven by nursing?

A Finding costs associated with nursing services is the challenge that every manager faces in being accountable. Costs are driven by nursing interventions, patient characteristics, and length of stay. In order to determine nursing's contribution to each DRG, you need to identify what nursing services are routinely provided to patients with a specific DRG and determine their costs. This can be done in the following way:
1. Select a DRG that represents a large percentage of patients admitted to your unit.
2. Develop a nursing care plan that includes interventions and expected outcomes for patients with the selected DRG for each day of hospitalization.

3. Use your patient classification system to assign time associated with implementing the nursing care plan.

4. Using the cost of 1 hour of nursing care provided on your unit, determine the cost per day of hospitalization for the average patient with the selected DRG, based on their nursing care plan.

5. Total the costs of nursing service over the length of stay and divide this total by the total DRG reimbursement to determine the percent of nursing service that contributes to the DRG.

These figures can be refined by adjusting the length of stay or nursing care hours to consider the percentage of patients who do not fall within the range of "average" patients with the selected DRG.

CE LOVERIDGE

Credentialing

♦ **WHAT ARE THE BASIC ELEMENTS OF CREDENTIALING?**

Q What are the basic elements of a credentialing and privileging approach in shared governance and how do we use it as a basis for defining performance and evaluating performance outcomes?

A Evidence of the basic credentials of the registered nurse such as licensure and validation of skills and experience is usually the function of the human resources department at the time of employment. References for professional competence and character should be obtained. Interviews with nurse managers and appropriate key personnel provide a basis for evaluating the applicant's "fit" with the organization, expected responsibilities, and personality of the department. Competence of the nursing staff should be demonstrated every 2 years. In a shared governance environment, all professional nurses have the privilege and opportunity to participate in the nursing organization. Annual performance evaluations should reflect competence of skills, sincerity, and a commitment to excellent patient care.

Credentialing is nationally recognized certification in a specialty area (e.g., critical care, intravenous therapy, or oncology nursing) that signifies that the nurse possesses advanced knowledge and should be used as a clinical resource person for patients and other health care workers. Shared governance environments are one way to empower nurses at the bedside to use those skills within the overall councilor structure or at the unit-based committee level. By participating in the writing of standards, policies, and procedures; defining the educational needs of the staff; and implementing the quality assurance and assessment activities of the nursing unit, the advanced nurse has ample opportunity to share and define nursing practice within the organization.

Many hospitals incorporate a levels program within the job description for the clinical practitioner. This provides the basis for performance evaluations. At St. Joseph's Hospital of Atlanta, the levels program defines three levels of performance for the staff nurse, with monetary rewards for achieving and maintaining the behaviors defined in the levels advancement program. Advanced educational degrees and credentialing are not part of this levels program because the nurse is compensated for them at the time of employment or as a bonus when they are achieved.

Performance-based evaluations are very helpful to the staff nurse to have clearly defined expectations of behaviors and for the nurse managers to have specific responsibilities and expectations of nursing practice already established for each performance level. All nurses begin at Level I and then have the opportunity to advance via a written process to the next level. Performances are based on behavioral criteria. Level I competencies as related to behavior or performance are nursing process, quality assurance, discharge planning, patient teaching, communication, and professional development. Level II behaviors are in addition to Level I; these RNs are expected to be preceptors and clinical resources to the staff. Level III registered nurses complete Level I and II requirements and are regarded as role models for their peers. An example is that the Level I nurses would understand the shared governance program; a Level II nurse participates in shared governance at the unit-based or councilor structure; and a Level III might chair a shared governance committee, council, or task force. Another example is that Level I nurses would participate in quality assurance (QA) data collection; Level II nurses would identify a unit problem and develop a monitor to document or resolve the issue; and a Level III nurse would identify a problem,

C

develop a monitor, identify trends in the data collected, and resolve the problem.

BH DUGGER

Crisis

◆ IN A CRISIS WHAT IS THE BEST WAY FOR A MANAGER TO SUPPORT STAFF?

Q How can a nurse team member best support the team in times of crisis?

A Crisis occurs frequently within the hospital environment. A manager who is calm, organized, supportive, and helpful can assist staff in managing a crisis effectively. *Helpful* is an important word. The manager who just walks out of her office and provides a supportive statement on her way to a meeting may not be appreciated by staff. Pitching in to help, rolling up your sleeves, and getting into the crisis is the best way you can show support for the staff. After the crisis is resolved, conduct a conference with the staff who were involved. Analyzing why the crisis occurred and how it could have been prevented or managed in a better manner can assist staff in future crises.

JG O'LEARY

Critical Paths

◆ HOW DO CRITICAL PATHS RELATE TO NURSING PROCESS?

Q How do critical paths relate to the nursing process?

A Critical paths are one way of using the nursing process in a practice setting. Assessment is done as the nurse compares what is supposed to hap-

pen, as defined by the critical path, with what actually happens. When the patient does not progress as anticipated, the resulting variance must be identified and analyzed to determine the cause of the variance. Following this, the nurse plans and implements new interventions that will result in the desired outcomes. These new interventions are evaluated against the critical path to determine their effectiveness in meeting outcomes defined in the critical path.

Data regarding types of variance, reasons for variance, and effectiveness of new interventions are collected and used in reviewing and revising critical paths for specific patient groups. In this way, critical paths and nursing process are also used at a systems as well as individual patient level.

JB COLTRIN ET AL.

◆ CAN WE SUBSTITUTE CRITICAL PATHS FOR POLICIES AND STILL MEET JCAHO STANDARDS?

Q Can we throw out our policies and procedures and substitute critical paths, care pathways, and standards and still comply with JCAHO?

A Before you decide to scrap all your policy manuals, you may need to have a better understanding of what policies and procedures do for your organization. Policies and procedures exist for many reasons other than to meet regulatory and licensing requirements or to provide clinical care rules. Often we think of policies as being only clinically focused or patient care oriented (chemotherapy policy, central line policy, and blood gas policy). However, many policies are purely administrative in nature (payroll policies, vacation policies, and holiday policies). Sometimes, policies apply to both the employees and patients, such as the JCAHO-required smoking policy. It is not unusual for organizations to have proliferated policies to the point that large, dust-collecting policy binders fill dearly needed space. However, the excess production of policies and the poor use of policies does not mean that policies themselves are useless tools. Policies and procedures exist as one means to provide structure in organizations. Well-written policies include a policy statement (the rules), purposes for the policy (why the rules exist), and clear step-by-step procedures (ways of behaving that allow employees to comply with the rules). Too often, policies are carelessly written, not current or timely, or inconsistently disseminated. Despite these policy management issues, organizations need clear, cogent policies to do the following:

1. Clarify infrequently occurring situations that pose significant risk to patients or employees (e.g., how to use an intraaortic balloon pump).
2. Clarify frequently occurring situations to minimize organizational risk (e.g., universal body substance precautions).
3. Restrict activities to specially trained or qualified individuals (e.g., medication administration policy).
4. Set out organizational rules to comply with federal or state law (e.g., blood-borne pathogens policy).

If these policies are clearly written and easily accessible, they become a valuable resource that will be used by new and experienced employees in nonroutine or unfamiliar situations. Clinical protocols and critical paths are different types of tools to provide organizational structure. Clinical protocols are usually carefully constructed descriptions of the routinely expected types of care provided to patients with specific and common health problems, for instance, decubitus ulcer protocols and falls protocols. These protocols communicate to the organization the standards of care that are expected for any patient with these conditions. Critical paths are a newer tool that carefully spells out the expected course of a patient's treatment and care for a given diagnosis such as diabetes, stroke, or MI. These paths outline what tests, procedures, and treatments can be expected to occur for each specified day of a hospital stay for most patients, excluding complications. Neither of these tools can replace the need for all policies, but they can work in tandem with many policies to reduce the volume of unnecessary paper. Your goal as a manager should not be to eliminate all policies, but to ensure that every policy that exists is clearly written and timely, and serves a useful purpose.

MC ALDERMAN

◆ HOW DO I ENCOURAGE STAFF TO ACCEPT CHANGE IN POLICIES?

Q We are trying to move from policies and procedures to critical paths as a way to define care. The nursing staff on our unit are very attached to their policies and procedures. How do we help to change their mind-set to more continuum-of-care thinking?

A This project is best approached as a pilot for just one medical diagnosis first. It requires an interdisciplinary approach. Development of a critical path is a project perfectly suited to the very popular continuing quality improvement process. Don't attack the policies and procedures—those will fall into line later. Concentrate on just building one critical path with staff and evaluating it. When you eventually need to revise policies, revisions will probably be less substantial than you now think. Perhaps adding one policy and procedure on use of critical paths during the pilot project will ease staff into the change.

D SHERIDAN

◆ ARE POLICIES AND PROCEDURES STILL RELEVANT IF WE SWITCH TO STANDARD-BASED PRACTICE USING CRITICAL PATHS?

Q We are finding that we serve about five to six DRGs 90% of the time. We would like to move from policies and procedures to standards-based practice using critical paths. Should we begin by emphasizing the major DRGs we serve and focusing less on other procedural processes that do not relate to our predominant DRGs?

A Focusing on standards-based practice by developing critical pathways is an excellent strategy. Critical paths are a way to standardize interventions for a specific diagnosis in a specified sequence to achieve optimal patient outcomes. Developing pathways for the major clinical diagnoses allows you to focus your efforts to achieve optimal results. However, the development of critical pathways does not necessarily eliminate the need for policies and procedures, which provide guidelines about how to perform a specific task. You could, however, guide your revision and/or development of specific policies and procedures based on those interventions identified in the critical pathway. For example, a critical pathway for the care of stroke patients might require that a swallowing evaluation be done before the patient is allowed to eat. A procedure would need to be in place outlining how to perform a swallowing exam.

C ST CHARLES

Delegation

♦ HOW CAN I CHECK ON DELEGATED WORK WITHOUT INTERFERING?

Q I am a well-organized nurse manager. I set priorities and delegate appropriate assignments to get the work done through other people. However, I feel like I have to constantly check up on projects and make sure other staff get their work done right and on time. I know I am offending some of the experienced staff who think I do not trust them. What are some more effective ways to follow up on tasks I have delegated?

A When you delegate assignments, delegate goals or desired outcomes instead of tasks. Then have staff simply report to you on goal achievement. Establish parameters or standards within which staff can decide how to achieve these goals, and make the goals specific, measurable, attainable, realistic, and trackable (SMART). Then check up on what staff are doing *right* rather than what they are doing wrong. You will get the behavior you expect, so if you expect them to complete their goals, they will; look for the positive outcomes. This will maintain and probably even build trust.

Allow staff more autonomy in determining how to achieve the goals you mutually set with them. This stimulates their creativity and provides a sense of accomplishment.

When you delegate a task, design the goal with the staff person and decide *together* on a date and time for accomplishment. Encourage staff to communicate with you if additional resources are needed or if something unexpected arises that changes the goal or achievement date.

In essence, you will be changing your role from director, supervisor, manager, and parent to that of facilitator, resource, coach, teacher, role model, and peer adult.

If goals aren't achieved as mutually agreed upon, you must immediately meet with that staff person to determine what happened. Was there full understanding? Did it seem important? Did the person have enough knowledge or resources to accomplish the goal? If you find a person who is consistently late or doesn't meet the goals, intervene quickly. Set tight standards and clear goals and help the person develop in her current role or help her recognize that she perhaps needs to consider a different role.

RM HADDON

♦ HOW CAN I HELP NEW GRADUATES LEARN HOW TO DELEGATE?

Q As a manager, how can I facilitate the acquisition of good delegation skills by new graduates?

A New graduates experience all types of difficulties adjusting to their new work world. The daily pressures are high, and these staff may need more nurturing and mentoring by their colleagues and their managers to refine their skills effectively and confidently. As any seasoned nurse manager knows, delegation is not an easy task. First and foremost it takes self-confidence. You have to be comfortable knowing exactly what you are delegating and what you expect as an outcome before you will be willing to delegate a task. This takes time with a new graduate. A nurse manager can nurture the new graduate's self-confidence with good orientation and solid continuing education offerings, and by providing for a supportive relationship or mentorship with an experienced staff nurse.

Second, you need to have confidence in the people to whom you are delegating. You need to nurture in your graduate nurses a feeling of responsibility for educating and supporting the staff that work with them. They need to see themselves as being of value to that staff. They need to learn that when they delegate they are helping others learn and they are sharing in the development of those other people's skills. They also need to be involved in the periodic evaluation of those individuals and feel accountable for their progress. Teaming a new graduate with the same support staff over a consistent period also helps create those relationships.

As a manager you must work with staff to help them appreciate the need for teamwork and the differences in roles on the team. Delegation needs to be seen as sharing, not dumping.

Third, education regarding delegation for the whole staff will further solidify the acceptance and practice of the skills.

CCC LEVENS

◆ HOW SHOULD I ENCOURAGE STAFF TO DELEGATE?

Q The staff nurses under my supervision have little experience in delegating to assistive personnel. What tips can I share that will help them in delegating?

A Fiscal constraints, increased involvement of nurses in quality-related activities, increasing patient acuity, complex technologic advances, reduction in nonnursing support, and sporadic nursing shortages are placing increased demands on the health care delivery system. In response, many health care organizations nationally are changing their care delivery systems and staffing mixes and in that process are increasing the use of assistive personnel. This has resulted in a diversity of types of assistive models and a proliferation of titles and duties, all of which has caused significant confusion about the appropriate use of assistive personnel. Professional nursing organizations have, in turn, made multiple public statements about the appropriateness of their use.

The most common definitions of assistive personnel today recognize any trained, but unlicensed, health care worker to whom the RN delegates or assigns aspects of nursing care and who functions under the supervision of the RN.

Keeping those elements in mind, the following are some tips for successful delegation.

1. RNs must be aware of, and delegate assignments consistent with, the practice parameters prescribed in their state Nurse Practice Act. These parameters do vary from state to state and are legally regulated by the state's Board of Nursing. Perhaps what is most critical is that professional and statutory provisions require that when the RN delegates and assigns direct nursing care activities to assistive personnel, appropriate reporting relationships are to be established; the RN is directly responsible for supervising the assistive personnel to whom the activities have been delegated. This means the RN may transfer authority and responsibility for the performance of certain activities from one individual to another but retains accountability for the outcome or overall care. Respecting this accountability, assistive personnel are not assigned to patients, but rather to RNs.

2. Specific written job descriptions and competencies must be defined for *both* the assistive personnel *and* the RN. It is important to note that which tasks are appropriate for delegation will vary from unit to unit, facility to facility, and from one part of the country to another. Tasks delegated depend on the type of patient population and the care needs, the care delivery system, the configuration of the staff mix and division of role functions, the amount of ancillary support staff outside of nursing, labor-relations issues, and the ability and willingness of the individual RNs to delegate to assistive personnel. Experienced RNs usually are more comfortable delegating than those relatively new to the profession or the specific clinical setting or unit.

3. Inservice education or other formal or informal training must be provided to ensure competence of the assistive personnel for the type of activities specified as appropriate for that unit. This type of care usually relates to either direct (clinical) or indirect (nonclinical) patient care activities. Direct care activities assist the patient in meeting basic human needs such as assistance with feeding, ambulation, grooming, toileting, dressing, and socializing. It may also include collecting, reporting, and documenting data related to these activities. Indirect care activities support patients and their environment; these include removing meal trays, housekeeping, transporting, performing clerical activities, stocking, and performing maintenance tasks.

4. Conflicts between staff, whether professional or nonprofessional, will surface despite clearly defined roles, training, and competency demonstrations. Having a process in place to air grievances about care assignments and delegation of tasks is helpful for each unit. Also, if your organization's clinical assistive personnel float from unit to unit, it is the receiving unit's responsibility to orient the assistive personnel to appropriate care responsibilities on that specific unit and provide the rationale for those responsibility variances.

BV TEBBITT

◆ HOW DO I INTERVENE WHEN A STAFF MEMBER IS NOT FULFILLING THE ROLE SHE IS ASSIGNED?

Q I have delegated a committee responsibility to a staff member. The staff member has handled other special projects very well and has been suc-

D

cessful. I have input from committee members that this project is not going well; they say the staff member is unorganized and the meetings are a waste of time. The project has some serious problems that are beginning to affect other areas that I am responsible for. When I asked the staff member how things are going, she responds, "Very well." What do I do now?

A First, review the steps of delegation. Did you:

1. Determine that the responsibility is truly one that can be delegated? (Be sure that you have not handed over an assignment that can be done only with the authority of the manager behind it.)
2. Make the assignment clear when delegating it?
   a. Are the expected outcomes specified?
   b. Are the time lines clear?
3. Determine that the employee is capable of completing the delegated work?
   a. Has the employee had this kind of committee responsibility before?
   b. Is the person truly qualified to do the assignment?
4. Follow up and oversee the delegated assignment consistently and in a timely manner?
   a. Have you attended a committee meeting and observed the work firsthand? (This is a good way to determine if the information you are getting from others is correct or if there are interpersonal issues between committee members that need to be confronted and resolved.)
   b. Have you met regularly with the employee to ensure that the work is on time and on target?
   c. Are you asking specific questions related to the outcomes desired rather than the general question, "How are things going?"

If you answered *no* to any of these questions, then it may be time for you to regroup, meet with the employee, and revisit the assignment, keeping the steps of delegation in mind.

If you answered *yes* to all of the questions, then it may be time to reassign the responsibility to another staff member or find another mechanism by which to complete the task. Your first temptation may be to do it yourself. Don't succumb to this temptation unless there is not one individual reporting to you that is truly capable of doing the task or if it is a task that relies on the authority of the manager.

LJ SHINN

Discipline

♦ **IS THERE A NORMAL COURSE OF DISCIPLINARY ACTION?**

Q What is the "normal" course or flow of disciplinary actions?

A The first thing that must happen occurs long before disciplinary action is begun. That is, as the manager, you must ensure that all staff clearly know and understand your expectations. For example, it is not enough to say, "I expect all staff members to show respect for each other." You should say, "I expect all staff members to show respect for each other. Some examples of how this would look on our unit are coming to work on time so others can leave on time and letting another person express her opinion without interruption before asking questions." It is useful to ask the staff to give examples, to assist in the setting of group norms.

If a staff member then does not follow through and, for example, is late to work, you should call that to her attention in a friendly but direct way. You should remind the staff member of why it is important to be on time and that it is your expectation that the staff member do so. Ascertain if there are any unusual or extenuating circumstances to be dealt with. Make an anecdotal note in your files. If the employee is not late again, the note is destroyed and no further mention is made.

If, however, the staff member is late again, request an immediate meeting with her. Restate your expectations and ask if she is willing and able to comply with the expectation. If she is unable, determine why and if this is compatible with continued employment, and take appropriate action. If she is unwilling, the staff member needs to be told that this is one expectation held of those who wish to continue working on the unit, and she must comply or look for work elsewhere. If the employee is willing and able, document your expectation in writing, the deadline for compliance, and any expectations that must be met. Document the employee's agreement to comply. Give the employee a copy and place your copy in the employee's file.

If the behavior continues, some organizations require suspension for a specified period of time, usually without pay. Continued failure to comply then results in termination. All of this must be documented clearly.

There is another strategy that encourages the staff member to take responsibility for her own actions. In this disciplinary process, the suspension is substituted with a paid decision-day-off. You and the employee meet and you remind the employee of your expectation and that the employee has the ability and has stated in the past that she has the willingness to comply. You then tell the employee that it is time for her to decide if she wants to continue working on this unit. Tell the employee that she must stay home the next day and decide if she will return to work and comply. If she does, then she must understand that if the behavior changes and improves and then returns again, that she (the employee) is deciding to resign. If the employee decides not to comply, you will want a letter of resignation on your desk by 9 AM the next morning. State that if there is no letter on your desk then you will know that the employee is asking you to process termination papers. In either case, it is the employee who is deciding, not you.

It is important to hold employees accountable for their decisions. The manager who follows these steps will not be acting like a parent, but will be expecting responsible adult behavior from her employees. Failure to deal with the employee who is unwilling to work with the team will undermine the manager. By dealing with this employee fairly and in a timely manner, you ensure that other employees will have a positive work environment.

JE JENKINS

◆ IS THERE A NEWER TYPE OF DISCIPLINARY ACTION?

Q Are there newer or different forms or types of administrative disciplinary action emerging to guide managers in a highly participative environment?

A Discipline represents one of the most demanding aspects of the leader's role. Just as the US health care system is examining prevention, so should managers with respect to discipline. Thus the question becomes: What systems and processes can be put in place to reduce the need for discipline?

Although there is no system that will totally remove the need for discipline, there are approaches available to managers to greatly reduce the need. The most powerful mechanism available to managers in preventing the need for discipline is to facilitate group norms that guide staff toward an accountability-based practice environment through socialization that engenders commitment to one another, the patient, and the agency. Self-managed teams are an example of such an accountability-based practice group.

Whereas most group norms are covert or informal, in an accountability-based practice environment professional norms would be overt and codified in writing so that self-regulation and group regulation are facilitated. The ideal self-managed team uses its overt group norms to socialize members to acceptable group and organizational behavior.

The role of the manager in molding an environment of self-regulation is one of facilitator and guide. The manager acts to help staff identify those group norms that assist them in regulating behavior and moving toward self-management. After the norms are established and agreed on, the manager guides the team in the process of implementation, self-monitoring, and evaluation.

Fully autonomous self-managed teams perform very different functions from those dominated by management. They select group members, they establish group rules (within the context of organizational norms), they are interconnected with the goal of individual and group accountability for outcomes, and they evaluate their collective and individual performance (peer review).

As self-managed teams become more plentiful, the need for discipline will diminish. The enlightened manager or leader will facilitate this process in the interest of professional nursing. The need for discipline can be greatly diminished in an environment of self-accountability.

GL CROW

◆ HOW DO I DISCIPLINE AN EMPLOYEE WHO ABUSES SICK DAY POLICY?

Q I have hired a nurse to work on a special project that requires community outreach and independent activity. Although she has been employed

D

for only a month, I have noted that she has called in sick for 11 days. This is excessive. To complicate matters, the nurse is a member of a protected class of employee whom my agency has been striving to employ in order to increase the diversity of staff. From some comments other staff have made, I suspect alcoholism is involved. What should I do?

A Excessive sick time is an employee issue that must be dealt with uniformly for all employees. Most organizations have an illness policy and a well-established disciplinary process.

Every manager should be familiar with the policy and review it with staff to ensure an understanding of the expectation. If there is not an existing policy, the manager should develop the parameters and a well-defined method for handling this issue. This should include the number of days acceptable in a year and the progressive disciplinary process. The manager needs to develop a method for tracking employee illnesses, looking at number as well as trends and patterns.

The purpose is not to question the validity of the illness. The manager should not imply a judgment as to whether the illness is warranted. The purpose for an illness policy is to address excessive illness and its negative impact on department operations.

The fact that this employee is part of a diversity initiative should not alter the way a manager would handle an employee performance problem. It is unfortunate that many managers do mistakenly believe that some employees have a "protected status." Diversity programs are aimed at increasing the number of employees from a particular minority. Mentoring and development strategies are utilized but should not be confused with decreased expectations regarding standard of performance.

The issue of alcoholism with this employee is a particularly sensitive area. Vague comments or rumors from staff do not provide sufficient evidence regarding the presence of alcoholism. The manager should refrain from labeling or diagnosing a problem without more concrete information. It would be more appropriate to address the behaviors. However, if specific behaviors are present, for example, alcohol on the breath or obvious intoxication, the manager should seek advice from the human resources department. Some organizations have employee assistance programs to which the employee could be referred for help. Many professional organizations as well as

the state Board of Nursing have resource information for the impaired professional.

Based on the history of the employee, the excessive illnesses may relate to difficulty in adjusting to the new role. More information should be gathered.
1. Is there a preexisting chronic illness?
2. Is there a recently diagnosed acute illness?
3. Are there family responsibilities causing the sick time?
4. Is this work avoidance related to the role uncertainty?
5. Are the role expectations clear?
6. Does the employee have the necessary skills and assistance?
7. What supports are available?

The manager may need to further assist this new employee with role and skill development.

SF SMITH

◆ WHAT SHOULD I DO IF A STAFF MEMBER HAS ENGAGED IN HOMOSEXUAL ACTIVITY WITH A PATIENT?

Q One of our team leaders found a male staff member and a male patient in a compromising sexual encounter. It appeared that both parties knew each other and that this behavior was not new for them. The patient indicated it was not a problem for him. However, it did occur during the staff member's work time. How should I handle this delicate issue?

A I assume that your hospital has strong policies that address this issue. It doesn't matter whether both parties knew each other or were agreeable to this behavior, or even who initiated it. In the interests of a patient's safety and rights and in regard to professional integrity and appropriateness, this behavior is completely unacceptable. Termination is the usual response to this kind of behavior. The hospital is a place where health care work is done with a belief and trust on the part of all parties, providers, and patients that healing and professional work and relationships will be maintained. There is a time and place for everything. A sexual relationship between a health professional and a patient is almost never acceptable in any circumstances and is usually handled with firm discipline.

Follow your hospital policy with regard to this issue. If there isn't one, inform your supervisor or administrator immediately. Make sure you ask about your state board requirements for reporting this behavior to them, and be sure you carefully document all information from staff and patients and make it available to the authorities in your organization.

T PORTER-O'GRADY

Discrimination

◆ HOW DO I ADMONISH STAFF WHO USE RACIAL SLURS?

Q As I walked past the staff break room, I heard one of the nurses using racial slurs against a minority member of our staff. Other staff members were supporting her comments. How should I handle this situation?

A There cannot be any tolerance for racial discrimination in the work place. You have a responsibility to act as a staff advocate when there are circumstances as you have described. Intervene as rapidly as possible. With all of the group present in the break room, state your expectation that such behavior should not occur and will not be tolerated. It is best to indicate that further evidence of such behavior will result in immediate disciplinary action that could include suspension without pay and/or termination of employment. Since several nurses were involved in the incident, you should counsel each one individually and inquire about the situation. What circumstances initiated the conversation and activities? Why were several nurses singling out one staff member in particular? Although there is no acceptable excuse for discriminatory language or behavior, you need to provide them an opportunity to explain their behaviors and to feel that you have listened to their concerns. Deal with any issues other than the discriminatory language separately. Clearly restate your expectations and the consequences of

further discriminating behaviors or conversations. Every employee deserves to be treated with fairness, respect, and dignity in the work environment, and management must immediately intervene in any breach of behavior that could be personally damaging to an employee.

JF STICHLER

◆ HOW DO I RESPOND TO UNFAIR ACCUSATIONS OF PREJUDICE ON MY UNIT?

Q I have a staff member on my unit who is a member of a minority group. She frequently implies that prejudice plays a part in her patient care assignment. How do I help her to understand that this is not true without appearing defensive?

A Dealing with suspected prejudice is one of the most challenging situations that a nurse manager will face in her career. Our work places are becoming much more culturally diverse, and with that diversity can come significant communication, interpersonal, and legal issues, all of which need to be treated with the utmost care and sincerity.

I will assume that you have thoroughly investigated the allegations and have reached an unbiased conclusion that prejudice is not playing a role in patient care assignments, for this person or others. It is your responsibility to ensure that all nurses have the right to care for any and all patients for which they are qualified without regard to race, ethnic origin, age, or sex.

If you are satisfied that prejudice does not play a role in patient assignments, then you should undertake the following steps in resolving this conflict:

1. Ensure that you have thoroughly informed your superior and the human resources department regarding the allegations, and seek their advice and support. Be confident in your facts; we are more likely to act defensively when we are unsure.
2. In a conference with the employee and a witness, present your findings in a direct and open manner.
3. Allow the staff member to respond and ask questions.
4. Answer each question or concern factually. Do not allow the employee to drift into nonrelated topics.

D

5. If the conflict is not resolved, institute the problem solving or conflict resolution process. However, this process can become habitual; therefore place a time limit on the issue.
6. Monitor and evaluate the outcome in terms of assignment patterns for all staff.

Issues related to prejudice can be very unsettling to all concerned. The situation must be dealt with openly and directly, with the message that prejudice, if found, will not be tolerated. Because prejudicial behavior can be either covert or overt, the manager must be very thorough in her investigation. Educational programs on cultural diversity and its impact on the work place are important adjuncts to the manager's role in creating a environment that celebrates diversity.

GL CROW

◆ HOW SHOULD I RESPOND TO WHAT I THINK IS DISCRIMINATORY HIRING PRACTICE?

Q I noticed that in our hospital two equally qualified candidates for a nurse management position were reviewed and the man got the position. When we looked more closely at the selected candidate's background, we discovered that he had a BSN, and the woman competing with him had a master's degree in nursing administration, as well as having held previous positions in nursing management. This appears to be clear discrimination to us. What should we do?

A This situation could be a case of discrimination, but things are not always as they appear. There may be issues in the background of the other candidates that you didn't know about, or the candidate selected for the position may have done his homework and presented himself in a more qualified manner. Don't get hung up on credentials.

It is unfortunate, but the law will not allow you to do much about discrimination unless it affects you directly. You can contact a representative of the Equal Employment Opportunity Commission (EEOC) or consult your human resources department to find out what options you may have. You should also contact the EEOC if you believe that *you*

are the victim of hiring discrimination, and consider contacting an attorney.

P MARALDO

Diversity

◆ HOW DO I DEAL WITH BIASED PATIENTS AND PHYSICIANS?

Q Nursing has become an increasingly culturally diverse profession. As we educate ourselves and our peers regarding these differences, our physicians and patients continue to exhibit previously held biases and prejudices. As a nurse manager in this time of increased emphasis on customer and guest relations, how do I support the staff while meeting the needs of physicians and patients?

A There are at least three different concepts embodied in this question, and it is extremely important to separate them.

The first is the obligation of the institution to provide a work environment that is free of discrimination and harassment regardless of an individual's race, religion, age, sex, presence of disabilities, or other protected status. This is an absolute right of the individual to be free from discrimination and harassment from anyone he or she may come in contact with in the work environment, including physicians, co-workers, managers, vendors, visitors, and patients. If you are aware of any occurrences, they must be reported to the appropriate individual in your institution and dealt with immediately. If you are aware of an occurrence and you do not report it, you may be subject to civil liability and, depending on your institution's policies, could be subject to disciplinary action up to and including termination.

In order to assist you, your institution should have specific policies in place regarding the rights of individuals and the institution's response if an event should occur. Training all employees and physicians regarding these policies should be mandatory.

The second issue is one of sensitivity to and understanding of issues of cultural diversity. Many organizations, as part of their commitment to ensure that cultural diversity is valued, have organized opportunities for groups to meet and explore cultural issues and differences. If physicians are the primary area of concern, it might be beneficial to set up groups with the medical staff and a trained facilitator. If you are having issues with patients, the institution might consider a statement that is given to patients at the time of admission regarding the institution's philosophy of no tolerance regarding discrimination or harassment.

The third issue is how to meet customer expectations or stated requirements when prejudice is the basis for the request. The most important concept is that an individual staff member's rights absolutely *cannot* be waived or negated because of increased sensitivity to customer service.

Physicians and patients, although both may be considered customers, should be approached differently. Physicians have a contractual obligation to the hospital as a part of their medical staff privileges. These privileges subject physicians to many of the same rules of conduct as hospital employees. If a physician makes any statements that are prejudicial in nature, you should explain the hospital policy regarding nondiscrimination and nonharassment and ask her specifically to refrain from making such statements in the future. You should also report the incident, ideally in writing, to the appropriate individual in your institution, generally the director of human resources. If you are uncomfortable approaching the physician directly, you must still report the incident. If a physician requests that her patients not be cared for by a certain individual based on a prejudice about that individual, you should inform the physician of the hospital policy and state that you cannot honor her request. You should then encourage the physician to talk directly to someone in human resources or the medical staff office if she has further concerns.

Patients may also make discriminatory statements and/or make requests that a particular nurse not care for them. This is not an easy situation; it may require administrative support. Make sure you use resources within your institution to help you deal with the situation.

Patients may exhibit myriad emotional and behavioral responses when they are ill, and nurses must work with and manage each one every day. Your primary goal should be to manage patients' expectations, if at all possible, in a way that ensures that the rights of staff are not violated. Talking directly to the patient about concerns and the hospital policy of nondiscrimination should be your first step. (Ideally, your hospital has developed an institutional guideline.) If, after you have talked to the patient, you feel his or her actions are discriminatory, talk to the nurse and explain the hospital's commitment to provide a work environment that is free from discrimination and harassment. The nurse may decide, for patient care reasons, to relinquish care of the patient. It is important, however, that the nurse understand that it is her decision and that the institution will support whatever decision she makes. If the nurse chooses to continue to care for the patient, the message should be delivered directly to the patient along with an offer to assist the patient in transferring to another unit or institution, if he or she so desires.

C ST CHARLES

◆ HOW CAN I HELP MY STAFF BECOME MORE CULTURALLY SENSITIVE?

Q My unit staff is becoming increasingly diverse. As a manager, what issues should I be sensitive to and how can I help my unit become more culturally aware and ethnically sensitive?

A In order for nurses to understand each other, they must first understand themselves—their individual values and biases, and the filters through which they view the world. Plan a few exercises at staff meetings to encourage nurses to begin to examine their own values and attitudes.

As nurses become more sensitized to their own biases and cultural differences, they become more open to understanding others' cultures. Brainstorm with staff about ways to share information about culture. Begin with cultures of staff members. International potlucks are easy beginning icebreakers followed by cultural stories shared by staff and then perhaps journal article discussions.

Moving from knowledge to practice is always a challenge. In transcultural nursing, this is especially true. It is important to avoid stereotyping by moving beyond understanding the culture to understanding the individual within the culture. Discuss a particular culture of several of your staff members and ask them to share how they differ within that culture. Holiday observance is an easy topic (Sheridan, 1993).

D SHERIDAN

Documentation

D

◆ HOW CAN I CONVINCE STAFF TO INCLUDE DOCUMENTATION IN THEIR DEFINITION OF NURSING CARE?

Q What are some ideas to motivate staff nurses to treat documentation as an important component of nursing care?

A Many experts report that motivation is an internal individual mechanism. Managers can create an environment that promotes a certain behavior. The valuing of documentation cannot be mandated. The manager's role is to facilitate objective examination by the staff of the purpose of documenting. Some possible strategies to create a motivational environment regarding documentation might include the following:

1. Assist the staff in exploring what they value in documentation. What is and is not important, and why?
2. Have them investigate how the information is utilized by others and what regulatory requirements exist.
3. Provide resources regarding documentation and the newer approaches and systems available.
4. Examine the barriers that exist in the documentation system.
5. Encourage the staff to revamp the documentation system to better provide quality care.

SF SMITH

◆ HOW CAN I GET STAFF TO ADMIT TO DOCUMENTATION ERRORS?

Q There is a reluctance of midlevel management to acknowledge defaults in documentation (chart reviews); they offer excuses (such as staffing and overcrowding) as justification. How can this attitude be turned around?

A First, invest some effort in restructuring your approach to one of continuous quality improvement rather than defense of the status quo. The clinical practitioners are primarily accountable for the quality of nursing care being delivered. This process starts with a clear definition of the standards of care for your institution as well as the characteristics of the caregivers. Care is measured and opportunities for improvement are identified based on this foundation.

Accountability-based professional practice models like shared governance provide the structure for fulfilling the responsibilities of the discipline, which include practice, quality, competence, research, and management. Clinical and managerial accountabilities are clearly differentiated, with control of the clinical issues of practice, quality, and competence resting with the staff. For quality initiatives to be meaningful, they must be staff driven and truly focused on opportunities for improvement. Give strong consideration to revamping your whole approach, beginning with some discussion of your purpose.

JE BEGLINGER

◆ HOW DO I MOTIVATE STAFF TO DOCUMENT NURSING PROCESS?

Q How do I motivate staff to utilize and document the nursing process in the medical record?

A In my experience I have found that the nursing process is too conceptual for many staff members to consciously use without great mental effort. Nurses tend to be literal. For instance, nurses still see "Doing an admission assessment" as another task, and do not necessarily see its relationship to care planning. They are pleased with task completion and flowsheets, data sheets, and lots of check-off boxes, but they sometimes lack the language for evaluation. The SOAP format for progress notes still slows nurses down, and performing "head-to-toe" or system assessments is perceived as a separate documentation function from the "real work" of the shift. In other words, nurses tend to feel they are slaves to documentation, rather than that documentation works *for them* in any immediate way. Documentation forms must be built to structure the phases of the nursing process without adding steps, and, if possible, even combining steps.

CareMap tools do support, guide, and structure the nursing process in a more streamlined method, whether on paper or automated. They replace Kardexes, nursing care plans, and routine progress notes about patient status. The only progress notes needed are when patients differ from the norm, and as such, they create a strengthened version of charting-by-exception. Charting-by-exception is currently being considered by disciplines other than nursing, including physicians. As the industry moves to managed care, the CareMap tools as a basis for charting-by-exception will become the core of the automated medical record, and the nursing process will be embedded in its use.

In the meantime, for your current system:

1. Be clear as to how staff's documentation should look to reflect a nursing process.
2. Evaluate if the process is actually missing in staff's practice, not just in their documentation.
3. Ask for educational assistance from clinical specialists or staff educators if the nursing process is actually not in practice.
4. Verbally point out when individual staff use aspects of the nursing process, or coach them to the next step:
   - "You really followed through on your plan for the day for Mr. X. Make sure your note lets everyone else know what worked for him."
   - "Let me know what you assess about Mr. Y's emotional status."
   - "Calling the social worker was a great move based on your ideas about Mr. Z."
   - "Do you need any assistance organizing the transfer to rehab?"
5. Institute a peer chart audit system.

K ZANDER

♦ HOW DO I MOTIVATE STAFF TO USE NURSING DIAGNOSIS WHEN THEY DOCUMENT?

Q How do I get my staff to document using nursing diagnosis?

A Staff tend to see nursing diagnosis as a conceptual burden imposed on them by academics. A nurse manager has to be very knowledgeable about nursing diagnosis and then make it useful to nurses' practice by

1. Making it part of dialogue in report, case consultation, and other group situations, as well as in one-to-one coaching.
2. Mounting poster boards of usual, high-volume diagnoses or procedures for care by the staff, along with the five or six nursing diagnoses that each kind of patient begins with.

For instance, a patient receiving a total hip replacement will always have the nursing diagnoses of:

- ♦ High risk for injury.
- ♦ Impaired physical mobility.
- ♦ Knowledge deficit about the procedure and self-care.
- ♦ Pain.

Remember that one of the inherent messages in the nursing diagnosis methodologies is that nursing is a distinct profession with a distinct language for how it views and intervenes regarding specific clinical phenomena. Language is powerful and transferable, and an advanced clinician must be accurate and facile in using it.

An advanced clinician and/or manager must also be prepared to translate nursing diagnoses into other disciplines' language, always keeping the patients' needs at the center of the need for a "word bridge." In other words, nursing diagnoses should build bridges of understanding rather than walls of difference between nurses and their nonnursing colleagues.

K ZANDER

♦ WHAT SHOULD I DO ABOUT AN EMPLOYEE WHO FREQUENTLY DOES NOT COMPLETE CHARTING?

Q There is a particular staff member on my unit who often does not complete her patient records in a timely fashion. If things are forgotten, she simply comes back days later and inserts them in the record. I feel this is a problem. Am I correct? If so, how do I resolve this issue?

A Timely, accurate completion of the patient record is both a legal and a professional requirement. You are absolutely accurate in your assessment that a problem exists with this lack of compliance to the established policies and procedures within your setting. However, your response as a nurse manager to this issue needs planning because the behavior of

D

this staff member may go beyond not documenting in the patient record.

As the nurse manager, you are responsible for the quality of patient care delivery, including documentation. It is important to review the current methods of monitoring documentation and the quality of patient care delivered by unit staff because you need to know whether this problem is limited to one individual or is more widespread and goes beyond the lack of documentation.

Gathering data related to this problem will provide information to be used in a staff meeting and educational session on documentation. Discussing methods for improvement of documentation based on current policies and procedures can be the vehicle to address noncompliance issues. At the same time, this approach can provide a forum to brainstorm for new strategies for improvement.

The nurse manager should also meet with the individual staff member to discuss expectations related to documentation. It may be necessary to offer specific examples of noncompliance and write a developmental plan related to improvement. This employee's commitment to changing her behavior is essential to this process, and ongoing evaluation should be instituted to ensure compliance. Although the staff member may protest this structured approach, the nurse manager should point out the seriousness of the situation and the willingness of the system to allow the individual to demonstrate professional behavior without formal corrective action.

However, if the staff member does not express willingness to comply and participate in a self-improvement program, then the nurse manager should be ready to explain the next steps, including termination.

AMT BROOKS

Downsizing

◆ HOW CAN I BOLSTER MORALE WHEN LAYOFFS ARE IMMINENT?

Q Our hospital is going through a layoff process. This has the potential to seriously affect staff motivation. What are some guidelines to implement the policy well and still keep staff enthused?

A Most managers hesitate to get staff involved during the layoff process, but it can make a real difference. Involvement in layoff decisions provides staff with a sense of responsibility and involvement in the organization and also indicates respect for their input and knowledge of the work environment.

Let staff voice concerns and figure out ways to address the need for downsizing. Establish a committee of the most respected staff to identify areas that can be cut without significantly reducing staff productivity. But remember, the final decisions probably rest with you, and you must consider new methods for motivating the staff that remain at the institution. One way to do this is to set up committees to establish new productivity measures, procedural committees to streamline activity, and reward systems for those who work harder and smarter.

P MARALDO

◆ WHEN NECESSARY STAFF CUTS ARE MADE, HOW CAN I KEEP UP THE MORALE OF REMAINING STAFF?

Q The director of nursing has told me I must cut four full-time budgeted positions but must still maintain the same occupancy rate on my unit. How can we continue to provide the same services with fewer staff who are now feeling demoralized and put upon?

A It is important first to know what kind of positions needed to be cut, and what the time frame would be for eliminating the positions. Will the positions be cut by attrition, or do you need to have a plan that recognizes seniority and/or tenure?

The next approach has to be putting the staff in charge of the solutions. Downsizing or "right-sizing" is the trend in today's health care environment, while at the same time maintaining a commitment to patient care delivered by the right level of caregiver. Involve your staff in auditing your present delivery system and redesigning a more productive and effective way to take care of the same number of patients.

Steps in preparing for this change would be:
1. Conducting a literature search to determine what other environments are doing in redesign or delivery models that have been effective in redistribution of care.
2. Empowering a task force from your unit to look at alternative methods of delivering care. Be sure to select some of your more positive employees and the informal leaders as well as the leaders.
3. Using the human resource guidelines for reduction in force, make every attempt to place those affected by the cuts into other positions. If this is not possible, then make sure severance or appropriate notice is followed with outplacement services and counseling.
4. Assuring your staff that the new delivery system has a trial period and giving them a date for responding with an evaluation. In addition, be sure they understand that you value their input, but also that there may be changes you will be unable to make.

As managers we need to understand how threatened the staff feel under these circumstances. Every person immediately fears for her job, then retaliates with anger. By allowing the employees to be a part of the solution, we often get better results and a much less demoralized staff.

MA SORENSEN

◆ HOW CAN I ENLIST MY STAFF'S HELP IN SOLVING HUMAN RESOURCE PROBLEMS?

Q We have an empowered staff and we have to downsize one full-time equivalent (FTE). How do I get staff involved in that critical decision?

A Human resources and staffing allocation is a management accountability, yet standards of practice and quality of care are staff accountabilities. This clearly should be a shared decision between staff and management.

The decision to downsize one FTE belongs to management. The implementation of the decision can be turned over to the staff for resolution.
1. Make it clear that one FTE must be eliminated. The salary amount must be identified so that the staff has an idea of the dollars as well as the hours that must be eliminated.
2. Since you have staff empowerment, you probably have a forum such as a practice council or staff nurse council that can be vested with the decision on how to cut the FTE.
3. Management should be a part of the work group that will decide how to cut. Management's role is facilitating the group process, staying on target, and mediating conflict while moving toward resolution.
4. The staff on the council or committee should be guided to come up with options for the elimination of the FTE.

Alternative options need to be identified:
1. Closing the next vacancy.
2. Merging two part-time positions to come up with the dollars and/or hours needed.
3. Retraining and transferring the last-hired FTE.

Once alternatives are identified, the staff should be brought to consensus on the best feasible option.

JM McMAHON

◆ HOW DO I CUT STAFF FAIRLY?

Q Budget preparation for the coming year reveals that, because of volume decreases, direct care hours will need to be reduced by several FTEs in our nursing unit. How should I decide which positions to cut? How should I present this information to the staff?

A The need to decrease FTEs because of decreases in volume is one that is experienced consistently by nurse managers across the country as inpatient utilization trends continue to decline. There is reason to expect that decreases will continue because of health care reform. Thus developing a systematic method by which to reduce FTEs on a nursing unit in a manner that creates minimal impact on nursing staff is important. The first step in this effort is to assess your staffing system. Where direct-care hours are staffed in accordance with volume, the number of full-time equivalents that require elimination is easily calculated. Should this not be the case, it is extremely important to review and develop a system as quickly as possible to ensure consistency in adjusting to change.

D

To determine which positions to cut, identify a targeted cost per hour. In viewing this standard, you can then make a determination of which staff mix will most likely assist you in achieving this cost per hour. Direct-care hours staffed by costly full-time equivalents may not meet the budgetary needs. One must assume that volume is directly related to revenue, which is directly related to dollars that are available to pay staffing expenses. Thus determining numbers of FTEs without identifying the overall cost per hour per patient day will only postpone further inevitable cuts since contribution margins cannot otherwise be achieved.

Staff input will be required to determine which positions can be eliminated. Before that communication, however, it is important to identify where choices exist and where they do not exist. For example, if you are limited in the overall dollars that can be allocated to salaries, that parameter must be communicated. Before communicating with personnel, it is also important to identify alternative placement options. Will some staff members be without jobs? If so, work with your human resources or personnel department to determine how unemployment benefits are accessed and what those benefits are. Identify alternative positions. Are there positions available for nurses in the community? If you are a part of a large hospital system, ask whether patient days have shifted to the outpatient or ambulatory care setting. If so, there may be positions available to personnel who would otherwise be without employment.

Communication will be extremely important. If you exist within a unionized setting, it will be necessary to inform union representatives of the need to cut FTEs, the positions that may or may not be available, which personnel may be unemployed, and verification of the layoff and recall procedures under the union contract. While communicating with staff, share information related to why volume has decreased. If personnel have not received continuing education on health care issues and reform, explain these issues to them. Invite their input regarding the most feasible manner in which patient care needs can be met given the budget that does exist. Again, it is extremely important that choices not be given where they do not exist. However, personnel frequently are as capable as managers in developing viable alternatives if they have all of the information. You may consider developing a small work group consisting of

staff representatives to assist you in identification of options.

Budget cuts are never an enjoyable experience for nursing managers or nursing staff. They are, however, a common experience in an environment where utilization of health care resources is increasingly challenged. Determining a mechanism by which budget cuts may be consistently achieved will assist nurse managers in making these cuts in a manner through which personnel are clearly aware of the alternatives and are less likely to react based on misunderstandings.

LM LENTENBRINK

Dress Code

♦ WHAT NEEDS TO BE CONSIDERED WHEN ESTABLISHING A DRESS CODE?

Q We are attempting to establish a balanced, appropriate, and meaningful dress code that will improve the patients' perception of nursing. What should be some of the fundamental elements we include in our discussion of dress code?

A Research shows us that we form opinions about people based partly on the way they dress. Given that this is true, the first question in forming a dress code is to determine what impression you want the patients to have of the nurses in your organization. In the business of "impression management," your policy will have to be specific enough to provide guidelines for the clinical nurse and for the nurse manager who will coach staff and enforce the dress code policy. Surveys of patients reveal that they prefer the nurse to dress in a white uniform, with white nylons and white shoes. If more variation is desired by your organization, then the questions and specifics listed below will help you deal with the issue of consistency versus flexibility.

1. What is the purpose or essence of the dress code policy? Below is an example of a stated policy.

   "All nursing services personnel are expected to

present a standard of appearance which promotes a professional, caring image while allowing for some individuality and which ensures the patients' right to identify their health care providers by name and position." The policy must always consider the community standards for persons employed in health care.

2. Do all staff have to dress the same? Perhaps a divisional dress code is possible. Some decentralized organizations have unit dress codes.

3. What are the absolutes that must be met because of hospital policies (such as safety and infection control)?

   ♦ Street clothes may never be worn within the semirestricted or restricted areas of surgical suites.

   ♦ Hospital photo identification card and name tag must be visible to patients at all times.

4. How specific do you want to make the policy? Some examples follow:

   ♦ Earrings will not extend below earlobes.

   ♦ Gum chewing is not permitted while on duty.

   ♦ Uniforms will be a proper size and underwear will not be visible under the uniform.

   ♦ If hair is long, it must be secured on top or in the back of the head.

   ♦ Lab coats will be worn over scrub dresses and scrub suits when employees leave their work unit. Isolation gowns and patient gowns are not appropriate as a cover.

5. Who should develop the dress code? A task force of managers and staff is typical (7 to 9 people). A draft is sent to staff and management for input. Communication of the change and its purpose needs to occur in multiple forms and must be presented in a way that focuses on the change as a positive.

6. Dress is often a reflection of one's view of oneself (self-respect); therefore, what other issues are important to consider in formulating a dress code policy? Anything the nursing department can do to raise the nurses' self-respect (e.g., clinical ladder and other recognition programs, stopping of physician verbal abuse) will support nursing personnel dressing appropriately.

In my experience, in organizations where the administration, physicians, and nursing management treat the clinical nurse with respect and appreciation, professional dress is the norm. A sense of personal pride, professionalism, and empowerment appears to lead to appropriate dress.

VD LACHMAN

♦ ARE DRESS CODES NECESSARY?

Q Should there be a dress code for nurses in the inpatient work environment or should dress be left up to the individual?

A The question of dress code poses an interesting dilemma for nurses within an inpatient environment. As we develop professional practice models and focus on empowerment of staff, we assume nurses will exhibit professional behavior. Communication of this professionalism includes demeanor and dress.

Unfortunately, a dress code is not usually the answer to the underlying problem. In some institutions where nurses adhere to a structured dress code, they may not exhibit professional nurse behaviors. However, the public seems to appreciate a professional appearance and ability to readily identify the nurse, and they usually comment on their appreciation of this standard.

In institutions where there is an open approach to dress code, there is usually confusion and dissatisfaction on all sides. The public complains that they don't know who does what and whom to go to with questions. In addition, they comment on the lack of professionalism exhibited by having a "do your own thing" approach. While some staff express satisfaction with control over what they wear, nurse managers usually get caught in a dilemma between individual freedom versus an acceptable standard of dress.

Building consensus among staff for professionalism exhibited through competence, communication, responsiveness to patients, attire, and participation in decision making usually is more successful than merely developing a dress code. However, the personal safety of staff and patients must be a guide in determining the attire for staff. Developing principles for professional behavior related to quality improvement may assist in addressing the problem and at the same time, may result in a cohesive policy related to standards of performance.

D

It is important for nurses at all levels to participate in any activity related to solving problems that affect them. Focusing on outcomes that could result from wearing name tags and attire reflecting maturity will help to empower staff and exhibit professionalism.

AMT BROOKS

◆ WHEN A NURSE DRESSES PROVOCATIVELY, WHAT SHOULD I DO?

Q In the hospital where I work we have a strict uniform dress code for the nursing service. However, one of the nursing staff, an otherwise very competent nurse, dresses in uniforms that are tight fitting and have often been described as "sexy" or "provocative." She is the topic of conversation of many physicians and other male staff in our hospital. What guidelines should I use in approaching this topic with the staff nurse?

A The manager should review the dress code in detail as it pertains to this employee before discussing it with her. It is important in this delicate situation to preserve the dignity of the employee. Although professional appearance is somewhat subjective, the manager has a responsibility to address the concern. The manager should approach the employee in private with a spirit of concern, interest, and assistance. It is not necessary and may unduly upset or embarrass the employee to relay the information that she is the topic of male conversation. It is only necessary to address the appropriateness of her tight-fitting uniform and the perception that it projects.

SF SMITH

DRGs

◆ HOW ARE DRGs IMPORTANT TO ME AS A NURSE MANAGER?

Q I am not altogether sure what diagnostic groupings mean to me. Should I be more aware of what they are? What impact do they have on me as a nurse manager?

A Diagnosis-related groups (known nationwide as DRGs) are part of the prospective payment system that determines the exact amount paid to hospitals for the care of Medicare patients. The rate of payment is fixed in advance for patients in any one of 492 diagnosis-related groups. The average length of stay of similar patients treated for a condition that on average utilized the same hospital resources was used to determine the specific rates. Although health care reform may well change the health care delivery payment system, it is helpful for a nurse manager to know there are cost-cutting incentives built into the current DRG payment system. For example, if a particular patient stays less than the average length of time, or uses fewer costly resources, the hospital collects the full reimbursement and keeps the difference. However, if the patient stays longer or uses more costly resources than the average, the hospital still gets the same reimbursement and has to absorb the extra cost. What nurse managers often experience, as a result of better understanding the DRG payment system, is the hospital's attempt to reduce the patient's length of stay and/or to use fewer costly resources in providing patient care. Health care organizations have also increased their emphasis on clinical guidelines, productivity, cost savings, cost avoidance, and coordination of care and systems to maximize their impact on the bottom line.

Some nurse-intensive programs that were tested with the introduction of DRGs related to preoperative outpatient teaching for surgical admission; surgery on the day of admission; early discharge with home care, particularly for obstetric patients; day hospitalization; selective treatment or screening procedures; increased involvement of families in the patient's care and treatment; and outpatient chemotherapy.

From another nursing perspective, a number of nurse executives, in their continued attempt to determine the cost of nursing, built the impact of DRGs, disease severity, and the average length of the patient's stay into their nursing acuity or classification measurement systems. Their studies concluded that severity of illness is a better predictor of charges or costs than is length of stay.

Perhaps the most valuable lesson nursing learned with the introduction of DRGs is the necessity for, and value of, initiating discharge planning at the time of admission. More than in the past, nursing is drawing all the involved disciplines and departments into the discharge planning process to facilitate earlier discharges, thereby generating not only increased income for the hospital but also increased organizational power for nursing services.

As a nurse manager, if you do not know your unit's most prevalent DRGs and how the unit measures up from a financial, quality, and satisfaction perspective, it would be helpful for you to obtain this information and share it with staff. This can be particularly useful information as you mutually plan the unit's quality improvement and productivity goals for the coming year.

BV TEBBITT

Drug Use

◆ WHAT SHOULD I DO IF I THINK ONE OF MY STAFF IS SELLING DRUGS?

Q I have a strong suspicion that a nurse is diverting drugs and selling them to other hospital staff. How do I proceed as a manager to investigate and confront this nurse in a constructive manner while considering appropriate human resource and legal guidelines?

A The first step in this situation is to be aware of your resources. If this suspicion is indeed true, the diverting and selling of drugs is a violation of the law. A legal investigation will be required; thus this is not a situation you should handle alone. On the other hand, our legal system is built on the principle of innocence until guilt is proven. You do not want to unjustly accuse someone. Ask your human resources and legal department for advice about gathering appropriate information to be able to confront the nurse. They may also refer you to your local law enforcement agency to see how they want to handle such an investigation. In any such situation, you must have careful documentation—in writing—concerning the facts that have led to your suspicion. If you

have not already begun such documentation, you need to begin immediately.

Another aspect of this situation is determining if the nurse is personally suffering from chemical dependency, and thus also in need of medical treatment in addition to the potential legal problems. Resources that will help you would be an institutional employee assistance program and the professional nursing organizations' peer assistance programs. If indeed the nurse also appears to be chemically dependent, your approach will be much the same, and when you confront the nurse be sure to have someone else present. The second individual might be most beneficial if she is a recovering nurse.

Once this background information is gathered, the confrontation should occur as soon as possible to minimize the adverse effects on the quality of patient care on your unit. The confrontation should occur in a private place with your "witness" present. Tell the nurse that you would like to talk with her at a specific time to discuss work performance. At the time of the meeting, lay out the facts and allow the nurse to respond. Realize that the natural response is to defend and make excuses, so do not allow the nurse to dwell on these. Let the nurse know that she is valued as a person and that you want to help, but that if the suspicions are supported there has been a violation of the law and you also must ensure a level of quality care for the patients on your unit.

Sometimes the nurse will be relieved that the behavior has been discovered and may be quite receptive to the confrontation. On the other hand, the nurse may become hostile. In either case, you will have taken appropriate action and gathered the appropriate documentation to obtain a successful outcome.

JW ALEXANDER

◆ WHAT SHOULD I DO IF I THINK AN EMPLOYEE IS STEALING DRUGS?

Q I think a staff member is taking drugs from the patient drug supply. How can I prove this is occurring? If I see it happen, what do I do with this person?

A When a suspicion exists that a staff member is taking drugs from the patients' drug supply, addressing this problem requires a great deal of work

D

on behalf of the nurse manager. To ensure that suspicions are realistically based and that personnel are confronted in a manner that enhances problem solving while protecting patients requires a number of actions.

The manager should consider the nurse's behavior. Does the nurse accomplish assigned tasks with accuracy and in an alert manner? Does the nurse appear sleepy? Is her gait steady? Are her pupils dilated or contracted? Has this nurse made frequent errors with patients? What is the nurse's attendance and tardiness record? Frequently, if a nurse is taking drugs from a patient's drug supply due to an addiction or to other personal problems, these discrepancies will be noted before drug shortages are discovered.

It is extremely important to communicate with the hospital's or agency's chief pharmacist. The chief pharmacist is usually given the ultimate responsibility for the dispensing of drugs. If controlled substances are involved, the pharmacist may be required to contact that state's drug enforcement agency. One might also discuss with the pharmacist mechanisms to validate suspicions. Is there a way in which one can keep track of drugs *sent* to the patient versus those *administered* to the patient? This may require frequent auditing of the nurse's records. Though this practice may not validate that the nurse is taking drugs from patients, it may validate, at a minimum, that the nurse is not following proper procedure for documenting and administering drugs, thus allowing the manager to confront the nurse on a concrete basis.

Should the state drug enforcement agency be involved, there may be standard procedures required for reviewing documentation on the patient records and/or interviewing of individual staff members. On some occasions, the drug enforcement agency may prefer that the nurse not be confronted. Rather, videotaping administration or preparation of drugs in a medication preparation area may be recommended.

The nurse who is under suspicion must eventually be confronted. Before this, validate policy and procedure. Where this behavior is directly viewed, most hospitals will require suspension pending investigation to ensure protection of both the nurse and patients. Nurses usually divert pharmaceuticals for one of two reasons: to sell drugs or to maintain an addiction. Frequently nurses who are addicted may behave in a manner that ultimately ensures that they will be caught. These nurses are asking for help that they cannot provide for themselves.

Corrective action that is taken with the nurse will vary with circumstances and with personnel policy and procedure. If a state agency is involved, that agency may choose to arrest the nurse where narcotics abuse or suspicions of "pushing" exist. In this case termination is likely. Always check the status of the nurse's license with the state licensing agency. Frequently, agencies will have a record as to whether a nurse's license has ever been under review for a similar action. If this nurse has experienced prior review due to diversion of drugs, a harsher action with the nurse than what might otherwise be considered may be necessary. In some cases, a leave of absence with a requirement that a drug rehabilitation program be entered may be appropriate. On return from leave, periodic drug screenings with restricted access to medications may be instituted. This option may be a preferred option if the nurse involved has an otherwise excellent work record and is experiencing a situational crisis in her life. Finally, the employee assistance program (EAP) may be an option considered by the hospital regardless of whether it is preferred that the nurse be retained as an employee. Most personnel who take drugs, either for selling or to support an addiction, divert pharmaceuticals due to additional problems in their lives. The EAP may provide alternatives in addressing such personal issues.

Confronting nurses who divert pharmaceuticals is a difficult task for the nurse manager since this nurse is most probably a very troubled employee. If the nurse has an otherwise commendable work record, it is possible to provide options that may assist in recovery. In all cases, the work must be done by the staff member—not by the manager—or failure is a predictable outcome. These situations are frequently emotional. Thus the nurse manager, while showing concern for the staff member, must always remember that prioritizing the staff nurse's needs seldom supersedes the manager's obligation to protect patients.

LM LENTENBRINK

♦ **WHAT SHOULD I DO WHEN A PHYSICIAN COMES TO WORK UNDER THE INFLUENCE OF DRUGS OR ALCOHOL?**

Q My staff and I have reason to suspect that a physician on my service is impaired by drugs and alcohol. I have documented the physician's behavior and taken this information and my concerns to my boss. At this time, I learned that this physician is a personal friend of the CEO and is in line to be Chair of the Board of Directors. I'm concerned for patient safety. What do I do?

A You must let your professional integrity and obligation to protect patients from harm guide you in this situation, regardless of the internal hospital relationships. You must pursue whatever avenues are necessary until you are satisfied that appropriate action has been taken and/or the physician no longer exhibits behavior that might jeopardize patient safety. Options you might consider include the following:

- Ask your boss if your concerns have been addressed and, if so, to provide you with assurance that they are being investigated. It is possible that follow-up has occurred but because of issues of confidentiality you have not been kept informed. It is important to discuss with your boss what action you or your staff should take if the physician exhibits similar behavior in the future. Be clear about your concerns regarding patient safety as well as your own personal liability.
- Look in the hospital's administrative manual to see if there is a policy regarding what actions should be taken if an employee or physician is suspected of being chemically impaired.
- Put your concerns in writing, detailing the specific behavior you and your staff have observed, and forward this to the chief nursing executive or the next individual in your hospital's chain of command.
- Enlist the aid of a physician you believe would be willing to follow up on your concerns with the medical staff leadership and/or administration.
- Talk to the physician directly about the behavior you have observed and your concern for patient safety.
- Report your concerns directly to your state Medical Disciplinary Board. The board is mandated by state law to follow up on any complaints and, in most states, the identity of the individual who reports is kept confidential.

It is important that you document and continue to report any further occurrences. If, at any point, you or your staff believe patients are in danger, you should institute your hospital's chain of command to report the situation and request that either an administrator or medical staff executive come immediately to deal with the situation.

C ST CHARLES

◆ TO WHOM SHOULD I GO FOR HELP FOR AN EMPLOYEE WITH AN ALCOHOL PROBLEM?

Q One of my peers comes to work with alcohol on her breath. When I mentioned it to her she told me to mind my own business. I'm new to the organization and reluctant to tell her supervisor because she is a long-term employee.

A You must realize that the peer with the alcohol problem, if indeed she is dependent on alcohol, is demonstrating the classic symptom of the disease process: denial. The statement that you should mind your own business is part of the disease process. You have a professional responsibility to your patients and your peer to help her if she has the problem you suspect. However, in the work situation, the supervisor, from a managerial position, often cannot do much unless the alcoholism has a negative impact on work performance. From a professional standpoint, the supervisor is in the same situation you are with the responsibility to provide help for a peer.

You need to carefully observe your peer and document situations that are indicative of alcoholism. Such symptoms include mood changes, being off the unit for unexplained reasons, excess absenteeism especially following days off, frequent trips to the bathroom, and tardiness. If these behaviors occur, in addition to the smell of alcohol on the breath, you should confidentially report your documentation to the supervisor. Do not be concerned about your tenure in the organization; the supervisor should accept this information without any repercussions.

It is inappropriate for you to confront the nurse yourself, though the management team may ask you to be involved at a later time since you have expressed concern for this individual. Because of the nature of the disease process of chemical dependency, confrontation should always take place with two people present. One of those individuals should be someone trained in interventions and/or a recovering person. This situation creates the environment of support for the chemically dependent peer and conveys the message of caring and willingness to assist in obtaining treatment.

Through your concern and careful documentation, this peer should be able to obtain treatment, enter a recovery program, and successfully return to the work force.

JW ALEXANDER

Education

♦ **ARE THERE COURSES TO TRAIN NURSE MANAGERS IN BUSINESS TECHNIQUES?**

Q Has anyone developed a successful educational program to train nurse managers in the business of health care finance, resource allocation, and human resource management?

A Programs have been offered in the area of nursing administration. "Successful" seems to be the operative word. A good way to determine this would be to ask those nurse managers who have an advanced degree in the field of nursing administration about their educational programs. Nursing administration as a specialty area has undergone a number of changes. During the past three decades, nursing administration was primarily seen as a functional area added on to a clinical specialty. Fortunately that has changed and the decision at this point for nurse managers is whether to obtain a Master's in Nursing Administration, an MBA, or a combination of the two.

Another source for this education would be through continuing education programs. From this aspect, you may have to separate out the three areas specified in your question and find the course best suited to your needs. For instance, in 1992 Steven Finkler, PhD, CPA, author of *Budgeting Concepts for Nurse Managers,* offered an intensive, 5-day workshop on Budgeting for Nurse Managers at New York University (Finkler & Korner, 1993). In addition, the American Hospital Association offers a number of

workshops around the country in the area of personnel administration.

SR. M FINNICK

♦ **HOW CAN NURSING FACULTY BETTER RELATE TO THE REAL WORLD?**

Q How can nursing faculty keep up to date in theory and practice applied to the real world?

A This is a common concern among nurses regardless of whether they are in practice, administration, or education. What we need is a shared understanding of nursing grounded in a conception or theory of nursing that has nursing practice at its heart. We need to understand a unique focus of nursing that supports and develops our practice and our discipline of knowledge. Florence Nightingale provided our first model of using nursing theory in practice. The South Florida Nursing Theorist Conferences have provided excellent examples of bringing theory and practice together (Parker, 1990). Most of the nurses at the conferences have been nurses in hospital nursing practice and management. The idea of the conferences can be carried out on a smaller scale in local settings.

Instead of a focus on nursing we are often distracted by outside forces and give attention to problems that take us away from our primary obligation to society and to ourselves. The day-to-day life of nurses in practice seems driven by financial uncertainty, organizational changes, patient acuity, and measures of quality. The day-to-day life of nurses in faculty positions seems driven by courses to prepare, proposals to write for research funding, and articles to get published. The obvious problem shared by both groups is budget and staffing constraints. Nursing is at risk of increasing neglect; nurses are at risk of replacement. These are the issues that may serve to bring us together, that may lead us to ensure that nursing theory and practice are relevant to the real world.

The future of nursing demands unity among nurses in various endeavors such as practice and education. Nurses in practice and nurses in faculty positions must come to some common ground of sharing. This common ground is the remembering that needs of society for nursing direct the development of nursing as a discipline and profession, and therefore the functions of nurses in practice and education. The reflection of this common ground is an explicit conception of nursing, knowledge of nursing theories, and the use of nursing theory in practice, education, administration, and scholarship.

Valuing the nursing practice situation is the key to problems we face. All discussions about nursing and all dialogues among nurses should revolve around illustrations of actual nursing situations from the real world of nursing. The description of each nursing situation should include attention to the one nursed and the need for nursing, the nurse, the mutual goals and activities of the interaction, and the environment of the nursing situation. Nursing practice is then ensured as the center of nursing, and nursing theory, research, education, and administration find places according to the contributions of each endeavor to nursing practice. Nurses can examine each situation from viewpoints of nursing theory and be open to new knowing of the situation. Each nurse has expertise to bring to the dialogue and each can be respected for that special contribution. The distracting factors also will find places in relation to essential aspects of clinical nursing.

ME PARKER

◆ WHAT CAN I DO ABOUT A NURSE MANAGER WHO SEEMS TO CARE MORE ABOUT ADMINISTRATION THAN THE PATIENTS?

Q Nurse managers are losing touch with the profession and seem more concerned with appeasing administration than with quality care of patients or commitment to nursing staff. Many of our managers lack proper education for the job—they came up through the ranks because they were good bedside nurses or via the Peter principle. As a concerned nurse manager, what should I do?

A The requirements for nursing management are still in transition, reflecting changes in the role of nurse managers. Head nurses of the past had to be the best clinicians on their units because that is what their role required; as representatives of a centralized

bureaucracy, they often seemed more committed to the concerns of hospital administration than professional nursing matters. Now many nurse managers have multiple master's degrees in nursing and business administration and a stronger identity with the nursing profession in general. Since both types of managers will be working side by side in the near future, these two backgrounds must be used to complement each other as a strength for nursing administration.

You can reduce these groups into a single qualified team by
1. Phasing in consistent academic job requirements for entry management positions by attrition.
2. Insisting on membership in professional groups such as the local Organization of Nurse Executives for middle managers.
3. Setting aside monthly meeting time for sessions on core management skills.
4. Hiring an outside consultant to assess and facilitate role delineation in your management team.

RG HESS

◆ WHAT WILL HELP CLOSE THE GAP BETWEEN EDUCATION AND PRACTICE?

Q The gap between education and practice seems to be wider than ever before. The most glaring problem is related to "professional" behavior and socialization. What strategies will help to bridge that gap?

A Here is a wonderful opportunity for you as a nurse manager to begin a dialogue with your staff nurses and a group of student nurses. You could contact one of the school instructors who has students on your unit and ask if she, with her students, would like to help you and the staff develop a position paper for your unit on "professional practice." This might take the form of several brown bag lunches, a staff meeting, a task force work group, or an all-day educational workshop planned by you and the instructor. The idea would be to develop opportunities for the nursing staff on the unit to hold dialogue with students about the meaning of "professional

E

practice." Outcomes you could expect from the group are that they come up with a definition of professional practice or develop a list of behavioral statements that reflect professional practice or a list of values that define this topic for them. This document could then become the basis for your unit philosophy and the driving force for orientation, policy decisions, care planning, and even performance evaluation. This is one way to develop a "culture" of professional practice, which could become a means to teach student nurses on your unit professional practice through socialization into your staff norms. Remember that behaviors are often a more effective tool for teaching others than discussion. Students who are exposed to your professional unit culture and values may learn stronger lessons of professional behavior by observing what values are acted out in the practice setting than from similar time spent in a classroom seminar on the subject. You really do have a wonderful opportunity to influence the future of nursing.

MC ALDERMAN

♦ HOW CAN WE OVERCOME FACULTY OPPOSITION TO WORK WITH STUDENTS TO DEVELOP A PROFESSIONAL FOCUS?

Q The staff on my unit are interested in helping develop the professional focus of the nursing students who undertake their practicums on our unit. The students have indicated that they would be interested in that process. However, the faculty member is not comfortable with the notion and has ignored the staff's interest and recommendations. How can we help the faculty person to overcome her opposition to this process?

A Negotiate the clinical outcome objectives with the appropriate school faculty member before accepting a clinical rotation for her students. The objectives may clearly state that included in the students' clinical experience will be the professional ethics, values, and culture of the practice setting. These are equally as important as attaining clinical proficiencies in patient care delivery.

LM JOHNSON

♦ WHEN SHOULD I BEGIN WORK ON MY MASTER'S DEGREE?

Q I'm a single mother of three and was promoted a year ago to nurse manager of a busy surgical unit. I know a master's degree will eventually be essential to advance my career. Should I start school now? How can I manage it?

A A master's degree is necessary for career advancement. It will also provide a strong professional skill and knowledge base that enhances effectiveness in the unit manager position.

If, when, and how to start in a graduate program is a very individualized question. No two individuals' circumstances are identical and only the individual herself can make the decision. It is recommended that various factors be assessed and a plan be developed with specific time frames:

1. Investigate the various types of programs available, including type of degree, curriculum, cost, financial assistance, class schedules, and part-time versus full-time options.
2. Assess family and child care responsibilities and their impact on school attendance.
3. Assess personal and financial resources.
4. Investigate employer support and financial assistance. Is it possible to have a flexible work schedule? Can you utilize work projects to fulfill school requirements? Is financial assistance available?

SF SMITH

Employee Assistance

♦ IS AN EMPLOYEE ASSISTANCE PROGRAM FEASIBLE IN A SMALL INSTITUTION?

Q We are interested in developing an employee assistance program at our small hospital. We have limited resources but feel the need for such a program. How do we begin? Are our expectations reasonable?

A Developing an employee assistance program in your hospital demonstrates a commitment to employees. Offering services to address work needs as well as personal needs communicates caring about people. Although you mention that your hospital is small, all organizations must consider the same questions when making a decision related to creating this type of program.

A committee within the hospital should develop the goals and expected outcomes. This group can determine the type of model based on the number of employees, services expected, and budgetary considerations. A full-time staff member to direct and provide services may sound reasonable, but the small number of employees may not justify this expense.

The list of services needed should provide the basic framework for designing the program. Then decide which services will be offered at your institution and which services might be offered by other agencies on a referral basis. Consulting other organizations of similar size will enable your organization to utilize information and experience of others in designing a program tailored to meet employee needs. The hospital should also contact state professional organizations to explore the range of services developed for each group.

Acceptance of the program or services will depend on its integration into the structure of the hospital and should demonstrate the support of the hospital administration in meeting employee needs.

AMT BROOKS

◆ HOW CAN I ASSIST A STAFF MEMBER WHO IS A BATTERED WIFE?

Q A nurse on my unit is repeatedly late, absent, or leaving work early, always in the middle of another family crisis. I have heard through the grapevine that this nurse is a battered wife. Although the staff is trying to cover for her, her performance is suffering and her obligation as a team player is lacking. What can I do?

A As a manager there are two considerations that you have to make in this situation. The first is the care of the patients under your scope of responsibility, and the second is the care of the staff who provide direct services to those patients. You must deal with the employee's absenteeism because it directly affects the quality of care the patients are receiving and it places an added burden of work on the other staff members. This situation provides you with an opportunity to discuss the employee's attendance issues, *and* to introduce a dialogue around the causes of the attendance problems.

As a manager you can and should set the expectations for acceptable attendance based on your organization's policy. However, as a health care professional, you also need to explore the issue of possible abuse. You may ask the employee to help you understand the reasons for the attendance problems and what role you can play in helping her to be successful in correcting the problem. If she does not disclose social problems that compromise her attendance, then you may prompt the nurse to verify or contradict the problem by asking if she knows that staff have been worried that she may have serious family problems, including a fear that she might be in an abusive relationship. If the employee feels able to admit to such a situation, a referral to your organization's confidential employee assistance program or to a local community abuse program would be appropriate.

Depending on the adult abuse regulations in your state, you may be expected to report the suspected abuse. If the employee denies such a problem, then you must refocus on the expected attendance improvement, and ask the employee to suggest means to accomplish this. Possible limited-time solutions to explore would be reduction in work hours, change of shifts, change of start times, and change of scheduled days. Despite the ability to make any of the above changes, it must be made clear that the attendance standard must be met. In addition, you must let the employee know that disciplinary action would need to be taken if immediate and sustained improvement in the performance does not occur. You should agree to meet with the employee again within several weeks to discuss progress, and continue to monitor the situation, giving the employee feedback on her accomplishments.

MC ALDERMAN

◆ HOW CAN I OFFER HELP TO A TROUBLED EMPLOYEE WITHOUT BEING OFFENSIVE?

Q There is a professional worker on the staff I supervise who is undergoing challenging and difficult times in her personal life. Although this situation has not yet affected her work, I suspect that, if left unaddressed, it will. We do have an employee assistance program. How do I encourage her to pursue it without being offensive and "nosy"?

A By all means, you should approach the employee privately, confidentially, and in a very nonthreatening and caring manner. Explain that you are aware of some issues in this person's personal life and although you do not want to pry and are not asking for any personal details, you thought it might be helpful if this person considered using the employee assistance program. After all, this is why organizations have developed such programs. Life is complex, and none of us are without times when personal challenges in our life make our work difficult at best. I am sure if you approach this nurse with compassion and concern, you will find a grateful response for having such a concerned manager.

KJ McDONAGH

Empowerment

◆ IS THERE HARD EVIDENCE THAT EMPOWERMENT OF NURSES HAS IMPROVED THEIR RELATIONSHIP WITH PHYSICIANS?

Q Are there any research findings that suggest that empowering nurses through shared governance has actually increased the collaboration between nurses and doctors?

A Much of the research conducted in hospitals that have developed shared governance structures in nursing has been qualitative or descriptive research. This research and other hospitals' experiences do indicate that as nurses develop in their professional roles and learn to collaborate with each other on professional nursing issues, these skills transfer over into the nurse–physician relationship as well. From a quantitative research standpoint, at Saint Joseph's Hospital of Atlanta, the semiannual physician satisfaction surveys have consistently

shown nurses and nursing care being rated as the top reason physicians practice at the institution. At Saint Joseph's Hospital of Atlanta, we have experienced an excellent level of collaboration between physicians and nurses. As nurses became more adept at their work and more sophisticated in their communication with physicians, the physicians respected the nurses more and began to rely on them more heavily for judgments while the physician was away from the patient's bedside. This has promoted the autonomy of the nursing staff and fostered a healthy interdependence between the nursing and medical staffs.

KJ McDONAGH

◆ DO EMPOWERMENT PROCESSES REALLY CHANGE ANYTHING?

Q Aren't all these empowerment processes just an illusion created by management to make the staff feel good without really changing anything at all in the organization? We have seen so much of this "stuff" come and go that it gets tiring to hear about it and see no real changes occur.

A If no real changes are occurring in your organization, you can be sure that empowerment has not happened there yet. Increasingly we are seeing organizations moving to empowering workers, not because there is an overwhelming desire to be overly humanistic, but because survival increasingly depends on staff investment. Because of the increasing dependence on technologically proficient workers for the success of organizations, there is a greater need for models of work that incorporate staff into decision making. The specialization of knowledge requires more decision makers involved in setting work place goals and processing work. With the advent of quality imperatives, the greatest influences on outcomes are the activities of those who do the work of the organization. The trend toward empowerment is simply the recognition that quality outcomes cannot be achieved without the investment of those who do the work.

The problem with the increasing dependence on worker investment is the paucity of available models that can structure a belief in empowerment into an organization operating within the context of shared decision making. It is one thing to say one believes in empowerment; it is quite another to create an organization in which empowered processes and behaviors are the modus operandi. This is where most empowerment processes first break down.

The real challenge to making empowerment a permanent ongoing operational process in most organizations is the limited skill levels of most managers to deal with an empowered worker. When workers were obedient, compliant, or just plain not interested in what the organization did as long as it left them alone to do their work, management was a relatively straightforward process. When workers have a share in the power, decisions, productivity, and work processes, it is hard for the manager to know how to behave. Further, managing such a staff requires a set of skills not always present in most managers. The trauma for all concerned in this scenario can be significant.

To be successful, organizations must make sure that the development of the manager keeps up with the process of restructuring work to empower the staff. Management development is critical to the success of such programs and can be the difference between a successful transition or a chaotic and noisy reaction to a change no one knows how to handle. Such changes in the organization are becoming more common and will be essential to successfully achieving the outcomes of the work place. Be patient; it is just a matter of time before such processes will become the way of doing work and will not disappear as they once did. Current social and work shifts simply won't let us retreat to yesterday's style of managing and relating.

T PORTER-O'GRADY

◆ HOW CAN I BECOME COMFORTABLE WITH STAFF EMPOWERMENT?

Q As a nurse manager, I am not comfortable with group problem solving and staff empowerment. Should I reconsider the decision to be a manager?

A Before you reconsider your role as a nurse manager, take time to truthfully explore your feelings about staff empowerment. What is it about staff empowerment that makes you uncomfortable? Is it

lack of knowledge, old baggage, fear of losing control, fear of the unknown, or something else? Find a trusted colleague who is well versed in staff empowerment and who has successfully implemented it, and discuss these issues. Attend some workshops on the topic or consult an expert in staff empowerment. When first confronted with the realities of staff empowerment most managers are anxious, apprehensive, and sometimes even hostile. True staff empowerment is a growth process. It doesn't happen all at once. The staff and the manager will develop and grow into their roles together, over time. It is very structured and requires quite a commitment to education and learning.

Also, take some time to explore your personal and professional goals. If a goal is to advance professionally in administration, empowering your staff will be a requirement, so you'll have to make the commitment to overcome your discomfort. If your goal is to move along another path that won't involve working through others, you won't have to place as great an emphasis on the empowering process.

Decide where you want to go first and then if necessary, be willing to confront and handle the issues that will prevent you from achieving your long-term goals.

RM HADDON

◆ HOW DO I MAKE EMPOWERMENT WORK?

Q In empowerment processes, I want to share accountability and power with the staff. The staff, however, finds it difficult to accept empowerment. They have indicated that they want accountability and a share in the power and are willing to do the work. However, we are all uncertain as to what that work is. How do we begin to shift power and make empowerment work?

A There is increasing pressure on anyone in a leadership role today to involve people in decisions. People expect to participate but may experience a fear of the unknown. Getting everybody into the pool usually requires someone to test the water first. The manager's role is to tell others, "Hey, the water's fine, let's get in." With fear, the first goal is usually to get others talking about it. Practice the vocabulary of fear—words such as *scared, anxious, hesitant,* and *afraid*—in a confident, supportive tone that assures your staff that you are not implying criticism. Lead discussions of the following questions:

- ◆ "What barriers keep you from being as successfully empowered as we would like you to be?"
- ◆ "What can we do to turn this cycle around?"

Remember that if you want people to disclose their fears, recognize and be able to talk about some of your own. If you want people to speak up about sensitive issues, demonstrate that you can communicate about such issues. Perhaps more importantly, show that you are willing to listen to the concerns of others. Be aggressive in seeking ideas and suggestions from committed members and assuring that prompt feedback regarding use of those ideas and suggestions is provided.

Before you proceed: Clarify your intentions with the group to move toward a consensus-based approach for decisions. Emphasize your faith in the group's competence and skills. Identify your reasons for wanting to move in this direction: the desire to help the group achieve even higher levels of teamwork.

1. Use an agenda. Meetings without agendas can drift intolerably. Know which areas are purely informational, which are discussion items, and which require decisions. Review the agenda at the start of the meeting and decide as a group how much time should be allocated to each of the items.
2. Keep tangents to a minimum. If they do come up, call them out or ask one person to keep a list of the tangential ideas that arise during the discussion. At the end of the meeting, review the list and decide how and when to handle each item on the list.
3. When you are brainstorming ideas, encourage creativity and participation. Focus on listing all the ideas with no comment. After ideas have been identified, shift to evaluating each idea.
4. When a decision has been made, have someone record it and read it back to the group. This will focus staff on what has actually been decided. It also gives them an opportunity to change any wording that might be misleading or unclear.

The empowerment process requires a large investment from professional clinical nurses and their nurse managers. They are required to put great effort into learning new skills and relationships. They must face increased ambiguity and uncertainty about the process until it is established and working. Everyone must also cope with the psychologic pain and discomfort related to changing beliefs and attitudes.

Building the skills and agreements that support collaborative decision making has represented a very tangible way to turn an environment of fear into one of enthusiasm, creativity, and commitment.

LG VONFROLIO

◆ HOW DO I INTEREST STAFF IN EMPOWERMENT?

Q I want to create a more participative, empowering environment, but the staff members feel that they are overworked and underpaid, and that the manager should do what the manager is paid to do. Currently, the staff do not have all the skills needed to make decisions. Where does a manager go from here?

A Find out on which decisions staff would like to have input. Does their work schedule belong to you or to them? Is there an issue that requires more institutional resources to accomplish such as continuing education time or money? Begin to build interest in staff decision making by selecting an example that appeals to the staff and is attainable within a reasonable time frame. Help the staff develop group decision-making skills through experience. Success attained on a small scale becomes a powerful incentive for further action.

Use your in-house resources in building an expanded perspective of what professional practice entails. Remember, you are paid to achieve management goals of effective operation. Your willingness to share authority reflects your respect for your staff colleagues' abilities.

CE LOVERIDGE

◆ HOW DO I ENCOURAGE STAFF TO DEAL WITH STICKY ISSUES THEMSELVES?

Q I am working toward empowering my staff, but they are very selective in accepting additional responsibilities, leaving those issues they are uncomfortable with for me to deal with. How do I change this process?

A It is important to try to determine why they may be resisting. Several reasons may exist.

1. They may not feel knowledgeable or skilled at assuming these new responsibilities.
2. They may have tried in the past and been unsuccessful.
3. Their level of authority may not be clear.
4. The system may not support them.
5. One or more individuals may be manipulating the situation to gain control and power.

If there is a knowledge or skill problem, it is important to set clear parameters, discuss options with staff, teach them what you know, coach them as they try out their options, and be a good supporter by cheering their successes and letting them learn from their mistakes without punitive actions on your part.

Let them know that if they don't succeed the first time, you will support them in trying again. This can best be done by asking, "What have you learned from this and how would you do it differently next time?" If you have previously recalled their decision-making authority when you disagreed or when they were not successful, you may have to prove that you won't do it this time. You may have to prove it several times. Don't be put off by this; just be consistent in your support of them.

Be sure that the issue of their level of authority is clear in your own mind and with your staff. Are you asking them to collect some information for you to make a decision? Are you asking them to make recommendations for you to consider when you make a decision? Is it their decision, with the condition that you want to be informed (or do you want them to negotiate with you or someone else) before they decide? Or is it their decision to make on their own or on your behalf? These questions should be asked and answered before the responsibility is given.

As manager you need to assess whether the system will support their taking on this new level of authority. If you authorize them to decide how to provide care, but others in the organization (administration, procedure committees, etc.) can contradict that decision, they cannot be successful and you may be unintentionally setting them up for failure.

Finally, if one or more of the staff are manipulating for power, you may need to coach other staff members in confrontation and limit-setting skills. Role-

play with them, play devil's advocate to help them anticipate the response of the manipulators, and help them script responses. If the behavior continues, you may need to initiate counseling with the manipulative individuals.

JE JENKINS

◆ IS EMPOWERMENT REALLY EMPOWERMENT IF DECISIONS ARE MADE BY ADMINISTRATION?

Q As a nurse manager, I'm becoming increasingly aware that the true power is located in administration and only functions are being delegated to the nurse manager. If the nurse manager makes an independent decision in the best interest of her unit, it is often criticized and constrained by those in administrative roles. Is empowerment really possible when legitimate authority is held only by those in administration? Isn't the nurse manager then really just a tool of someone else's power?

A In a fully empowered environment, legitimate authority, or decision making, is shared. The accountabilities of each level of management must be identified, and the individual must be given full autonomy, authority, and responsibility to meet those accountabilities. However, in an overall corporate system, there are many subsystems nested within the larger one, creating a synergistic whole. There must be balance and congruence between all subsystems if the total corporation is to succeed. Thus communication, shared vision, and joint decision making must be coupled with autonomy at the unit and individual levels. Candid and consistent communication and feedback are essential if clarity and consensus are to be reached regarding level of authority and autonomy for individuals and groups within the system.

J KOERNER

◆ HOW DO I CHANGE THE NEGATIVE ATTITUDES OF NURSES WHO NEVER SEEM TO BE SATISFIED?

Q What do nurses want? Nurses who have been working on this unit for years seem more than ever to be dissatisfied. We are working toward shared governance, salaries are good, and we agree on the scheduling. It seems these nurses have everything they could want, yet they seem to be in conflict with nursing. What can I do?

E

A You have a difficult situation—one that many managers have to face but few feel confident in handling. Not infrequently, a sort of subculture can exist among long-term employees. They often have a great deal of shared experience in the work setting. Unfortunately, the attitudes in this subculture are not always positive. This group, if they were directing their energies toward constructive ends, could be a tremendous asset. When the energy is negatively directed, that is, engaged in maintaining the status quo, they can function as a weight on the entire department.

The first rule for you to remember (post it on your bathroom mirror) is this: *Do not take the resisting and complaining personally.* It is not likely that their attitude is about you or your management style. This understanding will free you up to assess the situation and make decisions. Other pointers follow:

1. Make the vision for the department explicit, involving the staff in the process as much as you can. This will help to take the attention away from personalities and turf issues, substituting a more objective perspective. The emphasis on quality in recent years is an excellent tool to help break up "group think" and redirect the values system of the work group. Decisions made based on departmental goals, and measurements of quality and cost have a legitimate logic and appeal that can be powerful.

2. Involve these long-term staff members in projects that recognize and take advantage of their considerable expertise. This does not mean that you can or should give them license for negative attitudes or behavior in the process. Do not be afraid to confront them. You might say something like, "It seems hard for you to participate in this project wholeheartedly," or "You didn't seem to want to be at the meeting today." This could open up an interchange in which you can give and receive feedback. The employee is made aware that her behavior is noticed and that you are concerned or disappointed.

3. Reward positive behavior. Rewards do not have to be financial. Receiving thanks and acknowledgement for work well done is very rewarding to some people. For other personality types, a more tangible reward is necessary. This makes a mix of reward options (equally available to everyone) effective. A half day off work, with pay, is a powerful motivator in response to a major accomplishment. While this has financial impact, it can be a manageable sum.

4. It is unfortunate, but all of the positive interventions in the world may not move these employees in the desired direction. Document performance, both positive and negative, of the staff regularly. Be well prepared with substantive information and specific situations when a staff member must be confronted. Confront in a timely way, and document in the process used in your institution. If necessary, terminate staff who are not amenable to change. You may think you cannot do without them, and your actions may cause political fallout for a time, but it may be the only way to move forward.

5. Don't forget that fun and laughter can sometimes bring people together faster than anything else.

Remember that in your position as manager, you are entrusted to develop and oversee the most effective department possible. These are some ways of moving in that direction.

J HIXON

Ethics

◆ HOW SHOULD I ADVISE A STAFF MEMBER WHO HAS AN ETHICAL DISAGREEMENT WITH A TREATMENT PLAN?

Q How does a manager support a staff nurse who finds herself in an ethical dilemma, that is, at odds with the plan of medical care or treatment that the physician has ordered?

A Basic to working with any ethical issue in nursing is deliberation about the focus of nursing and use of this focus to guide the thinking and action of the nurse. The nurse can be assisted in this situation by clarifying the meaning of nursing and the domain of nursing practice. The meaning of medicine and its domain can also be described as a way to further clarify nursing concerns from those of a medical nature. The nurse might then assume the role of a general advocate for the patient, a role any citizen might take, and try to seek the best interest of the patient from this viewpoint. Consultation with colleagues in the setting as well as in other nursing situations may also be useful. In any event, the nurse must take the action she believes to be right, based on the focus of nursing, and remain open to growth as new information unfolds.

ME PARKER

♦ **IS NURSING ETHICS IMPORTANT TO MANAGEMENT'S POLICIES AND PRACTICES?**

Q To what extent does nursing ethics influence policies and practices in nursing administration and management?

A Nursing ethics really permeates all of our work in nursing, from both a clinical and a management standpoint. Not only do nurse managers and administrators need to be aware of the ethical dilemmas that nurses face every day in the clinical arena, they must also be cognizant of the business ethics that confront us daily in our challenging work. These ethical issues include how nurses are asked to handle complex patient issues such as end-of-life decisions and withdrawal of treatment. Managers and administrators need to be aware of the fact that nurses need support and the empowerment to handle these situations with physicians and others in the organization. From a business ethics standpoint, nursing administrators and managers have to be concerned with appropriate staffing levels to provide safe and effective patient care and many other issues. Ethics truly permeates all decisions because of the very critical balance of our work in health care.

KJ McDONAGH

Falsifying Records

♦ **WHAT SHOULD I DO IF I THINK A PATIENT'S RECORD HAS BEEN FALSIFIED?**

Q One of the staff members informed me that a colleague had allowed a patient to fall and picked her up, with the only result of the fall being a bruise. In the patient's record, however, she indicated that the bruise was caused by something other than a fall and did not document the fall. How do I handle this problem?

A Any time you receive information of this type, it is important that you follow up as soon as possible to ascertain the facts and, if necessary, institute disciplinary action. If the allegations are proved to be true, a serious violation of nursing practice has occurred. However, it is imperative that you investigate the situation thoroughly. It would be helpful to review the patient's record and if the patient is alert, ask the patient if he did, in fact, sustain a fall. Then schedule an initial investigatory meeting with the nurse to discuss the incident. When you meet with the nurse, ask her to provide information and/or an explanation of the events. At the same time you should convey, very directly and succinctly, all of the information you have gathered and your concerns. In general, you should not make any decisions at the investigatory meeting regarding disciplinary action. After the meeting, consult with your supervisor and the human resources department regarding an appropriate course of action.

C ST CHARLES

♦ **HOW CAN I PROMOTE HONESTY IN FILLING OUT TIME CARDS?**

Q The process of recording on time cards has changed from punch-in to a system of write-in. Employees (professional as well as nonprofessional staff) are asked to write in their start and ending time, sign their card, and calculate the hours. The process seems to have problems, not the least of which is honesty of the staff in reporting to work on time and signing in late if they do not report on time. It is impossible for the nurse managers to always be present to monitor this system. What do you suggest as strategies for monitoring? How can the managers ensure consistent and honest time reporting?

A Before determining strategies, it is probably wise to review the reasons why the time card system changed from a punch-in to a write-in system. Was this considered an appropriate system for professional as well as nonprofessional staff? If so, what were the expected benefits of using such a system? If the expectation was to achieve a higher level of professionalism, you must first determine whether the staff share this vision. It may be that this is not a viable system for all personnel.

If it is determined that keeping this system is important, it may be wise to discuss problems that are being experienced with the staff. Personnel must understand that privileges are earned. To retain such privileges, staff must assist in ensuring the system's success. Depending on whether you work in a unionized setting, you may or may not be able to involve personnel in monitoring write-ins. An audit system periodically conducted without prior notice for a sampling of staff may encourage personnel to accurately document their time.

Managers cannot be absolutely sure that all practices are happening consistently and honestly unless they themselves are in a position to validate write-ins every day for each staff person. Personnel need to be informed regarding the implications of dishonesty as related to fraud and misrepresentation, while the system for those staff members who truthfully report such occurrences as lateness should not be so punitive as to discourage accuracy.

LM LENTENBRINK

◆ HOW DO I DEAL WITH STAFF WHO ARE FALSIFYING TIME CARDS?

Q I am a new manager of a nursing unit. The charge nurse has pointed out discrepancies between a staff member's sign-in form and actual time worked, to the benefit of the employee. The charge nurse states that this is not the first occurrence with this staff member, and there are some records to support this claim. How do I handle this situation?

A Every manager will, at some time, have to deal with an employee who falsifies records. There is a range of responses on behalf of the manager. Managers may respond with an oral reprimand, written warning, suspension, or even termination.

Fraud is a deliberate act of deception. The goal of fraud is generally for personal gain, for either favor or financial benefit. Fraud can be prosecuted as a criminal offense; therefore, it is a serious offense and should be dealt with firmly. You should undertake the following steps:

1. Ask to see the evidence.
2. Consult with your supervisor and the human resources department to ensure that you follow agency policy in gathering and evaluating evidence.
3. Determine whether the evidence is credible and that this one employee is the only person engaging in the behavior. If this is a "normal" practice for other employees, then your investigation and strategy for resolution may be altered.
4. Ensure that you are consistent in your reaction to the offense. Consistency in action is an important quality in leadership.
5. Decide ahead of time what your course of action will be and clear it with the human resources department; thus you are ensuring that you are not violating any provision in a union contract with regard to collection of evidence, interviewing, or level of discipline.
6. If the evidence is deemed credible, call a meeting with the staff member, the charge nurse, and another witness. Be sure to read your labor union contract; it may call for a member of the union to be present on behalf of the employee.
7. State your findings and allow the employee to respond. If you are convinced that fraud has occurred, there is no evidence that will excuse the behavior.
8. State your course of action clearly and firmly.
9. Follow through immediately with your course of action.
10. Evaluate the process.

Fraud can be extremely damaging to group cohesiveness. Staff members need to understand the ramifications of their behavior. In addition, they must trust that when fraud is discovered, the appropriate action will be taken.

GL CROW

Floating

◆ HOW DO I DEAL WITH STAFF WHO OBJECT TO FLOATING?

Q Many of the staff I work with feel that it is inappropriate to float to other clinical areas in which they are not skilled. In many ways, I agree with their assessment, but floating is expected. As a manager, how do I handle this situation?

A These days, it is imperative that we operate efficient, cost-effective nursing units. We in nursing are challenged with a fluctuating census. Floating staff is a valuable tool to adjust staffing in order to match census. The staff should be able to verbalize their concerns and ventilate frustrations, as well as provide constructive feedback on the process. A basic orientation to general areas (medical, surgical, pediatric, etc.) should be explored. Each nurse who floats has the responsibility to limit her clinical performance to that which she is comfortable with. For example, expecting an adult nurse to give medication on a pediatric floor might not be a safe practice for the licensed professional or for the patient. On the other hand, if the nurse can't properly assess the pediatric patient and give medications, how productive can she be to the unit at her expensive hourly rate?

A concrete suggestion is to limit floating to like areas, for example, surgical and maternal/child.
1. Educate the staff of the need to flex staffing (reasons include budget and productivity).
2. Offer the staff alternatives to floating, such as when the unit is overstaffed, a unit staff member volunteers to take benefit time and go home.
3. Establish cluster units. Surgical staff float to surgical floors, and medical staff float to medical floors.
4. Formulate an orientation that meets the needs of the cluster units.

While the decision to float staff is a management accountability, the specific didactic and clinical orientations needed are staff nurse accountabilities. Use your Nursing Practice Council or pull together some staff nurses with inservice help to hammer out the details of the needed orientation.

JM McMAHON

◆ HOW CAN I MAKE FLOATING FAIR?

Q Floating continues to be a thorn in the side of the nursing staff. How can we make it acceptable and fair?

A You're right. Floating has long been, and continues to be, a thorn in the side of many nursing staff. Yet it also seems unfair to let one nursing unit remain understaffed when nurses are available elsewhere. Understanding a few key factors that influence attitudes of staff toward floating may help you in developing a workable solution.

First, nurses who object to floating are not being uncooperative or lacking in desire to be helpful and supportive of their colleagues on other units. Most nurses actually get a high level of satisfaction from feeling they contributed to meeting a need of a colleague or patient. Their reluctance is most frequently generated by fear; these fears can be conscious ones, as well as some that lie just below the surface of awareness.

Fear of being inadequate. The nurse fears she may be assigned to the care of patients whose diagnosis and treatment or the technology associated with the treatment are no longer familiar to her. This nurse may worry that someone may identify her limitation and embarrass her in front of others or cause her to feel incompetent. In the extreme, she actually worries that a patient may be harmed by her not knowing.

Fear of being mistreated. A previous floating experience in which the float nurse seemed to be given the most difficult assignment or caseload may prevent a nurse from ever wanting to float again. Lack of appreciation shown to the float nurse applies here as well.

Fear of the unknown. In many instances the *unknown* is the staff on the other unit. If the nurse enjoys a warm, friendly, supportive relationship with her colleagues on her own unit, she may worry that the unknown staff will treat her badly or that she will spend her shift feeling isolated because she has no bonds with these staff and no one will reach out to help her feel welcome and appreciated.

Unfortunately, these fears and others that cause nurses reluctance to float are not unrealistic. To make floating acceptable and fair, anything that will build the relational bonds between nurses on different units will help. Since most organizations can't expect this to be accomplished between all units, they attempt it by identifying clusters of units or sister units. Within clusters, such as medical/surgical, critical care, or maternal/child, nurses develop relationships by working together on writing care standards, Q.I. activities, and other projects that provide an opportunity to bond. Floating is expected within the cluster, but nurses are not necessarily required to float outside the cluster. Many nurses report that knowing someone on the unit they are asked to float to makes a major difference in their feelings about floating.

Another practice related to fairness is the method used to determine which nurse will float. Whatever approach is used, it will be most effective when nurses are involved in determining the approach, guidelines are documented in writing to ensure clarity and understanding, and the policy is used consistently.

SA FINNIGAN

♦ **HOW DO I RESOLVE CONFLICTS WHEN ARRANGING FLOATING STAFF?**

Q One of the most challenging problems I have as a nurse manager is floating my staff to another unit when my staffing levels are barely adequate and my unit is harmed through the process of floating. I recognize that the other unit is more compromised than mine under the circumstances, but do two wrongs make a right? What do I do with this kind of conflict?

A This is tough. I would hope that you have a managers' forum in which all of the nurse man-

agers can discuss this. Although I agree with you that two wrongs do not make a right, it is essential to identify safe ways to care for all patients in the hospital. I believe there are better ways to resolve this than by spreading the misery (or shortage) around. I suggest that you work with your manager colleagues to make new decisions about floating.

Nurses should be used to staff their own units to appropriate levels first. Do not spread the shortage. If E3 has ten nurses scheduled and needs ten, they all stay on E3. If E3 has six scheduled and needs ten and the PRN pool has four and no other needs, E3 gets four. If three units need two PRN nurses each, then the staffing coordinator or nursing supervisor or managers need to discuss patient needs and distribute the PRN staff accordingly. If E4 is consistently understaffed, floating staff from otherwise well-staffed units is dysfunctional; E4's manager needs to work on a plan to recruit and retain staff.

In the interim, long-term agency contracts or pre-assigning of PRN pool personnel to a unit that is understaffed are preferable alternatives to shorting all units in the hospital. Many facilities do not want to use agency personnel; however, the long-term traveling nurse contract can be helpful in supporting a unit with problems while they looking for other alternatives. Last, think about evaluating what the patient population on the unit actually needs. It is possible that you can use some personnel to assist the staff with clerical work or to assist patients with activities of daily living (ADLs), thus helping to relieve the shortage. Work with staff on the unit to identify problems and solutions so that the unit becomes a more positive environment; this makes recruitment easier.

Extreme measures include limiting admissions on the unit with inadequate staffing. This is a very last-ditch and temporary effort because if continued, it starts the downward spiral of fewer patients, fewer staff. Some facilities expect all new nurse employees to work for some period in the difficult-to-staff work area, but this creates turnover problems on the unit that also lead to a downward spiral.

Temporary admission limits, with a work redesign program, team building, and staff involvement in problem solving and department design, have provided the best results in the settings I work with.

M PECK

◆ HOW DO I BUILD A STAFFING SYSTEM TO AVOID FLOATING?

Q Our nurse management leadership team has decided to stop floating from unit to unit and to make each unit responsible for the coverage of their own clinical needs. What are some of the fundamentals of building a unit-based staffing system that does not include floating between units?

A There is strong evidence to suggest that this is a worthwhile objective for several reasons. It logically follows that nurses working in a familiar environment and delivering care to patients in need of their particular expertise are going to deliver the best possible care. In addition, most nurses can relate to a dislike of floating and the awkward feelings that accompany practicing in a strange environment with limited expertise. This is not a simple issue to address, however, because your plan must ensure that your managerial accountability to see that care is delivered is fulfilled by having the right person in the right place at the right time.

This is not a decision to be made unilaterally by the management team. Enlist a group of clinical practitioners in the development of the plan at the outset. This will allow for developing consensus on your objective and thoroughly considering managerial and clinical perspectives in your planning. Issues that should be addressed in your planning follow:

- What are the patient census fluctuations in each area?
- How adequate is the coverage of patient care needs by the complement of current staff?
- Are there units that couldn't possibly meet their care needs independently? (A good example to consider is a CVICU that runs full at ten patients all week and typically drops to two on weekends. What happens during those rare periods when the census stays at ten all weekend?)
- What happens when a unit cannot address its care needs and another unit is slow?
- What are the expectations of staff, if any, beyond their scheduled hours in cases when demands for care in their unit exceed resources?

These sample questions should serve as a springboard for asking yourself every relevant question you can think of in the process of developing a plan for autonomous unit staffing. Leave no stone unturned in defining your process. The time to discover problems is not when the unit is full on Saturday night. There are hospitals that have successfully implemented plans such as this; thus it is unnecessary for you to totally reinvent the wheel. Seek them out and learn all you can from them to avoid making unnecessary mistakes. Finally, when you feel your plan is developed flawlessly, pilot it on selected units so you can learn about what you didn't anticipate in a controlled environment.

JE BEGLINGER

G

Goals

◆ WHAT ARE THE BASIC COMPONENTS OF GOAL SETTING?

Q What are the basic components of goal setting with the staff, and how do I get them more fully involved in planning for and setting goals?

A Goal setting and action planning follow unit vision and value determination. Goals are set to more effectively manage the unit's future and to determine in advance what is to be done.

There are three parts to the goal setting process:
1. *Goal development*—Goals are global statements of intended outcomes over a specific period of time (usually 2 to 3 years) that define how aspects of the unit's vision will be accomplished and the values supported.
2. *Objective preparation*—Objectives are targeted results that meet defined elements of the goals and address how much will be done during a 12-month period. Objectives are usually prepared in conjunction with the organization's fiscal or budget year because achieving objectives most often requires resources such as money, people, and time.
3. *Action planning*—Specific activities or steps are identified that will lead to achievement of objectives. These activities address process questions

such as who, what, where, and when. A lead person or group is also assigned for each activity or step.

Goal setting, objective preparation, and action planning are to be written, communicated, and updated on a regular basis. This written process needs to be comprehensive, covering all of the unit's products, programs, services, facilities, and resources that are affected in the defined time frame.

In addition, goal setting should be both flexible and action oriented. The nurse manager needs to be cognizant of the amount of work planned, the responsible individuals or groups, potential conflicting priorities, and overlap or duplication in roles. Involving staff in this goal setting process is a good "reality and equity" check for the nurse manager, because staff often perceive work load and role responsibilities differently than their manager does.

Other opportunities for effective and necessary utilization of staff input into the goal setting process include when space will be allocated or reallocated; construction or remodeling will occur; equipment, technology, or supplies are to be added or deleted; systems are to be modified; work methods are to be redesigned or restructured; roles or jobs are proposed to be redefined; interdepartmental or interdisciplinary relationships will change; accreditation or regulatory requirements are affected in any way; and organizational or unit standards, policies, or procedures need development, review, or revision.

BV TEBBITT

◆ HOW DO I KEEP A GROUP FOCUSED ON RECOMMENDED CHANGES?

Q After a group has agreed to a concept or a plan, how do I keep them focused and not allow them to go off in so many directions?

A When a nurse manager launches a project or plan, the degree of constancy in the performance of the group is directly proportional to the clarity of the vision and specificity of the plan of implementation. Communication before, during, and after the plan is launched is the key to a successful outcome.

Some plans call for close adherence to the script, with only one acceptable outcome. In such a situation, clearly defined goals and objectives along with a well-developed time line are essential. Establishing a steering committee to oversee the project and requesting that participants provide quarterly reports on their progress regarding specific objectives is an effective way to keep people on track. Communication tools and systems that reflect the progress of the group back to the larger organization are another way to celebrate small successes and keep people's work highly visible. This also is an incentive to participants to maintain diligence in their efforts.

Other plans require more innovation and immediate response to issues that arise when a new idea is being formed and normalized. Here the individuals are given guiding principles that must be adhered to, but the actual method of meeting the goals and objectives can be numerous and diverse. In this time of unprecedented change, such a style of leadership and program development often creates solutions and outcomes that far exceed those of any individual. Standardization of outcome rather than process is increasingly popular as a method for innovation and change.

Any seasoned nurse manager knows of the opportunities and frustrations inherent in leading groups of individuals through changing times. An axiom that is essential to the health and well-being of contemporary leaders is to "maintain the vision but embrace the hybrid." With such an attitude and expectation, managers can inspire and lead others to pool their collective wisdom to accomplish more than any single idea or entity could. Group IQ is greater than that of the individual. Thus innovation and change that allow for some variance within clearly defined parameters and principles are best suited to this era of leadership.

J KOERNER

◆ HOW CAN I HELP NURSES AND NONNURSES UNDERSTAND EACH OTHER'S GOALS?

Q What is the best way to translate organizational goals to nurses and nursing goals to nonnurses? I often find that the conflicts we have are due to misunderstanding of each other's goals.

A Some hospitals seem to function like two competing organizations—one for nurses and one for nonnurses, whereas other hospitals run like one winning team. In nonunified hospitals, competition and conflict seem to permeate every interaction, but in others, cooperation and collaboration rule. One reason for this difference is that people who work in team hospitals are clear about the direction they are headed in and that they are going together. These hospitals have effectively aligned the goals of members with those of the hospital and frequently translate those goals into action for their different professional groups on all organizational levels.

Goals are easy to lose in the crunch of daily operations, but successful managers cultivate two mandatory managerial perspectives that ultimately benefit the organization. The first perspective, the long view, recognizes that what is done today determines where the organization will be in the future. The effective manager is mindful of the goals of the organization and keeps them in front of everyone who may potentially contribute to their attainment. The other essential view is how seemingly unconnected goals of different hospital groups must come together to maintain the organization's viability. Many professional goals wouldn't have a life without the organization. Effective managers carry this important message to their teams.

By promoting the following goal-oriented activities, you can translate nursing goals to nonnurses, and relay nonnursing goals to nurses:

1. As a manager, you must become an expert in both sets of goals.
2. Invite the participation of nonnursing personnel in the formulation of nursing goals, and vice versa.
3. Recognize and accept conflict between different groups' goals, but encourage discussion and search for middle ground. Remember that disagreement can be stimulating.
4. Promote nursing and nonnursing goals in everyday activities; make them a part of your conversation. Encourage nurses to talk about nursing goals among themselves so they can articulate them to others.
5. Encourage the discussion of goals between collaborative groups during multidisciplinary rounds.
6. Make a review of progress toward goal attainment a standing agenda item at unit staff meetings.

7. Formally communicate goals in writing to the staff and incorporate them in individual performance appraisals.
8. Connect organizational goals to your quality improvement program.
9. Periodically meet with key physicians and other essential health care professionals (e.g., respiratory, social services, dietary) to clarify each other's goals and mutual concerns.

RG HESS

G

♦ **HOW CAN I CONVINCE ADMINISTRATORS OF THE NEED FOR PROJECT EVALUATION?**

Q What are some recommendations regarding how to handle administrators who don't want to evaluate project and program outcomes?

A Nothing succeeds like success.

1. Hand-pick a program that is valued by administration.
2. Set specific, simple project or program goals with completion dates.
3. Make sure measurement criteria are clear and specific.
4. Be careful to keep them short—no more than 3 to 5 per project or program.
5. Circulate them to administrators.
6. Measure goal accomplishment at 30-day intervals and circulate the summary to each administrator. If a date is missed on a goal or outcome, footnote it with an explanation.

Chances are the feedback will be positive from those above as well as the staff involved in the project. Each person will know where the project stands. This should provide a template for future endeavors.

If it does not, offer to formulate goals and measurements for any projects you are involved with. Be sure to send copies of summaries to your boss and her boss to keep the notion of evaluation alive.

JM McMAHON

Grievances

◆ WHAT ARE THE STAGES OF A STAFF-BASED GRIEVANCE PROCESS?

Q What should be the appropriate stages of a legitimate staff-based grievance process, and how and when should it be used?

A The process of filing and responding to a staff member's grievance will to some degree be dictated by institutional policy and also whether your organization is unionized. In addition, the variety of situations that may create a grievance precludes an absolute standardized approach. Although the number of steps in the grievance process, who responds, and how grievance hearings are conducted are affected by the aforementioned factors, the basic elements should be the same in any organization.

The first step in the grievance process should be responding to the informal grievance. Most grievances can and should be stopped in their tracks at this stage by an alert and sensitive manager. By effectively listening and giving fair and prompt consideration to issues raised, the supervisor may stop a simple concern from magnifying into a formal grievance. Involving staff members in resolving issues or concerns furthers their commitment to the outcome and is less likely to result in a grievance. Nevertheless, the informal concern or complaint stated as, "I have been wronged" or "I have been treated unfairly," must be understood as the first step in the grievance process and should be treated as such. Careful and rigorous documentation of the complaint and the supervisor's response must be made and continued throughout the grievance process.

Should the employee choose to upgrade the complaint into a formal grievance, the institution's grievance procedure or union contract should be carefully followed. Failure to follow the contract or policy and to adhere to time lines may affect any future ruling or arbitration hearing. Whether the organization is union or nonunionized, at this stage the employee is required to put her grievance in writing.

A grievance form should be made available to the employee ascertaining the specific grievance, circumstances surrounding the grievance and, of course, what corrective actions are being requested. Human resources should be consulted to facilitate this process for both the manager and the employee. The human resources department must be capable of objectively supporting the manager and the employee at this stage. In a unionized organization the employee may request a union steward to assist her in preparing the grievance and to be with her in all matters pertaining to the grievance. Although the contract should be consulted, this is generally accepted.

The employee grievance is heard with both sides—management and the employee—presenting their cases. Witnesses, documentation of support and, in general, *any* factual information may be used in responses by either party. The appointed grievance officer in unionized organizations or the manager's supervisor in nonunionized organizations hears the grievance with all arguments and supporting information from both sides and after a defined time period, usually several days, rules on the grievance.

In the event the employee does not agree with an unfavorable ruling, she may choose to elevate the grievance to what is considered Step II. The Step II process simply carries the grievance to a higher level in the organization. The process of hearing the grievance is essentially the same. However, many organizations, including unionized organizations, will go the extra yard to remove anyone with the slightest hint of being biased from the decision-making process. Only those who can truly see both sides of the issue will be involved in an attempt to ensure a completely fair hearing.

In most organizations the ruling made in Step II is considered final. Some nonunionized organizations may allow an appeal to the CEO and, of course, in unionized organizations, depending on the issue, the union contract may allow the grievance to be arbitrated.

As noted earlier, in an organization in which management is sensitive, knowledgeable, and skilled in handling conflict, most issues should be resolved before the formal initiation of a grievance. However, employees may sometimes disagree with a management decision or organizational policy or may perceive that they have been unfairly treated. When this is the case, employees should be encouraged and supported to use the grievance process.

All too often management interprets an employee's initiation of a grievance as negative. Legitimate grievances should be an opportunity for the employee to challenge management's position and for objective dialogue and evaluation of an action or a position. When the integrity of grievance procedures is maintained, employees will perceive a fair and just work environment.

GA ADAMS

◆ CAN USE OF THE GRIEVANCE PROCESS BE OVERWORKED?

Q I have noticed that staff often use grievances indiscriminately when they have difficulty accepting a decision. In a union hospital such as ours, when is the use of the grievance process legitimate and when is it not?

A Access to and utilization of the grievance process is a defined benefit and right of any employee who is represented by a collective bargaining agreement. The union has an obligation to provide assistance and representation under the collective bargaining agreement, and under a legal statute called the "Duty of Fair Representation." Any grievance that is filed, therefore, is "legitimate," at least relative to the employee's right to file the grievance.

However, staff filing grievances when there have not been any violations of the collective bargaining agreement, but simply because they are unhappy with decisions, does require action on your part. Staff who do not feel empowered or feel that they do not have control over their daily work life will, like many of us, try to find control however they can. In this instance, they seek control by filing grievances.

You should first gather information from your staff to determine areas of dissatisfaction, then engage your staff in discussions about strategies or models to address their concerns. Staff can sometimes request more "control" but do not understand or desire the accompanying accountability. It's important in your discussions that both areas be addressed.

I would suggest that you also engage the union in discussions regarding your concerns about the number of grievances as well as your commitment to improve staff satisfaction. Invite the union to participate in both identifying the core problems and helping to find solutions. Development of a collaborative and

interactive working relationship between management and collective bargaining requires a paradigm shift by both parties. However, the benefits can be significant.

C ST CHARLES

◆ WHAT SHOULD I DO IF A NURSE INITIATES THE GRIEVANCE PROCESS ALMOST EVERY TIME A DECISION AFFECTS HER?

Q There is a nurse on our unit who files a grievance at every opportunity she gets. Whenever a manager gives her some direction, she simply files a grievance if she doesn't agree. As a manager, how can I handle this problem?

A First, discuss this with the nurse and offer other methods of communication and problem solving. If this doesn't work, seek help from your human resources director. It is inappropriate to continuously file grievances, but perhaps your response is not appropriate either. Human resources policies and procedures define grievances and their use. The human resources director should know how this would be best managed in your organization.

D SHERIDAN

Health Care Reform

◆ HOW CAN I PREPARE FOR HEALTH CARE REFORM?

Q What operational approaches should we be moving toward in order to meet the challenges of health care reform?

A In the evolving health care reform movement, nothing will be as certain as change. The nurse manager will play a key role in creating the necessary environment for change to occur and the stability to

H

manage it. Expected health care reforms are still relatively unstructured and continue to provide opportunities for a good deal of flexibility. One constant in all of the uncertainty is that some form of managed care will provide the basis for the models that emerge. This is largely due to the fact that economics is the driving force behind the current reform initiatives.

Trying to sort through all the information on work and systems redesign can be intimidating—even paralyzing. In planning effective operational approaches, looking at some of the key principles related to successful managed care can help focus your efforts.

1. Practitioners can no longer be separated from the financial aspects of patient care. Information regarding the costs must be made available to those who make decisions about patient care. Financial departments need to work with providers to present information in redesigned formats better suited to service line analysis rather than traditional cost-centered information.

2. All health related choices have a price whether the choice is made by the care provider or the patient. The greater the freedom of choice, the higher the cost to the individual or organization. Resources need to be focused on delivering care at the most appropriate, least intense level. Look for mechanisms (such as critical paths and other formats that look at common characteristics of care) to lend consistency to approaches.

3. Hospital care will be avoided; early primary care intervention and ongoing prevention and maintenance will be encouraged. Therefore the census will continue to decrease in acute care hospitals, and demands for practitioners will shift to the community. Assess what additional educational needs will be necessary to move practitioners from acute care settings into the community. Identify who is likely to continue to be admitted and at what point in the continuum, then develop cost-effective approaches for these patients.

4. Payors will select providers (institutions and clinicians) based on efficiency of performance. Unnecessary steps, which add to cost and prolong service time, need to be systematically searched for and eliminated. Look for outcome measures that can be used to indicate success to payors and patients.

5. Departmental segmentation, so traditional in hospitals, adds complexity and cost. New models of care need to be collaborative and multidisci-

plinary and must eliminate duplication of service. Regulatory bodies (such as the Joint Commission) will facilitate this move through the format of their requirements. Look for ways to focus efforts on meeting both cost containment strategies and regulatory requirements.

6. The public needs education about health care in order to be an effective participant. Look for programs in your organization and the community that currently exist to educate the community. With additional effort, information relating to current health care economics and reform may be added to these offerings. Expectations and priorities of patients and families need to be weighed in relation to available resources.

To achieve the level of cost savings necessary and provide quality care that achieves reasonable outcomes that are meaningful to patients, payors, and providers is a challenge of considerable magnitude. This is especially true if our point of focus is limited to past approaches. Share information, data, statistics, successes, and failures with staff and other managers. Connect learning with successful and unsuccessful outcomes so that risk taking is supported. All professional disciplines have their sacred cows. They need to be examined carefully and retired after long years of use.

B FOSTER

Human Relations

◆ HOW CAN I MEND THE HURT MY THOUGHTLESS COMMENTS CAUSED?

Q During a heated discussion with a staff member, I made some comments I now regret. How can I approach this staff member to maintain our relationship and deal with the comments that I shouldn't have made?

A Unless there are some truly overriding reasons not to do so—and these reasons should not include personal prejudices or personality differences—you should apologize for the "inappropriateness" of your remarks. Before you do this, however, carefully think through what provoked your thoughtless comments and determine how best you can convert this negative into a positive experience. Don't forget the laws of God, nature, and physics: for every negative, there's a positive, and vice versa.

Be honest and forthright and contrite with the aggrieved staff member and express your regrets as soon as possible (don't let the incident fester). Frequently, an unpretentious apology, followed then or as soon thereafter as appropriate by a small, sincere compliment, should reduce the incident's negative impact if not eliminate it entirely. The compliment can be about something genuinely positive that the staff member has done or may be considering, or about something completely unrelated to the job.

The idea is to earn and keep your colleague's professional and personal respect by demonstrating a sincere interest in her as a person. If you haven't already done so, this is a practice you should develop and follow automatically, regardless of circumstantial need.

GA ADAMS

◆ SHOULD I HELP AN EMPLOYEE SOLVE PERSONAL PROBLEMS?

Q What is my responsibility as a nurse manager toward my employees in solving their personal problems?

A Staff can have complex personal problems that compromise their productivity at work. In fact, "workforce 2000" is forecasted to challenge managers to an ever greater extent as societal changes affect the traditional work ethic within this country.

Most managers do not have the educational background in counseling, nor do they have the time to devote to solving employees' personal problems. However, managers do have the right and accountability to monitor the productivity and performance of each employee. When that performance is not up to par, it is important for the manager to discuss this with the individual staff member. That discussion should include the following:

1. Clear examples of the performance behaviors and their consequences and effects on the work being performed. (It is helpful to link this with the job description, evaluation, job expectations.)

2. If the employee cites a personal problem as the reason for poor performance, listen but do not attempt to counsel.

3. Refer the individual to the employee assistance program (EAP) or related resources for further assistance in solving the personal issue.

4. Depending on the situation, assure the employee that you care and are willing to see her through this difficult period.

5. Outline the behaviors that will be monitored for improvement and make sure they are understood.

MT SINNEN

◆ IS THERE ROOM IN NURSING FOR THOSE WHO LIKE TO BE IN CONTROL AND MAKE DECISIONS?

Q Is there a place in nursing for people who need to be in control and who prefer making decisions themselves?

A Of course! There are many opportunities for individuals with different goals and styles to find a niche for themselves within the profession. The essential components of the nursing role demand a blending of dependent, interdependent, and independent role functions.

However, there is no place in nursing for individuals who are self-centered or seek isolation. The focus of nursing and nurses is collaboration and partnership with patients, colleagues, and others, and it requires a commitment to excellence and competence, and a willingness to be involved.

In the past, the emphasis on structure may not have allowed the diversity of thinking and acting that we strive for today. The richness of opportunity in nursing and health care allows individuals with different backgrounds, training, and goals to work together harmoniously in addressing the needs of the patient, managing complex programs and organizations, and advancing the profession of nursing.

With the emphasis on creating centers of excellence, it behooves the nursing profession to ensure that there are opportunities for creativity and innovation. It is hard to imagine that motivated and talented people who want to be in control of their own practice and prefer decision making themselves

H

would not find opportunities to influence the growth of the nursing profession.

AMT BROOKS

Incident Reports

◆ ARE INCIDENT REPORTS CONFIDENTIAL?

Q Are incident reports considered confidential information that cannot be accessed in court?

A Each hospital should have a written policy regarding incident reports. The policy should be developed with consultation from the hospital attorney or the attorney representing the insurance company. Laws regarding discoverability vary from state to state. In many cases, if the incident report is filed in an attorney or legal file with no copies made and distributed, the incident report is nondiscoverable. The incident report should be factual, avoiding any possibility for subjectivity.

The incident report should be completed by the person involved with the incident if at all possible. Although the incident report may be considered nondiscoverable, this does not mean the person involved in the incident or witnesses to the incident will not be subpoenaed for deposition or to testify in court.

SH SMITH

◆ ARE THERE WAYS TO MANAGE WORKERS WHO EXPERIENCE DIFFICULT PROBLEMS AT HOME?

Q What is the most effective way to manage a work force—particularly when many are single parents who must support and manage households—and encourage them to be motivated in the work setting and free from the troubles that they may be experiencing at home?

A In today's "learning organizations," management must recognize the importance of relationships. One of the relationships is that of work life and personal life. Part of your role as manager is to help facilitate a balance between the two. You can do this by becoming more flexible with your structures, less tied to policy and procedure, and more focused on goals and outcomes. It is no longer acceptable or appropriate to ask staff to leave their personal lives at home. As managers we must be sensitive to the holistic nature of our staff, just as we recognize the impact one aspect of life has on another in our patients. We must do the same with our staff.

For example, you may want to periodically ask individuals how things are going; is there anything you as manager could do with scheduling or work load that might help them? You might want to consider things like self-scheduling, flex scheduling, partnering, support groups, child care or elder care services, and diversionary activities. We have to begin thinking in new paradigms that are more responsive to the personal needs of our staff.

Explore with your staff the practices within the work environment that add to the stress of their lives, and then brainstorm ways of improving these practices. Remain open to new ideas. Try to find ways to make these new ideas work. As nurses, it is especially important that we learn to create a "caring environment" for our colleagues as well as our patients.

RM HADDON

Interviewing

◆ HOW SHOULD I PREPARE TO CONDUCT AN INTERVIEW?

Q What are the basic credential "check-offs" that I should begin to develop before interviewing a candidate for employment?

A First, review the job description of the position you need to fill. Does the description adequately describe the job to be done? If so, you should be able to identify the educational and experiential qualifications for the job in the description. Does the job description list any special skills needed for the position, such as dexterity with computers, monitors, or other equipment? Does the job description mention any special licensure (e.g., licensure as a registered nurse) or certification requirements (e.g., certified in advance life support)? These items are essential to any preinterview screening of a candidate and can readily be set forth in a checklist format.

If no job description exists for the position or if the job description is inadequate, then a new description should be developed. Managers should be able to describe the jobs that they are responsible for. Job descriptions should include the following requirements:

1. Education.
2. Licensure (certification or registration).
3. Experience.
4. Responsibilities and duties.
5. Reporting relationship.

Adequate descriptions of a job and related credentials and other requirements are requisite to candidate screening. Such descriptions can save time and energy, and eliminate frustration. Such descriptions ensure that the candidates who are interviewed meet the basic job qualifications.

LJ SHINN

♦ WHAT ARE GOOD QUESTIONS TO ASK DURING AN INTERVIEW?

Q I am interviewing candidates for staff nurse positions for a unit in the hospital. What are good general questions to ask? What are good questions to ask to decide whether a candidate would be a good staff nurse for a specific area?

A The following are general questions frequently asked during an interview:

Warm-up questions:

1. What made you apply for this position?
2. How did you hear about this job opening?
3. How would you summarize your work history and education?

Work history:

1. What special aspects of your work experience have prepared you for this job?

2. Can you describe one or two of the most important accomplishments in your career?
3. What kinds of supervision have you received in previous jobs?
4. What kinds of supervision have you used with your subordinates?
5. What kinds of supervision are best for the job you are seeking?
6. How would you describe one or two of the biggest disappointments in your career?
7. Why did you choose to pursue this career?
8. Why are you leaving your present job? (Or, why did you leave your last job?)
9. What kinds of co-workers do you like best? Why?
10. Of all the jobs you have had, which did you like best? Why?
11. What kind of an organization do you prefer to work for?
12. Where does this job fit in with your overall career plan?

Education and training:

1. What special aspects of your education or training have prepared you for this job?
2. How has your education or training helped you?
3. What courses in school have been most helpful to you in your job?
4. What areas would you most like additional training in if you got this job?

Career goals:

1. What kind of job do you see yourself holding 5 years from now?
2. Why do you feel that this is the best career path for you?
3. How will this job help you achieve your career goals?
4. What would you most like to accomplish if you got this job?
5. What might make you leave this job?

Job performance:

1. Everyone has job strengths and weaknesses. What do you feel are your strengths regarding this job?
2. What are some areas needing improvement?
3. When you become aware of a weakness in your performance, what do you typically do? Please give me an example.

Lateness and absenteeism:

1. How do you think problems of lateness should be handled?

2. How do you think problems of absenteeism should be handled?

The following questions relate to specific aspects of nursing practice:

Clinical practice:

1. Describe your clinical experience.
2. How do you feel about being a nurse? Why did you choose nursing as a career?
3. Why are you applying for this position?
4. Describe your nursing process in delivering care to a patient.
5. What do you feel are your strengths?
6. What are your long- and short-term goals?

Quality assurance:

1. To whom do you feel an obligation to assure quality?
2. Describe a method of quality assurance in which you have participated.

Shared governance:

1. Describe your experience with shared governance.
2. How do you lead others?
3. How do you view the role of the nurse manager?

Patient and guest relations:

1. Who are guests in your unit?
2. How do you approach guests in a patient care unit?
3. How can family members be incorporated in the plan of care?

Professional practice:

1. Describe your views of professional organizations in nursing.
2. How do health care team members interact to achieve optimal patient outcomes?
3. If you could change anything about nursing practice, what would you change?

K KERFOOT

♦ WHAT QUESTIONS DO I ASK IF I WANT TO FIND OUT ABOUT A PERSON'S ATTITUDE AND PERSONAL OUTLOOK?

Q It is often difficult to discern from an interview whether a prospective employee has the right "soft skills," such as attitude, energy, and personal skills to succeed in a job. What questions or assessment tools can I use to acquire this kind of information?

A Before any interview, you need to take a good look at the job description and list the skills and behaviors needed for the candidate to be successful. As you analyze the job, you will need to determine the kind of behavioral questions that will establish these characteristics in the applicants. Look over this list of "soft skills," and rank them in order from most to least important to you:

♦ Hardworking
♦ Good judgment
♦ Organized
♦ Team player
♦ Trustworthy
♦ Versatile
♦ Helpful
♦ Creative
♦ Diplomatic
♦ Willing to learn
♦ Flexible
♦ Independent

The best predictor of future behavior is past behavior. Formulate questions that will require the prospective employee to draw from performance in previous circumstances.

For example: the open position is in utilization review. You need an independent, detail-oriented, flexible employee. The director is very autocratic, and you want to make sure the applicant will fit. You might use the following questions: "Describe to me how you handled great census and work fluctuations in your last position in UR. Tell me about a time when you felt that if you had been able to accomplish the tasks in your own way, the outcome would have been better. What kinds of processes do you think staff nurses should be involved in to make your work more productive?"

Or, perhaps the open position is in the cath lab, and the physicians have been known to be demanding and unreasonable. You feel you need assertive, decisive, but tactful nurses to cope in this environment. You might ask, "Tell me about an incident you had with a physician when you would have approached the matter differently the next time. How did you convey this interaction to your supervisor?"

If you are hiring for a medical-surgical unit that has a history of communication problems on the night shift, you might be seeking a charge nurse who is a team player, enthusiastic, and forward-thinking. You could ask, "Your past experience as a staff nurse put you in charge occasionally. Tell me how you responded to an older nurse who challenged your ability."

Interviewing is not easy for a novice, but once you have established the questions needed for determining whether the applicant has the right skills, you will find it a challenge and most rewarding. Remember: the best predictor of future behavior is past behavior.

MA SORENSEN

♦ WHAT ARE KEY QUESTIONS TO ASK SO THAT I HIRE THE RIGHT PERSON?

Q As a nurse manager, I have the authority to hire personnel within the personnel department guidelines. I have two positions open but the last person I hired was the wrong nurse for the job and for my unit. What are some interviewing guidelines that I can use to help me fit the right person to the job and to the culture of my unit?

A Interviewing is the least scientific part of the selection process and often results in our wondering whether we have hired the right person for the right place. If you have experienced hiring the wrong person, you may want to reevaluate the knowledge, background, skills, and personalities of those nurses who have been successful on your unit to better understand what makes them successful. Having done that, it would be helpful to construct a somewhat structured interview process to help discern that the applicant has those needed skills and attributes.

Think of the interview as having four distinct parts, and know that each of those parts will lead to your making a better decision if executed well.

1. Develop mutual trust and goodwill. The quality of the interview really depends on your ability to do this. Using your own natural style, develop a few opening questions to welcome the candidate and make her feel at ease. You may choose to ask about her trip to your hospital, or the weather, or your city . . . just informal chatter to make her

comfortable. You may choose this time to offer a cup of coffee, a cold drink, or a tour of the unit.

2. Before the interview, you should review the application and have specific questions in mind regarding the applicant's demographics, past history, and career progress. Often, however, the first time a manager sees the application is when the recruiter escorts the applicant in, so you may have to improvise. Use this review time to give the applicant the time to "fit into your space" while you peruse the papers. This is a perfect time to continue the informal questioning of "What brings you to our city?," or "Tell me about your present position," or "Why are you looking for a change?" This may be a good time to question a long gap in employment or many career changes or frequent moves. If the trust has been established, this exchange can be invaluable to determine cultural fit as well as clinical fit. Most applicants want the opportunity to present themselves with integrity and forthrightness, and if this time is unrushed and open, you will both exchange much information.

3. The third step is one for which you must have prepared well in advance. Having reviewed the background of your successful employees, develop a series of open-ended, structured questions that you will use with every applicant to establish whether each has the knowledge, skills, and attitudes you have found to be successful on your unit. For example,

   ♦ "Describe a typical day in your present job." (attitude, skill level)
   ♦ "What do you like most about your job?" (focus)
   ♦ "What did you have the most trouble with?" (problem solving)
   ♦ "What kind of a manager do you like to work for?" (organizational match)
   ♦ "How does this job fit into your long-term career goals?" (goal oriented)
   ♦ "How have you handled this kind of a problem before . . . ?" (behavioral question)

   These questions will vary depending on the needs of your unit and the attributes most important for successful fit.

4. Last, closure needs to give both the applicant and you some time to determine whether this is the right position for the right person. Always invite the applicant to give some thought to the position and to call back with any further questions, and

reserve the opportunity for yourself to see all the other applicants before making a decision. *Never* say you just need to check references before making your decision, but do give applicants a time frame in which to expect a decision.

I would encourage involving the staff in the interview process. They have a unique sense of fit and may also "buy into" supporting your decision if they are involved in the interview and selection process.

MA SORENSEN

◆ WHAT ARE APPROPRIATE QUESTIONS TO ASK A CANDIDATE FOR A MANAGER OR DIRECTOR POSITION?

I

Q When I am interviewing candidates for a manager or director position in the hospital, what should I as a nursing manager focus on and what are appropriate questions for a nurse manager to ask the candidate?

A Nursing leadership positions will be key to the change process as hospitals move toward a more cross-functional empowered work force in the new century. Leadership behaviors directly influence job satisfaction, productivity, and employee turnover. Goals for today's nursing leaders must include effective communication, staff morale improvements, promoting interdisciplinary relations, and maintaining or reducing expenditures while continuously improving patient care (Meiglan, 1990). Questions that determine "organizational fit" include those that determine the candidate's unique characteristics such as values, temperament, conflict resolution approaches, and decision-making style.

It is acceptable to question the candidate about previous management experiences in past positions. What were these experiences? Did they include fiscal responsibility? Question specific ways that budgets were managed, including cost savings programs that were implemented. With the emphasis on professional practice models of nursing today, ask the candidate if she either implemented or worked in a professional nurse practice model. If so, what were the successes, barriers, and outcomes? Glean other questions from the job description as appropriate, and ask for specific examples of how each job requirement would be fulfilled.

It is helpful to define questions before the interview to be used primarily as guidelines. Try to avoid rigidity and allow a free flow of conversation; valuable information often can be gained informally and outside of the predetermined questions. Leadership ability may be perceived differently. Generally, nursing staff seek a leader who is more knowledgeable, competent, experienced, and confident than they are. They expect a leader to be effective without being pushy, unreasonably demanding, or forceful (Meiglan, 1990). Asking a candidate situational questions may assist in identifying leadership potential as well as the candidate's leadership style and ability to make a positive impact and a "good fit" in the new position.

J TORNABENI

◆ WHAT QUESTIONS SHOULD A RECRUITER ASK?

Q What questions do personnel and recruitment people have a right to ask prospective staff who are being interviewed for employment?

A Employment law is constantly changing. Nurse managers need to be familiar with federal, state, and local employment law. Corporate counsel and human resource professionals are invaluable in helping managers to become knowledgeable about the law and the do's and don'ts of candidate interviews. In addition, the nurse manager should be familiar with the provisions of collective bargaining agreements that relate to positions within the manager's jurisdiction. Be sure you know the job description (be certain you have one) for the position you are to fill. A description that sets forth the qualifications for and responsibilities of the job will make interviewing much easier.

Do not ask:
1. Questions related to age, race, creed, color, religion, or national origin.
2. Questions regarding marital status or plans to marry or have children.
3. Questions related to child care.
4. Questions related to a spouse.

It is permissible to ask about the citizenship and visa status of the applicant (if the person is not a US citizen). Federal law states that employers must have proof of citizenship status for all employees.

There is much confusion subsequent to the passage of the Americans with Disabilities Act about what questions can be asked related to handicapping conditions. The safest ground is to ask questions related to the job, that is, you can describe the job to be done and ask the candidate if she can do the job.

Prepare a list of questions before the interview. Have the human resources department review them. Sequence the questions from simple to complex. This puts the candidate at ease, builds trust, and gets the interviewer in a listening mode. Do listen—listen for the clues the applicant gives about the job. Ask about:

1. Relevant job experiences.
2. Communication skills.
3. Professional goals.
4. Skill sets—computers, statistics, fluency in a foreign language.
5. Likes and dislikes.

Finally, be observant. Body language can tell you a lot. For example, does the applicant maintain eye contact with you or look at the ceiling, floor, or out the window? Ask questions that do not lead to automatic answers. Don't ask "How do you get along with people?" Do ask "Describe your working relationship with your manager or team members at the Metropolitan Nursing Center."

LJ SHINN

◆ WHAT QUESTIONS MAY I ASK OF CANDIDATES' REFERENCES?

Q I need to check references on potential candidates for our nursing staff. What questions do I have a right to ask, and how should I ask them?

A The reference check is a strategy managers can use to confirm (or dispel) observations made during candidate interviews. Although a manager can ask almost any question she wants, the litigious nature of employment today means previous employers are likely to give out minimal information. In fact, many employers refer all requests for reference to a centralized department such as human resources. The human resources department may only verify employment dates and salary history.

To make the most of a reference check, prepare a list of questions. This will save time for both of you.

A predetermined list of questions will ensure that the reference check is systematic and comprehensive. Questions will come from candidate interviews, job descriptions, and your knowledge about what it takes to do the job to be filled.

When checking a reference, do the following:

1. Be sure the person has time to talk with you. Consider scheduling an appointment to talk. (This strategy can backfire and result in no information, because the person has time to contemplate the interview.)
2. Tell the person who you are, the health care facility you represent, and the purpose of the call.
3. Listen carefully—to what *is* said and what is *not* said.
4. State what you have observed while interviewing the candidate and ask if that matches the person's own observation. (You may want to share negative observations as well as positive ones.)
5. Ask how long the person has known the applicant and in what capacity and if the person would hire the candidate again.
6. Give the person a chance to offer additional observations when you have concluded your questions.
7. Give the person your phone number and encourage a call back if she thinks of other information to share with you.
8. Get to the point. Describe the job and ask open-ended questions. Such questions are less threatening and do not tend to lead the person to a specific answer.

Typically candidates will give you the names of persons they believe are most likely to give good references. Ask for the names of former colleagues, subordinates, or bosses. Then call people not on the candidate's reference list. Ask the candidate for copies of past performance appraisals or personnel files. Ask for copies of presentations given or articles written. All of these documents will help in determining if the candidate is right for the position.

Be sure to know your organization's policy related to reference checking. (Some organizations centralize the process.) Failure to check references can be disastrous. Reference checks should be documented and kept in personnel files if a candidate is hired. A reference checklist might be used, but it is also important to have space to take notes and record observations and information.

LJ SHINN

J

◆ WHAT QUESTIONS SHOULD BE ASKED AT THE EXIT INTERVIEW?

Q Whenever staff resign from our facility, we routinely conduct an exit interview. What are some of the most important questions we should ask during an exit interview?

A I firmly believe that exit interviews work best to retrieve information regarding the work environment if the employee is leaving due to job change or relocation. When an employee is leaving due to work dissatisfaction, an exit interview is obviously too late to save the employee–employer relationship. If the employee has complaints about X, Y, and Z, why were they not addressed during employment? Where was management? During an exit interview may be a difficult time to ascertain why the employee is leaving, especially if it is due to work dissatisfaction. An individual may take the attitude, "I'm not going to help you out." Also the employee may hold back negative information because she may fear that a poor employee recommendation may be given to future employers.

If exit interviews are conducted on all employees, then the following questions may elicit valuable information:

1. What kinds of changes would keep you employed here?
2. If we could go back to when you were employed here, what was the turning point to make you consider a job change?
3. Please identify two exceptional work practice conditions.
4. Please identify two unsatisfactory work practice conditions.

LG VONFROLIO

JCAHO

◆ HOW CAN I COPE WITH CHANGING REGULATIONS?

Q It seems the more change occurs, the more regulations emerge. I feel deluged with changing state, federal, and Joint Commission on Accreditation of Healthcare Organizations (JCAHO) regulations. How do I deal with all of the new regulations?

A To avoid the frantic activity just before a JCAHO survey and to be prepared for a possible unannounced survey by JCAHO or your state, set up a system to continually update your policies and practices.

1. Appoint a person or committee to review new regulations and recommend changes. This may be your quality improvement nurse or your nursing quality improvement council or committee.
2. Have recommendations, usually in the form of suggested policy drafts or revisions, on the agenda for review by your management team or shared governance nursing council.
3. Make changes a part of your daily operational systems, and incorporate regulatory demands as they arise.

D SHERIDAN

◆ ARE NURSES INVOLVED IN DEVELOPING JCAHO CRITERIA?

Q Are nurses involved in development of JCAHO criteria? If so, why do the criteria appear so medically dominated?

A Nursing has always been involved in writing the nursing criteria for JCAHO, but only recently has nursing been invited to participate on the JCAHO board to review JCAHO criteria for patient care. The JCAHO criteria are not necessarily "medically dominated." A medical reviewer is a member of the review team, but the team also includes a nursing reviewer and a hospital administrator. The medical and nursing team members review the administration and clinical practice of their respective professions for compliance to JCAHO's standards. The JCAHO team reviews patient care within multiple departments in the hospital setting for compliance with predetermined standards for each department.

There has been some concern voiced that JCAHO has not kept abreast of recent changes related to the administration of nursing service. JCAHO criteria have not reflected the organizational changes often seen in shared governance systems or in decentralized departments in which the nurse executive is the director or vice president of the division, reporting to the chief operating officer or chief executive officer. In the latter example, there may be multiple nurse executives rather than one chief nursing officer as required by JCAHO.

JF STICHLER

◆ HOW DOES JCAHO'S "QUALITY FROM THE TOP DOWN" STANDARD AFFECT QUALITY COORDINATORS?

Q How have the new JCAHO standards dictating "quality from the top down" affected the positions of quality coordinators?

A JCAHO has indeed changed its focus, to include not only the assurance of clinical practitioner quality but also quality organizational performance. This change stems from the belief that even the most effective quality assurance program can be limited by a lack of top administrative support and system or organizational barriers to change.

If you are a quality assurance coordinator, you must be feeling the stress of transition from quality assurance to quality improvement. Indeed, your role is in transition along with your organization! The chart below outlines the key elements of each system that will require your leadership to become integrated within a new quality program:

Professional Quality Assurance	Quality Improvement
Individual responsibilities	Collective responsibility
Practice expectations and standards	Organizational process and performance standards
Professional practitioner leaders	Manager leaders
Autonomy	Partnership
Administrative and professional authority	Full organizational member participation
Response to complaints	Benchmarks

The opportunities for individuals working in quality programs have increased in number and in significance. Problems may arise in the knowledge, skills, and preparation of the quality coordinator relative to new role demands. In the past, successful quality coordinators came to the position with a solid record of quality performance and good interpersonal skills.

They had or developed a working knowledge of professional practice standards and the 10-step process. Today, the knowledge and skill demands have multiplied. For example, skillful work with very diverse groups has intensified the interpersonal component of the role. Today's quality coordinators are expected to understand and apply the methodologies used to track organizational performance, as well as more sophisticated evaluation models. In addition, you must have a strong foundation in systems theory and concepts of organizational performance. Competence in computer applications is also important.

These new role demands require, for most individuals, intensive continuing education or a return to school for advanced preparation. Indeed, there are schools of nursing considering offering advanced degrees in quality assessment. The next several years will be challenging for you as the quality coordinator. You will be counted on to lead the organization into greater sophistication in its quality assessment and to facilitate needed systems changes.

The quality coordinator is indeed a role in transition. Role requirements will continue to expand as health care organizations evolve their systems in response to quality demands. It is probably time to pursue your professional obligation to continuing education.

CK WILSON

◆ DO JCAHO STANDARDS APPLY TO AMBULATORY AND INFIRMARY HEALTH CARE?

Q Do the continuous quality improvement (CQI) standards of JCAHO apply to ambulatory and infirmary health care?

A The current JCAHO standards apply to hospital-sponsored ambulatory care, which means freestanding medical office buildings, surgi-centers, infirmaries, and urgent care settings are not currently covered. If, however, your organization operates a same-day surgery center in the hospital setting, then there is a chapter in the acute care hospital standards that applies, as do all other chapters. As to CQI, the Joint Commission has indicated that they will not make CQI techniques a mandatory part of their requirements, but it is evident from the changes in the quality standards that many of the theoretic concepts central to CQI are embedded throughout the JCAHO standards. For example, multidisciplinary and inter-disciplinary teams to do monitoring and evaluation, use of aspects of care (the prospective focus), 1 year or more of comparative data (continuous improvement), and change to functional chapters (focus on organizational systems, not departments) are all reflections of CQI values. Whether or not the total CQI methodology is adopted by JCAHO, the techniques and tools for quality improvement are ones that will be useful for you to obtain.

MC ALDERMAN

♦ **WHAT IS JCAHO'S POSITION ON NURSING CARE PLANS USED IN DOCUMENTATION?**

Q Please help me with clarifying JCAHO's position on the nursing care plan in nursing documentation.

A I have selected key statements for you from *An Introduction to Joint Commission Nursing Care Standards* (1991), pp. 29 to 31.

1. Do the new standards require a "care plan"? What is the difference between a "patient care plan" and a "plan of care"?
Answer: Technically, the new nursing care standards do not require a separate document called a "care plan," unless there is some other regulation, state requirement, or hospital policy that requires such a document. However, nursing care interventions must be planned. This planning is usually documented in the patient's medical record by the conclusion(s) stated at the end of the nursing admission assessment process and the selection of a standard of care or the designation of nursing diagnoses and the interventions that will be used to meet the patient's defined nursing care needs, and by subsequent revisions as required by hospital policy and warranted by the patient's condition.

There is relatively little difference between a "patient care plan" and a "plan of care." The key is that such plans need not necessarily be in a separate document—whether called the nursing care plan or the plan of care—as long as the planning is evidenced in the patient's medical record.

2. How do the new standards affect the use of multidisciplinary treatment plans?

Answer: The standards do not affect the hospital's choice to use a multidisciplinary treatment plan. Again, the hospital determines whether it will use such care-planning processes and how they will be documented. The standards focus on what must appear (referenced either directly or indirectly) in each patient's medical record.

3. May licensed practical/vocational nurses participate in the care-planning process with or under the supervision of an RN?
Answer: Licensed practical/vocational nurses may participate in the care-planning process, as well as the nursing admission assessment process, to the degree permitted by applicable state law, nurse practice acts, and hospital policy.

K ZANDER

Job Descriptions

♦ **WHAT IS BASIC CONTENT FOR A JOB DESCRIPTION?**

Q We are considering rewriting our job descriptions. What should be the basic content included in all job descriptions?

A Each institution has its own format for the finished product, but there are several commonalities to be found in all job descriptions.
1. Statement of purpose or job summary. Why does this job exist, and what key functions does the employee do that are not performed by others in the organization? What are the interrelationships, and how will the described job be affected by the positions above and below it? Will there be common functions between this job and others?
2. Time frames. The normal amount of time in which the employees could be expected to perform this function, either by hour, shift, day, or week. This can be important when determining if this can be a part-time, full-time, or shared position.
3. Status. Is this job considered a management or exempt position in which the employee fulfills the requirement of the job within broad time frames using her own judgment, or an hourly

position in which the employee has no choice of hours and times worked?

4. Titles. The title chosen should reflect a relationship to others within the organization at comparative levels so that there is a uniform understanding.

5. Education required to perform role and functions. The minimum educational level should be spelled out with qualifications, for example, a minimum of a bachelor's degree or completion of degree within 1 year of accepting the position. Credentials and/or certifications required for hire or within a certain time after employment should also be spelled out.

6. Experience. The amount of experience required or basic aptitude should be noted. If experience will be accepted in lieu of advanced education, this should also be stated. Essential experience in a particular clinical area should be listed.

7. Personal aptitudes. If the job requires collaboration, communication, and negotiation skills beyond those expected of all employees, these can be specifically spelled out. In addition, if the position requires business writing skills and public speaking, these should be noted, for example, formal teaching sessions for patients, families, and community, or perhaps marketing and public relations.

8. Evaluation criteria. Most job descriptions today are being written so that the evaluation criteria either are the identical statements found describing the work or are easily obtainable from the content.

9. Job duties. All functions that the employee must perform are listed under this heading. In the current atmosphere of increased productivity, job descriptions are most currently reviewed when jobs are being redesigned, therefore the following questions need to be asked at the beginning of all job description review and redesign:
    ♦ What is the employee to do that is not or cannot be done by someone filling an existing job description?
    ♦ Why do you need this new position, or why are you writing in new functions?
    ♦ Will productivity and/or costs increase or decrease, and will problems be resolved or created?
    ♦ What is being done in terms of functions at the level above and below this position?

♦ Will those jobs need revision if you alter or create a new position?

10. Essential functions. With the introduction of the Americans with Disabilities Act in 1991 there has been a great emphasis on determining the "essential functions" of a job that an employee can perform with or without reasonable accommodations. To establish a job function as essential, certain requirements must be met. Because the guidelines for compliance with this act are still evolving, guidance from the human resources department must be obtained before the job descriptions are complete to avoid discrimination complaints.

S LENKMAN

♦ HOW DO I ESTABLISH OUTCOME-ORIENTED JOB DESCRIPTIONS?

Q We want to establish outcome-oriented position descriptions that define accountabilities rather than functional responsibilities. How should we begin to approach this task? Do they make any difference?

A Yes, there is a difference. The purpose of the job description is to establish a contract between the employer and the employee. The contract should outline duties, responsibilities, and reporting relationships so that a fair and equitable distribution of the work to be done can be maintained. The position description serves as the foundation for designing a system that provides a measure of performance of the worker and includes safeguards for quality patient care. Not all tasks can be identified in a position description; therefore functional models that focus on task responsibilities are inadequate.

Outcome-oriented descriptions place the duty to perform professional nursing practice in a position that authorizes as well as obliges the staff member to examine the entire context in which care is delivered and perform at a higher level. In today's environment, which includes multidisciplinary workers, it is essential to have clear and public lines of accountability.

You can approach this task by identifying a staff nurse group to design the position description. They

J

are the experts who can best describe what is expected behavior at the staff nurse level. They should review the literature for articles related to job descriptions and performance evaluation and select those elements that best fit your organization. Once a draft or a position description has been developed, it should be circulated to the staff for comments and modifications. After revisions have been made, a period of pilot testing should be established to further refine the description and process.

CE LOVERIDGE

♦ **HOW CAN I HELP STAFF REDESIGN JOB DESCRIPTIONS FAIRLY?**

Q My staff want to redesign their job descriptions to better identify their roles and accountability. I am happy that they are interested, but as their manager, I am concerned that they will fail to address some of the accountabilities essential to their role and protect the interests of the organization. How can I make sure that doesn't happen without appearing to limit or direct their activities?

A It is always encouraging when the nursing staff want to take an active role in the revision of their job descriptions. This is an indication that they are accepting more accountability for the quality of care and nursing performance in the organization. Most of the time, nurses will be very critical and include high performance expectations for each level of clinical nursing practice, but as a manager you can provide direction to them. You may want to consider the development of the job descriptions as a shared responsibility and work with them in the revision and development of the new job descriptions. Take this opportunity to assist them in identifying performance criteria that every nurse should integrate into professional practice. By working with the staff in the revision of the job description, you will have an opportunity to develop shared expectations for performance and develop a greater sense of collaboration with the staff.

This will be a good opportunity to introduce the concept of performance-based job descriptions, which will weight specific performance standards ac-

cording to the importance that staff and/or management wants to emphasize for professional growth or improvement. If a system for shared governance has been established in the nursing organization, one of the councils may provide the direction to the revision and development of the job description with the draft copy ratified by a coordinating and/or executive council.

If you are not directly involved in the revision process, list the behaviors that you believe should be included and share them with your staff. This will clarify your expectations for them and help them to be successful in their task.

JF STICHLER

Knowledge Workers

♦ **HOW CAN I HELP IMPROVE MY STAFF'S PERCEPTION OF THEMSELVES AS KNOWLEDGE WORKERS?**

Q What can I do to help my staff see themselves as knowledge workers who need to think critically and continually evaluate and improve their practice?

A Seeing nurses as knowledge workers is not as difficult as assisting them to see themselves that way. Some people in the nursing profession go so far as to say that nurses really are not knowledge workers and that we should stop acting as though they are. I believe that the perception of whether they are knowledge workers has less to do with their educational preparation than with how they are utilized in the practice arena.

For many nurses, there has been a long-term focus on functional proficiency and technical expertise. This commitment to the mechanical has been facilitated by the models of care available in most institutions that permitted that pattern to be maintained and have even facilitated it at times. Supporting this has been the heavy focus on mechanics by physicians and administrators who saw the role of the nurse as a doer rather than a thinker. It has never been the belief of the profession of nursing or in the hearts of most nurses that this perception was accurate or even appropriate.

As the health care system changes, increasingly there will be a stronger need for the thinking and doing part of the nurse's role to work in concert. As patients move from inpatient bedbound care to broader more community-based, noninstitution, and home-related care models, nurses will move to address those care issues. Nurses will have to exhibit independent judgment, work with a variety of health professionals, manage an increasingly complex array of health variables, and do much more support and advocacy than what has been done to date.

The nurse manager getting ready for this transition should prepare staff for this kind of health care milieu. The nurse will have increasingly less supervision of her work. She will work more interdependently than in the past. The nurse will have to constantly and confidently exercise her good judgment and link her decisions with those of other professionals in separate disciplines. Some initial steps in this process are the following:

1. Make sure nurses are familiar with the changes occurring in health care that are demanding a change in role, location, and behavior. Information about changing expectations and expanding roles will facilitate nurses' response to newer expectations.

2. Create a work milieu that supports increasing independence and provides expectation for more involvement in decisions that affect what nurses do. Continue to "push" the staff into those issues that they find most challenging and are afraid of addressing. It is only when they know that they can handle them that the fear of taking them on will be reduced.

3. Accept fewer excuses for not being involved in decision making related to professional practice. If you let staff escape ownership of clinical decisions or create the impression that such ownership is optional, you will delay buy-in and investment.

4. Create a few critical events that force staff to think and act on their own instincts and skills. Don't protect them from risk or try to act in their place. Be there to make the risk taking safe as they respond to critical issues (problems in caregiving, a "problem" doctor, self-scheduling, change in care delivery, etc.). By creating opportunities to own issues and develop skills to deal with them, you

present tools to the staff that they can rely on in taking their own risks and solving their own problems.

5. Increase the complexity of issues they take on for problem solving. Continuously challenge them to dig deeper into their own thinking and skill base for dealing with issues that affect what they do. Stop distinguishing between what the manager is able to do and what they do. Partnership behaviors facilitate ownership and staff response.

We continually talk about accountability as though it were an intangible process that can't be clearly enumerated. That viewpoint is simply incorrect. Staff and the manager must define expectations and roles in problem solving, solution seeking, and opportunity finding, to which each contributes. When that understanding is achieved, high levels of performance should be expected, and growth in the role, improvements in care, and staff ownership should result. That is how knowledge workers behave. When that happens the issue of whether they are knowledge workers becomes a moot point.

T PORTER-O'GRADY

Leadership

◆ HOW DO I DEVELOP A VISION FOR EMPLOYEES?

Q Part of leadership is described as providing a vision for employees. What are the steps in this process?

A Providing vision is a process often misunderstood by managers. First it is helpful to say what it is not. It is not goal and objective setting or action planning. Visioning does not require charisma, vivacity, brilliance, or innovation. It also does not necessarily mandate dramatic change. Visioning is simply how the manager defines a desired future or preferred destination for some point in time, usually 3 to 5 years from the present. Vision changes at each level in an organization. At the highest level, it is quite broad. At the unit level it is more focused on the specific specialty or area of responsibility; however, the unit vision always builds on the larger organizational vision or picture in some way, if a vision currently exists.

Visioning has three major combinations of characteristics:

1. Visioning combines hindsight, insight, and foresight. The nurse manager envisions where the unit has been, where it is, and what it has, and identifies the driving force for what it needs or wants to become.
2. Visioning is focused, connected, and balanced, yet flexible, individual, and opportunistic. Visioning requires the nurse manager to continually examine her personal thinking and to test that thinking against organizational reality. In that process of testing, the nurse manager listens to others and is open to their perceptions with the purpose of enlarging her thought process and objectivity.
3. Visioning builds on knowledge, skill, experience, intuition, and faith. Visioning is a whole-brain experience using the nurse manager's analytical skills, experience, and "gut" feelings about the future. Ultimately it is the nurse manager's faith in herself and others that allows release of old thoughts and creates new insights, thereby transforming restraining forces on the unit and in the organization into driving forces.

Steps in the visioning process for the nurse manager follow:

- Identify current and future issues, trends, and events that will provide opportunities for change for your organization and your unit.
- Define and accept reality about how those issues, trends, and events will affect your organization and your unit. From that reality, determine the preferred yet possible future.
- Identify and relate what you believe, value, and desire about the issues, trends, and events. That is, determine the values you believe are necessary to achieve the vision.

To more effectively picture your vision and values, answer the following questions about your unit 3 to 5 years in the future:

- What is the philosophy of management?
- How are decisions made?
- How do the professional practice and care delivery models function?
- What do the systems for unit information and data look like and how do they interrelate?

- How and where do your quality initiatives and resource utilization efforts fit?
- What are the roles and relationships of nursing with medical staff? With other professionals? With support and ancillary services?
- How do you perceive nursing staff performance? Outcomes? Behaviors? Attitudes?
- How do performance standards reflect changed or newly defined responsibility, accountability, and authority?
- What type of orientation, inservice, and continuing education as well as personal and professional development systems exist?
- How are recognition and reward given?
- What is the role of the unit's nursing staff in the community?

Remember, too, that initiating visioning is the rightful role of the leader, not the followers. It is the leader's responsibility to ensure that:

- The vision and values fit with, and are developed in response to, those of nursing services and the organization.
- There is a process in place for agreeing on the unit's vision.
- The unit's vision is operational, realistic, and not in conflict with other like units' vision.
- The vision is clearly defined, shared, known, and understood by those affected so that it can and will, in time, be accepted and owned by the unit's nursing staff.

Usually it is best to begin the visioning process in the nurse manager's mind with one or two major changes that may need to occur on the unit in response to an issue, trend, or event. Visioning can be a simple process; however, it is never a simplistic one. Visioning requires listening, negotiating, asserting oneself and one's values, persuading, supporting, and paying critical attention to timing. Because of the human element necessary in articulating and selling the vision, visioning takes significant time and commitment on the part of the nurse manager. If as a nurse manager you question your commitment to your position, your unit, or your organization, do not disillusion yourself or your staff by starting this process and aborting it along the way. Visioning gives rise to both hope and action. Once lost, it is not easily recovered by the individual who will follow in the departing nurse manager's footsteps.

BV TEBBITT

◆ HOW DO I CREATE A VISION?

Q Everyone agrees that the ability to create a vision along with managing change are the benchmarks of successful transformational leadership. How does one go about creating a vision? What are the essential skills and process steps?

A "Vision implies the ability to picture some future state and to be able to describe the state to others so that they begin to share the dream" (Tichy & Devanna, 1990).

Bennis (1989a) says the first basic ingredient of leadership is a guiding vision. He states that the leader must have a clear idea of what she wants to do—professionally and personally—and the strength to persist in the face of setbacks, even failures.

DePree (1989) writes that the single defining quality of leaders is the capacity to create and realize a vision.

Nursing managers must be able to articulate a clear and challenging vision that inspires others to focus attention on the overall direction of the organization. It is the nurse manager's responsibility to create a description of what the unit looks like when it is fulfilling its purpose. Leadership involves envisioning a desirable future and enabling others to get there (Poscarella & Frokman, 1989).

The nurse manager must explore a variety of internal and external factors that influence the creation of a vision appropriate to the organization and its mission.

External factors include:
1. Trends and assumptions you can expect in your specialty, including technologic advances, medical discoveries, and reimbursement changes.
2. Trends or changes expected in your customers.
3. Trends or changes affecting your customer base.
4. Trends or changes expected from your competitors. Where might new competition come from?
5. Trends or changes that threaten your competitive edge.
6. Opportunities to take greater advantage of current competition's advantages or strengths emerging from anticipated trends and changes.

Internal factors include:
1. Your organization's stated mission and values.
2. Your organization's strategic plan and your unit specialty's relation to it.
3. Trends or changes expected in your organization's financial and physical resources.
4. Changes or trends anticipated with regard to your work force—number, age, skills.
5. Your work group's values.

Peters and Waterman (1982) say visions come from within and from outside, and must be inspiring, clear, and challenging.

Bennis (1989a) further states that vision is dynamic, not static, and must be renewed, adopted, and adjusted. When it's too dim, it must be abandoned and replaced.

In *The Transformational Leader,* Tichy and Devanna (1990) describe the following exercise designed to enhance commitment of staff to the vision.
1. Engage staff in writing an article describing the unit 5 years from now and the role they played in the transformation. Use words that paint graphic pictures—what the environment looks like, what people look like, and what they are saying and doing.
2. Identify common themes—personal and organizational.
3. Create a common vision.

This exercise serves as a springboard for consensus and tends to focus attention on the overall direction of the unit and organization.

K KERFOOT

◆ WHAT LEADERSHIP BEHAVIORS ARE EFFECTIVE IN ENCOURAGING DEVELOPMENT OF TALENT?

Q What leadership behaviors have been proven most effective in liberating talents in the workplace?

A A leader who can balance both the business and the human side of her work is usually an effective one. A skilled communicator always has an edge over one who cannot listen well or cannot clearly define the issues. A successful leader has a vision and will role model the vision in her work and the way she approaches her challenges. The style of the leader may vary, but the following behaviors are likely to be the most effective:
- Providing a model for risk taking and providing challenging experiences.

♦ Coaching and mentoring.
♦ Offering rewards and encouragement for creativity.
♦ Sponsoring new projects, new committees, and new networks.
♦ Celebrating their successes when they display their knowledge and skills.
♦ Providing individualized attention for problem solving and skill development.
♦ Demonstrating acceptance of a wide variety of individuals.

JB COLTRIN ET AL.

♦ HOW CAN I ENCOURAGE STAFF TO TAKE CHANCES?

Q What strategies can I use to help the staff to experiment and accept the risk of trying new ideas and work methods?

A Personal attitudes, behaviors, and strategies of nurse managers that support risk taking include the following:

1. Opening lines of communication to yourself and, through you, to top management. This means allowing and expecting participation and collaboration in unit-related or organizational issues or problems. Opening lines of communication also means that you tolerate confrontation of personal attitudes and behaviors by employees. You must value differences of opinion on the unit and give specific feedback frequently regarding individual performance, contributions, and attitudes.

2. Providing support to staff by clearly defining expectations plus allowing and learning from mistakes and failures, rather than instilling the fear of punishment. You can also demonstrate support of risk taking by being oriented to experimentation, encouraging idea sharing, and making available to employees the data, equipment, supplies, or other budgetary resources necessary to achieve the suggested new idea or work method change.

3. Identifying and developing rewards that because of budgetary constraints probably will not include more money. Rewards may be in the form of training and development opportunities, access of the idea to a higher level of management, and perfor-

mance evaluations that respond to the employee's contributions that have required risk. Also, praise employees for risk taking whenever possible. Identify specifically the risk the employee took and the positive outcomes on the unit; or state what was learned from the employee's idea that benefited unit or organizational quality, productivity, or cost reduction, or increased customer satisfaction. It is important for the nurse manager to remember that what is perceived as a reward by one individual on the unit may not be perceived as such by another, because of personal differences and needs. It is honest praise, however, that is the nurse manager's most universally powerful tool to foster continued staff risk taking.

BV TEBBITT

Liability

♦ IF I'M COVERED BY EMPLOYER'S LIABILITY INSURANCE, DO I NEED MY OWN POLICY?

Q My employer informs me that the institution's liability insurance covers me. Do I need my own professional liability insurance?

A Institutions carry liability insurance to cover employees while those employees are performing job-related duties. This coverage assumes that employees are following the institution's policies and procedures. Ask to see the policy that the institution carries. This policy should be reviewed to determine the extent of such coverage for the employee. During this review, it is important to note the policy type and limits to determine coverage and assumable risks.

An advantage to having your own liability insurance is that your insurance company will work primarily to defend you in the event that a suit occurs. Frequently these insurance companies will work with the institution's insurer. If you are employed in activities that result in liability outside of the work you perform within the institution, you may also require liability insurance to cover those activities. If you are an independent contractor rather than an employee, you should definitely purchase individual insurance.

If the institution's liability insurance is extensive and sufficiently covers your liability, purchasing your own insurance may merely prove to be an additional expense. Some people believe that having insurance may encourage a lawsuit should a potential plaintiff learn you have independent insurance and, thus, available funds.

The choice to purchase additional liability insurance is personal. Policies available may provide coverage for claims reported during the policy's duration ("Claims Made Policies") or for claims that result from acts that occurred during the policy period ("Occurrence Policy"). The nurse should consider the type of policy preferred, services provided outside the employment arena, personal assets, advanced practice activities, suits within the nurse's practice area, and her own security needs (Feutz-Harter, 1989).

LM LENTENBRINK

◆ IS IT LEGAL TO REFER PATIENTS TO OTHER HOSPITALS FROM OUR EMERGENCY ROOM?

Q One of the problems that frequently occurs in our emergency room is that patients who come to us are directed to other hospitals in the local area. I've noticed that poorer patients, those without physicians, and some high-risk patients are sent without first being assessed in our emergency room. Is this legal? If not, how can I as a nurse manager best address this issue?

A One of the key responsibilities of any manager is to be well versed in any legislative or regulatory requirements that affect one's area of responsibility. The situation you describe is in clear violation of the federal law known as the Emergency Medical Treatment and Active Labor Act. This law was enacted to provide assurance that patients truly in need of urgent or emergent care or pregnant women in imminent danger of delivering would not be denied access to care on the basis of inability to pay.

Although this law does require that emergent care be rendered to all patients in need regardless of ability to pay, it does not require that hospitals treat any

and all patients who come to the emergency department requesting care. This would potentially place an undue burden on an emergency service, clogging it with individuals who may choose this route rather than the appropriate primary care route for basic care.

The key issue for the caregivers is having a system in place that allows you to expeditiously differentiate between the emergent and nonurgent situation. The most effective approaches involve an initial professional nurse assessment to determine the urgency of need for medical care. This *must* be followed by a physician assessment to be in compliance with the antidumping law.

It is a pretty safe assumption that no one in your institution is deliberately violating federal laws pertaining to care of emergency patients. The consequences of doing so could be fatal to an organization because they include loss of designation as a Medicare provider. I would recommend that you address this situation promptly and in a straightforward manner with the appropriate individuals in your institution. First, fully familiarize yourself with all federal, state, and local statutes that may pertain to the services you deliver. In addition, review the accreditation standards of JCAHO and any other standards that may be helpful to you such as those described by the Emergency Nurses Association. Evaluate your institution's current policies and practices in light of professional standards and legal requirements. Identify areas where you have deficits and think through your recommendations as to how to remedy the situation. Approach your immediate supervisor first with an overview of the situation and your recommendations for corrective action. Make it clear you'd like to take a lead role in solving this problem in collaboration with other key leaders such as the medical director of the emergency department. Together you can develop a plan to involve other appropriate parties in rectifying the situation.

Although it is hard to believe that the situation you describe could be anything other than a serious oversight, it is imperative that immediate action be taken. If for some reason there is an unwillingness on anyone's part to address this issue, you must pursue it to the highest level of the organization. If it remains unaddressed, an employment change for you would be well advised. Beyond that, in terms of communicating this violation of federal law, let your conscience be your guide.

JE BEGLINGER

◆ IS IT LEGAL TO GIVE PHONE ADVICE TO DISCHARGED PATIENTS?

Q After discharge, our previous patients often call asking us for advice regarding continuing clinical care in their homes. We have given advice freely and hope that it has been helpful. However, we have been concerned about legal liability. What is your advice?

A First, check with your hospital risk management department and hospital legal counsel regarding your current practice. Their input and guidance will provide a framework for your protocol. It is essential that the responses be consistent and clinically grounded.
1. Establish a small group of RNs and physicians to draft clinical protocols based on symptom diagnosis and providing the standard response and protocol. An example might be:
   Fever:
   ◆ What other symptoms are present?
   ◆ What is the age of the patient?
   ◆ Has the patient made a recent trip to the doctor or emergency department?
   ◆ How many days has the fever lasted?
2. Write responses based on the various answers, for example, if the fever persists in spite of aspirin, come to the emergency department.
3. End each phone inquiry with this standard response: If the symptom persists or worsens, call your doctor or come to the emergency department.

JM McMAHON

◆ CAN I BE HELD LIABLE FOR A CLINICAL SPECIALIST'S PRACTICE RELATED TO PATIENT CARE?

Q The clinical nurse specialist assigned to my unit has little credibility with the medical and nursing staff, yet as part of her role responsibility, she is asked to precept nurses orienting to our unit. In addition, the clinical specialist does not report directly to me. Am I at risk for potential liability for the clinical specialist's practice related to patient care on my unit?

A Yes. The complexities of this situation are numerous. However, as the nurse manager, you are accountable and responsible for the care delivered on your unit and for the team of people providing that care. Whether it is a patient transporter who lets a patient fall from a gurney while traveling down the corridor of the unit or the CNS precepting the unit's nurses, the manager is accountable and responsible.

That does not mean that the accountability is not shared with the employer; and it does not mean that the licensed individual is not accountable. All who are licensed have varying degrees of joint accountability and responsibility based on the scope of practice of the profession, the standards of the profession, and the institution's position description and listing of responsibilities and the hospital's operating procedure (and manual, if applicable). If an untoward event occurs, it is likely that the injured or aggrieved will look to all involved for recovery. (Be sure you carry liability insurance!)

While you note that the CNS does not report to you, you have not indicated whether she is an employee or staff member of the hospital or an individual working under a contract. Given the facts presented, I cannot discern her status; however, if she is on contract, with discrete duties that require no supervision from other staff, your liability may be minimal. However, you need to have the hospital clarify the role of the CNS in relation to your responsibilities, and indicate in writing, whether she is a staff member or contract employee, to limit your responsibilities for her actions.

However, as long as the CNS is interacting with staff under your direct supervision, you may be responsible for her performance as it relates to your unit. You have a responsibility in the example cited to document the performance of the CNS and draw the problems to the attention of the CNS's supervisor. You may counsel the clinical nurse specialist and identify the areas where improvement of performance is needed. Depending on the situation, you may ask that the specialist not be assigned to the unit. You can handle your accountability best by taking definitive action to document all questionable activities and incidents, clarifying the role and responsibility of the CNS, and communicating all concerns to your superiors.

All nurses, whether managers or not, should keep records of any adverse or inappropriate incidents carried out by others within the work setting for which the nurse may be held accountable. Notes do not have to include every aspect of the incident, but the date, time, adverse occurrence, and inappropriate actions taken are essential. Narrative should include enough information for the nurse to recreate the incident and for others to get a sense of the malfeasance. By keeping a personal log, the nurse provides additional protection against others' recollections of events that may be the basis for suit.

LJ SHINN

♦ **WHAT HELP SHOULD I OFFER A STAFF MEMBER WHO IS GIVING A DEPOSITION?**

Q Several of the staff nurses on my unit have been involved in giving a deposition. How can I best support them during this process? What specifically do they need?

A Depositions are anxiety-provoking ordeals for staff members who have never before experienced them. You can best support them by ensuring that they have the information they need relating to what is expected of them and how the information they share will be used. Explaining the process and the reason for depositions should assist in diminishing the anxiety that results when staff members are informed that they must give a deposition.

Depositions are a method of discovery in the litigation process. A question and answer process is used in an effort to seek out information. When staff members are asked to provide a deposition, they may be asked to provide information either because of their experience with the incident in question or because of their knowledge as nurses of nursing policies, procedures, and practices. In general, when a deposition is taken, legal counsel representing both the plaintiff and defense are present. Questions and answers are frequently recorded by a stenographer. Following the deposition, the questions and answers are transcribed to written form.

To support your staff, provide them with preparation time before the deposition. Facilitate contact with hospital legal counsel and/or a risk management representative before the session. Encourage staff to ask that legal counsel outline what they can expect

during the process of the deposition. Staff members may ask what case they are involved in and why they must give the deposition. Staff members should be encouraged to note questions before meeting with hospital legal council. During that time, they should also inform legal counsel of their desire to have a copy of their deposition once it is documented.

Hospital legal counsel will most likely provide some general tips that staff members may follow during questioning. These tips may include:

1. Be truthful.
2. Answer the question but say no more than asked. Elaboration can be misinterpreted and misused.
3. Require that questions be asked concisely. If the staff member does not understand the question, she needs to ask that the question be restated.
4. Attempt to answer all questions with a simple yes or no.
5. If the staff member does not remember or doesn't know, she should say so.
6. If the session becomes too tiring or anxiety provoking, it is okay to ask that a break be taken so that the individual can confer with legal counsel.

Although participating in a deposition is seldom a pleasurable experience, anxiety can be reduced by providing information to staff members before the actual procedure. Encouraging discussion and contact in preparation for this event may diminish anxiety caused by fear of the unknown.

LM LENTENBRINK

♦ **IF A NURSE REFUSES TO DO A PROCEDURE BECAUSE OF RELIGIOUS BELIEF, WHAT SHOULD I DO?**

Q A nurse working on our medical unit in the hospital is a Jehovah's Witness. She does not agree with the practice of giving blood to patients and does not wish to take part in carrying out this procedure. Where does she stand legally and morally if she refuses to do this procedure, and how shall I advise her?

A In reviewing various legal books written for nurses I was unable to find a case that exactly replicated this situation. However, there are cases in which a person's religious beliefs were upheld when refusing to participate in professional activities that contravene the nurses' religious beliefs (Cushing, 1988). (These cases dealt mostly with abortion.) This right of refusal is not an absolute right because it is contingent on the fact that the patient's condition not be jeopardized because of the nurse's failure to act. Legally, she would be required to carry out the procedure to save the patient's life. However, you as nurse manager should make an effort to obtain the services of another nurse to start the blood transfusion if time and other factors permit. This expectation needs to be clearly communicated at the time of discussing conditions of employment during the initial interviews. This nurse needs to reassess where she could best work that would not include assisting with blood transfusions to the degree that would be commonplace on a medical–surgical unit.

A good practice in the future would be to make sure that persons who have this concern be made aware that it is not always possible to have someone substitute for them. This is especially true in the smaller, rural hospitals.

SR. M FINNICK

L

Licensure

♦ WHOSE RESPONSIBILITY IS IT TO ENFORCE LICENSURE REGULATIONS?

Q The licensure validation process in our hospital is usually slow and not always effective. Are we creating increased liability in our organization by not strongly enforcing state licensure regulations, or is the obligation of the individual licensed professional to ensure that licensure is recorded in a timely and effective manner?

A In order for the employer to do business, the employer most likely will have to meet certain state laws or regulations. Hospital licensing laws and attendant regulations, for example, usually require the hospital to validate the credentials of those who must be licensed by the state to practice certain professions. In addition, any facility that is accredited by the Joint Commission on the Accreditation of Healthcare Organizations (JCAHO) will have to meet the requirements set forth in the JCAHO manual. Among these requirements is that each member of the nursing staff be competent to do her job, including clinical assignments that are based on relevant licensing laws or regulations. Further, the accreditation manual requires that an organization that uses nurses from external sources (an agency, registry, or pool) document evidence of licensure before engaging the nurse to work in the facility. Various reimbursement laws may also require nursing personnel to have a license or other credential in order for services to be reimbursable. Thus a facility engages in risky behavior when not validating licenses of its professional workers.

Adequate job descriptions, clear qualifications, and good interview and reference checking processes will assist in hiring appropriately credentialed nurses. Shoddy reference checking and failure to ask for and keep up to date licensure records are courting disaster. Impostors do attempt to work as registered nurses.

Finally, a word about the obligation of the individual. The individual licensee also has an obligation to be currently licensed to practice as a registered nurse. Practicing on an expired or invalid nursing license is akin to driving with an expired or invalid driver's license. It is against the law and jeopardizes public safety.

The nurse manager should be familiar with the licensure validation process of the facility in which she works. As a part of the management team, the nurse manager will work to be sure the institution's processes are relevant and timely.

LJ SHINN

♦ CAN I WORK AS A NURSE MANAGER EVEN THOUGH MY LICENSURE PROCESS IS NOT COMPLETE?

Q I have been hired as a new nurse manager in another state. My employment begins before the completion of my licensure process. Can I function as a nurse manager without completing my licensure?

A The answer to this question depends primarily on state licensure laws. In most states a nurse must be duly licensed in the state in order to practice (this may not be true if you are working in a military or veterans hospital). The appropriate state board of nursing should be contacted as soon as a job move is contemplated to determine the licensure requirements and to begin the licensure process. Each April the *American Journal of Nursing* includes a directory of nursing organizations. The issue includes the name, address, and phone number of the licensing board in each state. Keep a copy handy.

Many states will issue a temporary permit while the licensure application is in process. This permit allows the nurse relocating from another state to begin work while waiting on the license. The permit is usually valid for 60 to 90 days and may be renewable once or twice.

A prospective employer should be able to tell you the state's requirements. In addition, the employer may have policies that govern the employment of a nurse before licensure in the employer's locale. Be sure to ask.

Keep in mind too that JCAHO requires that each member of the nursing staff be competent to do her job, including adherence to applicable licensing laws and regulations. A facility accredited by JCAHO will want to meet this requirement and will seek documentation that the nurse is licensed in the jurisdiction in which she is to practice.

LJ SHINN

Managed Care

♦ WHAT KIND OF DEPARTMENTAL SUPPORT WILL I NEED AS WE INITIATE MANAGED CARE PROCESSES?

Q As we move to managed care processes in nursing, what kinds of support do we need from the other departments of the hospital?

A The supports needed do not change. What changes is the intensity with which you work with some of the departments. With managed care the bottom line becomes a more important focus than it has been in the past, partly by decreasing patient days. As a result, the coordination of services provided to the patient becomes more intense because services are provided in a shorter period of time. Administration can function as a support system by updating the management team on changes, being responsive to changing needs, and listening to frustrations as the organization moves toward a new care delivery system.

DD GILES

♦ HOW CAN I PREPARE STAFF TO WORK WITH MANAGED CARE WORKERS?

Q How do I prepare the staff I work with for the ongoing influx of managed care workers who have not traditionally been a part of the unit-based health care team?

A Many staff nurses are unaware of the forces driving health care today, and they do not realize the importance of welcoming the managed care worker to the health care team. A first step in changing the attitude toward these new members is to make sure you as the manager understand how the managed care worker fits into the unit-based health care team. Once a contract has been negotiated, the manager must be made aware of who will be the key person from the managed care provider that the unit will be working with.

Clarifying what information the managed care worker will need and why, and what assistance the managed care worker may expect from the staff will help to avoid unrealistic expectations from both parties. The next step is to help the staff understand what managed care is, how it works, why the institution would enter into a managed care contract, and how to continue to provide quality care under the perceived constraints of managed care. Setting time aside in your monthly staff meetings to inservice the staff on these issues is important. As the staff begin to understand these issues, they begin to understand the language of managed care, and they begin to understand how their practice may have to change in a managed care environment, including the welcoming of nontraditional team members. In some cases, inviting the managed care worker to a staff meeting to meet with the staff and answer questions might be helpful. Collaborating with the finance department in setting up inservices to explain the different types of reimbursement that the institution is receiving (e.g., a per diem reimbursement versus capitated reimbursement) also helps the staff to understand how welcoming the managed care worker to the unit-based health care team will facilitate movement of the patient through the health care system in a timely manner while continuing to provide quality care.

DD GILES

◆ UNDER A MANAGED CARE CONTRACT, DOES MY ROLE CHANGE?

Q How does my nurse manager's role change now that my institution has managed care contracts and critical pathways?

A Managed care is providing quality care with effective resource utilization. There has never been a better time for both managers and staff to become knowledgeable and involved in both the business and the art of caring for patients.

First, it is important to understand how the role of the nurse manager is changing on a global level. The role of the traditional nurse manager who had only to worry about how the nursing care on her floor was being delivered has passed. The descriptor of management has changed. Not only are nurse managers expected to understand how nursing care is being delivered, but they are also expected to understand utilization, capitated market demands, continuum of care, integrated delivery systems, CQI, networking, and wellness. Never before has it been as critical for the nurse manager to have an understanding of the big picture.

No longer is the health care delivery system the hospital; rather the hospital is now viewed as a cost center that—to be successful—should not be filled. The hospital is no longer a stand-alone entity; it is now part of an integrated delivery system supported by physician groups, health plans, and a continuum of services that ensures the wellness for a given population. The nurse manager's role requires knowledge about all elements of health care the patient may need in order to access the expertise and resources available. This is necessary to effectively move the patient in and out of all continuums of care in the most appropriate and expeditious manner. The inability to ensure the appropriate level of wellness for that population could mean the financial downfall of hospitals that successfully survived in an old paradigm.

Health care is rapidly moving into an environment of capitation in which hospitals and physicians will receive predetermined dollar amounts to care for a given population. Physicians and hospitals will need to form partnerships to care for this population and will need to be motivated to keep this population healthy because illness will affect a health care system's ability to be financially successful. Therefore the nurse manager's perspective must be focused on the maintenance of patients' health rather than on their illness. Nurse managers must understand the health care needs of their patient population and the service costs of providing that care. They must be up to date on current health care trends and state and federal policies that continue to affect how care is given and compensated. The bottom line is that the manager in this environment is not only a nurse manager, but a global general manager who keeps her finger on the pulse of both her care area and also the entire health care delivery system to keep them healthy and fit for reaching current and future visions.

So how does this global understanding relate back to the day-to-day activities of the nurse manager? The nurse manager will need to move from the traditional managerial functions of directing, controlling, planning, staffing, and evaluating to a role of leadership. The manager's role becomes much more encompassing of all aspects regarding the patient's stay in the hospital and is not limited strictly to the nursing care provided. The nurse manager must be able to lead and manage multidisciplinary or cross-functional teams and staffs. To facilitate quality, efficient health care service, the manager must be aware of all disciplines and how their interactions are integrated on behalf of the patient's care and the patient's perception of that care. The team must be empowered to make decisions about patient care to ensure their ownership of the care being provided. The nurse manager role requires that the manager and her staff see themselves not as being encumbered by traditional barriers between and among disciplines and departments, but rather as working together as a team, recognizing and utilizing the expertise of each discipline in the most appropriate manner to ensure positive patient outcomes. All professional staff are expected to deliver and held accountable for the same high level of practice for patient care. The nurse manager must facilitate professional growth of nurses and other health care providers to be innovative, creative decision makers and risk takers, and she must role model that behavior herself.

Critical paths provide the health care team two essential elements to make all this happen: a multidisciplinary plan of care and measurable expectations, both of which have been absent in the past. Critical paths provide the platform for nurses, physicians, and other disciplines to collaboratively plan for the needs of the patients. They get all disciplines focused on outcomes desired for the patient and timeliness associated with those outcomes. They also move caregivers away from tasks to focusing on patient outcomes through well-designed pathways of care. Critical pathways can demonstrate aberrations in care and point out areas for improvement.

Critical pathways provide the mechanism to clearly understand both the care and the service that are being provided. In industry, the cost and the production steps are known and therefore are measurable. Efficiency becomes a question of knowing the product and its production time, and capitalizing on efficiencies to produce the product at a cost that will provide a profit. To put it simply: produce the right product at the right time for the right client at the right price. Health care has great difficulty in defining itself, its product, and its cost, and therefore it has difficulty becoming more efficient. Critical paths create the tool to measure the care provided to a known and somewhat predictable population.

The nurse manager working closely with the clinical nurse specialist and professional staff must assist the staff to use the critical paths in the way they were designed. The caregiver must focus on the outcomes desired for the patient and on the activities that will move the patient to the next level of care. The staff nurse cannot continue to focus on tasks and view critical paths as yet another thing to do. Rather, critical paths should change the way the nurse manages the patient's care. Having the caregiver now focus on outcomes, length of stay, costs, and barriers or differ-

ences in care and the impact of those differences gets the frontline staff involved in the success of the institution as well as improvement of patient care. This change in how the nurse functions needs to be supported by providing the staff with information that traditionally has not been shared. The staff needs to see the outcomes—financial as well as clinical—in order to remain committed and stay enthusiastic about the changes associated with critical paths.

Critical paths and their outcomes will be, and in many places currently are, the way in which hospitals are gaining managed care contracts for specific groups of patients. Payors want to see patient outcomes and costs associated with care, and critical paths provide a way to compare organizations. These quality indicators and measurable outcomes become a marketing backbone in a competitive "everything else is equal" market. Sophisticated information systems will need to provide reliable, frequent, on-demand reports that meet payor and clinician needs. The nurse manager will need to let go of the concept of "routine" quality indicators for quality improvement seeking indicators.

J TORNABENI

◆ HOW WILL CAPITATED CONTRACTS AFFECT PAYMENTS?

Q How can nurse managers prepare themselves for the changes in payment and expected outcomes associated with capitated contracts?

A Nurse managers must first understand the dynamics of managed care and how capitation works. Capitation means that the payment for care is fixed and paid up front, and the institution is "at risk" for what happens to the patient. The goal is to keep that patient healthy and not in need of more expensive health care services. The fewer resources consumed by the patients, the greater the likelihood that the institution will have some money left over at the end of the year. This means a hospital can make more money by keeping patients out of the hospital.

Nurse managers can take several steps to ensure that they are prepared for managed care and the changing reimbursement environment:

1. Understand *all* of the costs associated with the care of your patient population. This should include everything that occurs from the moment

the patient enters the hospital to any postdischarge care needs. Begin to evaluate what is essential to a positive outcome for the patient and design care to include only those things that make a difference. You may find that a "critical path" will be helpful in this.

2. Explore and understand the critical processes that ultimately put that patient in your hands. In other words, what occurred before admission that resulted in the admission, and is there any aspect of care that could have been provided early on to avoid the hospitalization? You may also need to develop outpatient services in order to allow the patient to be discharged sooner. This presents great opportunities for nurses.

3. Develop good relationships with those physicians who care for your patient population. Understand what reimbursement risks exist for the physicians. Influence their practice patterns positively by providing data to them regarding the effectiveness of their care in a nonpunitive manner.

4. Expect your staff to assume responsibility for understanding the individual reimbursement issues of each patient they care for. Help them understand they are "spending" either the patient's money or the hospital's.

C BRADLEY

M

◆ CAN I PARTICIPATE IN MANAGED CARE CONTRACTS?

Q How can the nurse manager be an active participant in managed care contracts?

A There are many opportunities for you to contribute to a managed care contract. First and foremost you need to be able to identify your patient population. Determine if your patient population is funded by case mix, DRG, or nursing diagnosis. Determine through the business office the expected length of stay (LOS) for your patients. Through multidisciplinary collaboration, develop critical paths that can delineate on a daily basis the expected outcomes for your client population. Tracking your patients' outcomes on a daily basis allows you to care for your patients within the allotted length of stay. Note that many of the insurance companies reim-

burse your hospital for just the allowable length of stay. If patients stay longer, the patient could fall into an outlier class, and the reimbursement to your institution is less.

Track achievements and variances. Find out what causes variances, and through total quality management (TQM) or through your continuous quality improvement (CQI) committee (may be called quality assurance) you can eliminate the variances.

Your financial management department keeps LOS data. Request monthly information regarding your patient population and the average LOS for those clients. Always remember that a hospital receives managed care contracts because care is provided in a cost-effective efficient manner. We want to hope that contracts are negotiated based on quality outcomes, but the reality is that most contracts are actually negotiated based on who can provide the care in the fastest, least costly manner.

JG O'LEARY

◆ HOW DO NURSE MANAGERS ADVOCATE FOR CLIENTS IN MANAGED CARE CONTRACTS?

Q How can I as a nurse manager role-model advocacy for clients in managed care contracts?

A The goal of managed care is to provide high-quality care at a fair and reasonable cost. The nurse manager functioning in this environment must understand the financial impact of this new financing model and share that openly and frequently with the staff. No longer can the financial information be revealed to management alone; everyone in the organization should have access to and understand the realities of the organization's financial performance. The nursing manager must gain a solid understanding of the different financial reimbursement mechanisms and determine ways to manage those dollars effectively and, at the same time, ensure high-quality care.

Managed care challenges health care providers to utilize dollars appropriately and to ensure that patients are receiving their care in the most appropriate arena. The nursing manager must know the proper ways to reroute patients to centers of the most efficiency, no longer viewing the hospital as the only choice.

As the nurse manager, you must role-model innovation and willingness to take risks. You must continually seek new and better ways to deliver high-quality care within the reality of the organization's resources and challenge your staff's thinking on how to do things differently. Role-model a clear understanding of what the patient's needs are and ensure that staff are providing for them in a highly competent and efficient manner. What requires a nurse, and what can be done by other caregivers under the direction or supervision of nursing? The manager must be able to think outside the confines of nursing, to recognize the needs of the patient and determine who is best suited to deliver those needs. Utilization of resources in the most cost-conscious fashion is critical.

You must be able to role-model team values, advocate, and initiate a multidisciplinary team approach to patient care. Recognize the unique contribution each discipline brings to the task and take a leadership role in structuring the patient care delivery model around the contributions and abilities of each team member. Nursing will need to let go of being all things to the patient; managed care no longer affords us that luxury. Rather, the nurse manager must be able to put nursing in a leadership role of coordinating and delegating the care to the most appropriate level of caregiver.

J TORNABENI

Management Development

◆ HOW DO I AVOID BEING JUST A "FIRE FIGHTER"?

Q I find that I spend all of my time as a nurse manager "putting out fires." How can I get beyond this?

A This is hard for most of us. One part of your job *is* fire fighting. To some extent, it will always be part of the job. However, I find that most of us are quicker to go after the fire than need be. Often someone else can fight the fire. For instance: an angry family member may need your intervention, but not before the staff person has had a chance to try to resolve the problem. Often staff requests for schedule changes or last-minute family issues become the manager's problem. Let the staff deal with those issues as colleagues. If you inherited a "disaster area unit" and have *nothing* but fires, you need to develop a work plan so that you are clear about where you want to go and how you plan to get there. You will still fight fires, but you will be focused on some proactive work also.

Define where you want the work area to be in 1 and 2 years. Write the plan down. Talk to your supervisor about your plan. Outline the steps you will take to accomplish the plan. There is a saying: "If your job is to eat an elephant, you have to do it one bite at a time." So it goes with managers and fire fighting. There are some fires you must put out, but if you have a goal and a work plan, you will be clear about what you are working toward and how to avoid just fire fighting.

Here is an example from one of my colleagues. She was responsible for a work area with very high turnover. It was consistently understaffed and had excessive salary expenses because of outside agency use and overtime. Burnout was a major problem, and quality of care was a concern. There was no way to fix the area overnight. The manager worked with the staff to develop a recruitment plan, retention plan, and a plan to optimize scheduling so that some core people were on duty at all times. Traveling nurses (outside agency nurses who make long-term commitments for 1 to 3 months) were hired. The manager used available resources to help: her supervisor, human resources (the person responsible for helping with nurse recruiting), the staff, and other department managers (not just nursing) who had had similar problems and worked them out. It took 3 years, but the work area is staffed, turnover is below the national average, and staff are using a shared governance model to manage the unit; they report a high level of satisfaction.

Planning in this way lets you focus on a program to proactively address unit problems. It moves you away from hopping from one problem to the next.

I would also suggest you work with the staff to set goals for the department each year. Just have a cou-

M

ple, especially if you are doing a lot of fire fighting. Goals help everyone take a more proactive stance in working together.

M PECK

◆ HOW DO WE TRANSFORM HEAD NURSES INTO NURSE MANAGERS?

Q Our organization has experienced tremendous change in role expectations of the nursing leaders at the unit level. We have gone from head nurses to nurse managers, with increased responsibilities. Our staff, who are predominantly prepared at the diploma or associate level, are having difficulty understanding and accepting the difference. How do we go about helping them to help us make this a successful endeavor for everyone concerned?

A The issue of the professional development of nurses and nurse managers is a critical one for our profession. As nurse managers moved out of the traditional head nurse role, many had difficulties migrating from the concept of being an additional pair of hands or a part of the staffing ratio in their previous role to being a fully integrated manager, role model, and coach for the staff. Assuming a full-time management role and balancing the clinical needs of the unit have been challenging in these transitional times. Education and having good role models and mentors are essential to this process of developing nurse managers. Concurrently, intensive education for staff nurses is necessary to help them understand the changing role of nurse managers as well as their own role. Nurses should be assisted in becoming more independent in their work and more collaborative with each other to make clinical decisions. Helping to move staff nurses from a role that is dependent on a manager to be independent and interdependent with their colleagues is challenging. The most successful strategy is joint education sessions with staff nurses and nurse managers, as well as meetings and opportunities to discuss the operational issues that arise from role conflict and role changes. Intensive education is essential to this growing process.

KJ McDONAGH

◆ WHEN SHOULD I CLARIFY MY RESPONSIBILITIES AND AUTHORITY TO FULFILL THEM?

Q How do I approach clarifying my responsibility and authority when I am often given added responsibility without authority to accomplish what is requested?

A Clarify expectations at the time that they are assigned so that the requisite authority accompanies the obligation. If you discover after beginning your new role that you do not have sufficient authority, renegotiate with your supervisor what can be expected with the authority that you do have. Think through the processes you will use to complete your responsibility, even using decision trees or program evaluation and review technique (PERT) charts, and discuss these plans with your supervisor. Identify areas in which you lack sufficient authority, and get it!

CE LOVERIDGE

◆ HOW CAN I IMPROVE MY REACTION TO ANGRY PEOPLE?

Q As a nurse manager, when someone is upset with me, I become "tongue tied," incoherent, and not very responsive. What can I do to get over this kind of reaction?

A Even seasoned nurse managers with exceptional self-esteem initially lose their sense of "inner balance" when confronted with negative emotions, particularly another person's anger. There are three positive actions a nurse manager can take in this type of situation:

1. Listen intently to determine what is making you feel "off balance." Mentally ask yourself: Is it the situation or the interaction itself? Is it a specific person with whom I'm working? Is it staff members' expectations of me? Does my discomfort relate to unit standards or work rules? Is it related to my skills or lack of them, or those of others? Is it related to the fact that I may not have enough data or the type of data or information needed? Is it

lack of cooperation from employees? My supervisor? Top management? Is it fear of failure related to my self-esteem level or job success? Is it due to procrastination in doing something because the task was distasteful or difficult, leaving me indecisive?

2. Ask specific questions of the individual confronting you at the time, or repeat what he or she has said to ensure your understanding. People usually become more even tempered, particularly when displaying negative emotions, if they are asked for additional information. It gives them an opportunity to continue release of negative energy and provides the nurse manager a chance to regroup and formulate an appropriate response. Ways to get more information and "buy time" might include saying, "Tell me again what happened from your perspective." "Did I hear you correctly when you said . . . ?" "How did what happened affect patient care or the patient care team?" "Who else was affected by the incident causing you concern?" "In what way was that disconcerting to you?"

3. Stick with objective facts when you do respond. Avoid using absolutes such as *always, never,* or *none.* Also, avoid double-barreling by bringing in unrelated incidents or behaviors. And finally, name your emotions without acting them out. An example of this might be, "When you say or do . . . I feel . . . Then I say or do . . . What I need from you is . . . What I am willing to do is . . ."

BV TEBBITT

◆ SHOULD I GIVE UP MY ROLE AS NURSE MANAGER?

Q How do I reconcile my self-perception of being an excellent clinician with that of being only a mediocre manager? How do I know if I should give up my management role?

A Translation of skills and techniques, such as the nursing process utilized by a quality nurse clinician at the bedside, to the ones needed to become a quality nurse manager can be problematic.

This is particularly true if preparation and skill enhancements for the role of nurse manager are minimal.

It is unfortunate, but this practice of promotion from good clinician to a position of increased responsibility, authority, and accountability (nurse manager) has existed in our system for a long time. Limited opportunities for the quality bedside nurse to advance through the nursing hierarchy contributed to this practice—a practice that is changing rapidly.

The role of nurse manager, on the other hand, continues to expand into additional areas of accountability. More is expected than ever before.

Your perception of mediocre performance may come from both realities. An excellent clinician does not necessarily make an excellent nurse manager.

A conscious attempt to separate the roles, their definition, expected behaviors, accountabilities, and outcomes will be a starting point to more accurately and fairly analyze your performance as a nurse manager.

Validation of your perceptions from peers, subordinates, and superiors will provide guidance regarding areas that need strengthening.

Consider the various opportunities available in the management development area and internal sources for additional skills development workshops. Your personal commitment to alter your perception will determine your success.

Another way to look at it is that when the "fire in the stomach" is no longer burning to eagerly do the job, it's time to reassess, make decisions, and take action.

LM JOHNSON

◆ ARE MANAGERS STILL NECESSARY?

Q First line management continues to be shot at from all sides. The way we once managed is no longer acceptable. We must now coach, facilitate, and sponsor our employees. A lot of what we used to do is now being done by teams of our staff. Even information is easier to access these days without going through traditional management. Is management disappearing? Is it really no longer necessary?

M

Management is not disappearing, but it is evolving into different roles. Staff are taking on scheduling and clinical issues. Managers are taking on the roles of strategic planner, business manager, guidance counselor, and marketing representative, as well as coach, facilitator, and sponsor. As health care reforms come into play, the manager role will be critical to the implementation of these reforms. The manager will be pivotal in getting staff professionals to accept the necessary changes reform will bring about.

K KERFOOT

◆ HOW DO I BALANCE THE NEEDS AND EXPECTATIONS OF MY JOB?

Q As a nurse manager I find myself juggling the needs of many constituencies: staff, administration, physicians, patients, and self. How can I find balance in meeting all these needs and demands?

A First, you must recognize that you are only one person and have only so much time in a day. Each day, you must allow yourself time to play. If you do not permit yourself to do this, burnout will occur quickly.

Second, you must prioritize needs. Those items that can be delegated should be delegated. Schedules should be juggled to allow time for yourself. No one is indispensable, and if you continue to think that you are the only one to do any job, you can burn out quickly.

Third, reflect back on each day to review the day's events. Dwell on the positive events, not the negatives. Negative thoughts can be helpful when reviewing the events if you treat them as learning experiences. Everyone will have hectic days and busy days. When reviewing the day's events, look at better ways to handle situations in the future. Always find something positive, and congratulate yourself on that.

Finally, incorporate play into your work. Some people find playing with "electronic toys" restful but also useful for work. This can be playtime as well as completion of work. Using travel time wisely to and from work is also helpful. Listening to tapes, dictating notes, or simply putting the day's events in order

allow you to take advantage of needed quiet time when at home. You must tell yourself it is okay to spend time on yourself. This is important to avoid burnout.

Balancing many demands and needs requires good time utilization skills, delegation skills, and prioritization skills. Just as finishing work-related projects and tasks is important, taking care of yourself is also important.

K KERFOOT

◆ HOW CAN I AVOID DUPLICATION WHEN MANAGING MORE THAN ONE UNIT?

Q I am responsible for managing two separate nursing units and constantly feel pulled in two directions. I often feel as though I am duplicating my work. Are there some strategies to reduce the duplication yet provide each area with equal attention?

A As a nurse manager you should be focusing primarily on three main areas:
1. Management of human resources—facilitating hiring, orientation, and scheduling, as well as being a delegator and motivator to get the job done.
2. Management of fiscal resources—budgeting.
3. Management of material resources—making sure that supplies and equipment are available and ensuring that the physical environment is conducive to working.

The best strategy I can suggest to you to reduce your feeling of duplication is to begin to view your responsibilities differently. Rather than viewing yourself as responsible for two units with duplicative responsibilities, I suggest you view yourself as a professional manager who is responsible for managing a set of processes. You just happen to divide your human, material, and fiscal resources into two distinct units. When you view the situation from that perspective, it is not necessary for you to make sure each area receives "equal" attention. What is necessary is for you to make sure that the management systems—human, material, and fiscal—are in place across all levels of your responsibility. Once those systems are in place and are operating efficiently, you should intervene based only on need. Your staff should be able to operate day-to-day business without your constant presence. If that is not the case, you may need to do some more work on developing your management systems: fine tune your scheduling system and back-up contingency plans, educate your staff more, involve them more in the fiscal issues related to your units so they feel accountable for budget targets, and negotiate with materials management to ensure adequate levels of supplies so that you don't have to intervene at the point of a problem. The real challenge of a manager is to develop processes and put systems in place so the unit operates without constant management interventions. By focusing on developing these processes you will find less duplication of your efforts and at the same time develop a more autonomous staff.

CCC LEVENS

♦ **WHAT SHOULD I DO TO ENCOURAGE MANAGERS TO BE MORE APPROACHABLE?**

Q How can I foster an attitude of approachability among managers?

A Managers differ in their personality styles, comfort level with management, and interactional abilities, which ultimately affect how approachable they will be to their staff and to each other. The executive level of management needs to role-model the behaviors that they expect of their managers by being approachable themselves. "Approachable" may mean available for assistance, input, or direction; open to criticism of current policy or procedure for the sake of improvement or change; or available for personal interaction for relationship building and/or team building.

Staff input about the manager's style and effectiveness should be periodically assessed, with feedback presented to the manager in a constructive manner. Some managers may need the assistance of a facilitator or coach to help them develop new skills in interacting with staff and behaving in a more collaborative manner. If they are insecure in their management skills or in negotiating conflictual interactions, continuing education on topics such as conflict man-

agement, team building, group interactions, basic management skills, or other related topics may be useful. Role-playing specific management and staff interactions that may be uncomfortable for the manager can also be helpful in skill building.

Staff can help the manager to be more approachable by altering their own interactional styles as well. For some managers, it might be helpful for a group spokesperson to meet with the manager to represent potentially conflictual feelings, rather than the group "taking on" the manager in an open forum. No one likes to defend herself from a hostile group in a public forum. The representative spokesperson approach facilitates the positive management of a negative message and improves negotiations for change. Collaborative environments are developed from a belief in the interdependence of the staff and manager to create a successful unit. Both parties need to feel that they are valued as people and for their expertise in clinical nursing and/or management.

JF STICHLER

♦ **WHAT DO I DO WHEN I DON'T KNOW THE ANSWER TO A STAFF MEMBER'S QUESTION?**

Q Sometimes when the staff ask me an important question they expect me to respond to, I simply do not know and have no answer. How do I respond when I really don't know?

A You can't know the answer to everything. The processes affecting your role and the pace of change make it impossible for you to have all the answers at your fingertips. Much of change is risk and timing, and there are times when what is occurring in one place or role is not communicated or is unclear. When you don't know, say so. There is nothing wrong with not knowing. If you need to know, find out and keep working with the system until you get what you need from it. There is no more important role for the manager than that which relates to the effectiveness and the proper use of information. As a leader, gathering and generating information may be one of your most important activities. Therefore accessing, interpreting, and generating it becomes a

M

major role expectation of managers. It is incumbent upon the manager to be open to information and innovation so it comes as no surprise; the manager must act as a conduit for it. Even so, there are times when you just don't know the right answer and need to let the staff know that what you can do is find out or assist them in finding out. This way you partner with them and build a stronger basis for generating and managing information.

T PORTER-O'GRADY

♦ **HOW VISIBLE SHOULD A NURSE MANAGER BE?**

Q What are the best ways for a nurse manager to be "visible" to caregivers, and what is realistic regarding visibility for today's nurse manager?

A One of the most important contributors to staff satisfaction is visibility of the "boss." Staff expect the manager to stay in touch with what is happening on the unit, to be available for patient and physician problems, and to demonstrate interest and concern about the staff and their work.

Hospitals are now and will continue consolidating management layers and departments. This means managers will no longer manage just one unit, but they will have multiple units and multiple disciplines to oversee. In addition, there will be decreased levels of management necessitating redistribution of work to the remaining thinned out layers. Therefore the manager will have more areas to manage, increased responsibility to administer those areas effectively, and less time to spend directly with staff than in the past.

With the changing and expanding role of today's nurse manager, it is no longer possible for visibility to be maintained in the traditional manner of being physically present. However, visibility extends beyond the senses and into the mind. In this context, the nurse manager's presence can be manifested throughout the culture of areas she manages. This presence is woven into the core values of the unit and is reflected in the mind of each staff member. This can be a positive, cohesive force that binds a staff into a team, holds them together during times of uncertainty, and encourages them toward growth and maturation. The manager's presence is really the flame that keeps the vision illuminated; it is a covenant that should not be taken lightly by anyone entering or staying in management.

The successful manager of the future will have expanded knowledge, skills, and responsibilities yet will be readily accessible to staff when needed. The only way this streamlined structure will work is if the manager is able to create an environment of empowerment for staff. Only through empowerment can staff truly assume responsibility and accountability for their practice. The role of management then becomes one of accessibility and availability when the staff need it. This is all balanced by a clear vision and is supported by well-articulated values and performance expectations.

Visibility does not necessarily mean the amount of time the manager spends on the unit, but rather how the time is spent. In other words, it is not the quantity, but rather the quality of time that matters. Staff must feel the presence and know it is readily available, but they must also feel there is a deep sense of trust in what they can do on their own. This trust means the manager doesn't hang out, intervene, or control activities. The manager needs to develop a sixth sense to recognize when the staff is in need and to be there to support or mentor as appropriate.

Managers need to communicate with their staffs, sharing with them some of their responsibilities and activities so there is enhanced appreciation of the scope of their role. It is also important for staff to recognize the contributions their leader makes to the organization as a whole. Staff must realize that as they become more and more empowered, the role of management changes. They must also realize that as managers become responsible for more areas and other disciplines, the availability of the manager changes. In other words, staff must learn to stop hanging onto the past when managers were "mother hens" watching over their "brood." The new manager is to be recognized as a resource to the staff who are functioning at a much higher level in the organization. As a result of this higher level, the nurse manager also has a much greater impact on the day-to-day operations of the hospital. The nurse manager's role will become much more visible and instrumental in the strategic direction of the organization. Staff need to recognize and appreciate the enhanced role nursing is playing as a result of their expanded role.

When making rounds, which must be done at least daily, the manager needs to utilize the time effectively. If 15 minutes a day could be set aside just to be on the units, talking with staff without a planned agenda, a large amount of information could be shared. The concept of not having a planned agenda is important in that staff often have contact with manager only when she has a message to deliver to the staff. Rounds should be spent seeking input from staff, finding out what is going well and what they need help with, what is getting in their way, and what they need from the manager in order to do their job more effectively and efficiently.

No matter how busy the manager is, it is important that the staff feel listened to and valued for their comments and concerns. When staff share information, concerns, questions, or suggestions, the manager must commit to some form of follow-up. Getting back to staff with answers to their questions or concerns is critical. This needs to occur on all shifts so that everyone feels valued and appreciated. Sitting down with the staff and discussing concerns is an excellent way to role-model and mentor staff. It also demonstrates the value you have for them and solving their problems.

Other high-profile methods of visibility include unit retreats, staff and shared governance meetings, and the posting of office hours. Just as university professors establish office hours for student contact, so too could nurse managers. The nurse manager could also maintain visibility through written communications. A note placed in a mailbox for a job well done, or even for failing at trying something new, praising the staff member for accomplishments, or just for taking a risk and trying, would go a long way to establish visibility. During times of high stress, such as high census, high acuity, or short staffing, a pizza delivered to staff at mealtime would convey a powerful statement.

Honesty about issues is appreciated and accepted. The manager who is seen as honest and forthright gains the respect and trust of staff. The manager who skirts the issues is readily seen through and quickly loses the respect of staff. When making rounds, staff need to see the manager as focused on them and not preoccupied or just making an appearance. A hurried approach or rushed answer or vacant smile can be read through, and the effort to be visible is lost.

Finally, the manager should talk to the staff about their expectations of visibility. There should be discussion about what staff expect and what the manager can consistently provide. If for some reason the staff's expectations aren't feasible, there should be negotiations to agree on attainable expectations. Staff need to let the manager know what their needs are when she is available and to communicate with her if there are issues that cannot wait. An open and honest environment in which issues are discussed openly and freely is essential. Conflict should be viewed as a healthy way to look at things differently and as a springboard to creative problem solving.

The degree of visibility of a nurse manager is really limited only by the imagination of the manager and the time and effort she is willing to invest in maintaining it. Yes, it is time consuming, but perhaps the manager needs to examine the reasons for entering management. Was it to manage units or people? Without people, units are only rooms and equipment. Management should focus on achieving positive patient outcomes and customer satisfaction in a cost-effective manner. The way to achieve this is through the empowered, integrated health care team. Focus on development of that team, and they will achieve the outcomes.

J TORNABENI

◆ WHAT'S THE BEST WAY TO MANAGE HIGH PERFORMERS?

Q How do I best manage high performers (such as clinical nurse specialists) with strong wills, minds, and spirits?

A Not all nurses who are high performers thrive in the corporate world. Some have great abilities, interests, and talents, and they enjoy expressing them through the collective efforts of groups and systems. Others have the same abilities but thrive in a more autonomous setting. These nurses experience more difficulty with the time and politics involved in moving large groups forward. They feel restricted by the cultural norms and corporate policy found within well-defined systems and structures.

M

The first task of any manager hiring a high performer is to ascertain her world view along with her clinical competence. This can be accomplished in the interviewing process with several thoughtful questions and observations. Does the language of the individual reflect past accomplishments through a joint effort with others, or independently? What are the individual's attitudes and feelings regarding authority and well-established parameters of corporate systems? What are the individual's expectations of the organization? How does the individual see herself in relation to the larger universe?

The manager must then clearly outline the vision, mission, and short-range and long-range goals of the organization for the practitioner so that an informed career decision can be made by both. It is important for the manager to explain the corporate culture along with the philosophy and norms of the nursing practice. She must also describe to the high achiever the method of management and leadership that motivates this particular group of nursing practitioners (group needs and responses to others will vary depending on their level of maturity). Finally, the manager must state specific expectations of this practitioner, along with the degree of autonomy and authority the individual will be granted. Accountability and evaluation outcomes must be explored along with continuing career development opportunities that exist for advanced practice.

This dialogue must also be carried out if this is a new manager who has "inherited" a high performer. To prepare for the discussion, the high achiever may be asked to create a "talking points" paper that entails her career aspirations along with short-range and long-range goals. A similar document should be prepared by the nurse manager, with goals and objectives for the unit or the organization. As the two individuals explore their common and divergent ground, one of three outcomes may occur. They may find a great deal of congruence and excitement in a shared vision for their collective work. They may also find a broadening of perspectives as each incorporates pieces of the other's vision into a revised and enlarged vision for the unit or organization. Or they may find that there is little that is shared, freeing the high performer to look for career opportunities in an environment or setting more congruent with her long-range career goals.

J KOERNER

◆ HOW CAN I CONVINCE STAFF THAT I CAN BE LOYAL TO THEM AS WELL AS THE ORGANIZATION?

Q The staff I work with feels that my primary loyalty is to the organization. How can I help them understand that I am a nurse advocate for them, too, but I must also have an organizational viewpoint? Also, how can I assist them to develop a better organizational perspective and interdisciplinary approach to patient care?

A This first question pulls at the heartstrings of every nurse manager from time to time. Practically speaking there are a number of suggestions:

1. Evaluate your own needs and values. How satisfied are you with the divergence and polarities of your role as a nurse manager? You are accountable for patient care management, operational management, and human resource management. Do you prefer one over the other? If so, are you giving incongruent messages about your role to your staff? Is the staff clear about how your role differs from theirs? Make no assumptions about this. They may not like or appreciate the role difference; however, they have a responsibility to understand that difference. It is the nurse manager's responsibility to continually and consistently educate the staff. This is more effectively done by modeling than by telling.

2. Know what your staff members need and value. As a manager you should remember that staff do unto others what they perceive is being done unto them. It is also wise to be aware that staff want the facts to fit their preconceptions. When the facts do not, it is easier for them to ignore the facts than to change their preconceptions. Therefore, it behooves you, as the nurse manager, to be consistent and clear about where you are spending your time. Set your priorities weekly to address at least one item that staff perceive they need or value in order to be more effective in their work. Tell them what you are going to do for them. Do it. And then tell them how what you did made a difference in their work lives. Be specific in identifying what efforts you make for them. Don't assume they know where you, as the nurse manager, put your time and efforts and why. On the other hand, a nurse manager does not need to justify to staff

where or how she spends time. However, being defensive when asked only adds to the staff's negative perceptions and emotions.

3. Be visible. This can be translated into being meaningfully present, even though not always personally visible. It means being available when it really counts to the staff. When it really counts depends a great deal on staff maturity and morale. Visibility includes designing and implementing effective communication systems with *all* the staff. Visibility also encompasses maintaining a vital and viable nursing philosophy and "cutting edge" clinical knowledge, even though your clinical skills may not be at that same level. Staff need to be confident that you as their nurse manager can talk both their clinical language as well as the language of management and/or administration. Get feedback to determine how well they perceive you can, and do, effectively speak both languages.

4. Build trust. Listen to staff individually and collectively. Seek to understand where they are coming from. Tell them the truth as you know it. Clarify their expectations. Ask for their input. Keep your commitments. Avoid surprises. Be fair, respectful, and courteous, even if they cannot, or do not, return in kind. And finally, acknowledge and appreciate their accomplishments and contributions to the goals of the unit and to the patients they care for and serve. Give them specific examples of their successes so they know you know they have made a difference.

BV TEBBITT

♦ **WHERE CAN I GO FOR HELP WHEN I AM DISSATISFIED WITH MY MANAGEMENT SKILLS?**

Q. How and where do you go when you are frustrated with your management skills and are being perceived by staff as continually policing them?

A. When your management skills seem inadequate and you are continually cast in unwanted managerial roles, it may be time for a self-assessment as well as a shared assessment with some trusted peers. Through contacts within and outside their immediate work environments, managers establish needed networks that support and validate them in their dynamic roles. Managers also need to update and revitalize their skills.

Here are some actions that can not only sustain you as an effective and satisfied manager, but can also relieve you of law enforcement duty with your staff:

1. Seek out a special person to help you with your managerial development—a mentor, or at the very least, another manager who possesses skills more advanced than your own and who is willing and able to coach you on an ongoing basis.

2. Cultivate your own network of other nurse managers. Check in often with these peers, learn from their experiences, and contribute your own expertise when you are able.

3. Find managerial professionals outside of nursing for fresh perspectives about your work situation.

4. Maintain contacts with *staff* nurses outside of your work environment. They can provide you with an alternate view to your management situation and allow you to realistically examine your behavior from your staff's point of view.

5. Become introspective. Debrief yourself after critical incidents that you might have handled more effectively, examine alternate strategies, and develop plans for the next time.

6. Attend workshops where you can refine your interpersonal skills in areas such as assertiveness and conflict management with the assistance of professional trainers.

7. Routinely read nursing management journals such as the *Journal of Nursing Administration, Nursing Management, Nursing Administrative Quarterly,* and *Nursing Economic$.* Browse through the nonnursing management section at your local bookstore.

8. Stay in touch with the clinical area by reading the literature that your staff reads.

9. If possible, work occasionally in a staff role to develop a staff perspective.

10. Maintain administrative certifications. They encourage you to participate in continuing education and give you a reason to attend professional conferences. Pick a broad scope of sessions, including presentations that you wouldn't normally choose.

11. Go back to school; it will renew you.

12. Monitor your style of supervision. You might be supervising the professional group too closely. Remember that as professionals, they were socialized to supervise themselves.

RG HESS

◆ IS THERE A LIMIT TO HOW MANY EMPLOYEES A GOOD MANAGER CAN MANAGE SUCCESSFULLY?

Q Can a unit manager really be effective when her scope of responsibility may include 60 or more staff members?

A At first I was tempted to respond *no* to this question. However, there is no magic ratio of managers to staff, just as there is no perfect ratio of nurses to patients.

The response to the question depends on a number of factors. How has the manager organized the staff—5 teams of 12 each with the team leaders reporting to the manager? 6 teams of 10 each with 6 team leaders reporting to the manager? Does the manager have responsibility for 60 plus staff over 3 shifts, 7 days per week? Have definitive performance goals been agreed to with all direct reports? Does the manager have a regularly scheduled time to meet with each direct report to keep abreast of work? Does the manager surround herself with competent people? Are there time lines established for work? Is delegation occurring, with related follow-up? If the answer is *yes* to these questions, it is likely that the answer to the question of whether the manager can be effective is also *yes.*

In addition, the manager can be more effective if she has a single focus: *management.* If the manager has patient care responsibilities, for example, it's likely her effectiveness will be diminished. Similarly, if the manager has a major role in managing operations of the facility, for example purchasing, then the manager's effectiveness is likely to be lessened. In other words, what is the complexity of the manager's job and what kinds of relationships does the manager *need* and *have* to do the work?

In today's work environment management is beginning to be viewed very differently from in the past. Employees are expected to be more self-directed and more accountable and responsible for themselves. Managing knowledge workers like registered nurses calls for a different management approach, as well. Layers of middle managers have been eliminated in many work settings and larger groups of employees are reporting to senior executives. Sophisticated information and feedback systems are keeping senior executives and employees in touch. Thus the answer to the question can be *yes* or *no,* depending on the circumstances. It is critical for today's manager to keep in mind that the concept of management is changing, and the smart nursing manager will change as well.

LJ SHINN

◆ SHOULD A NURSE MANAGER ALSO BE EXPECTED TO WORK AS A CLINICAL STAFF MEMBER?

Q How can I convince a nurse executive or other members of administration that a nurse manager should be given time to work administratively without being expected to work as a clinical staff nurse?

A Most nurse managers do not spend the majority of their time doing direct patient care. Although it is important that the nurse manager keep current on the clinical issues on her unit, a manager may make more effective use of her time by coordinating and facilitating the work on the unit. It has been suggested in our organization that nurse managers spend about eighty percent of their time on the nursing unit. This may be spent at the bedside in direct patient care, but it is more effectively spent interacting with the staff about clinical, budgetary, and administrative issues; with physicians in developing collaborative collegial relationships; and with patients and family making sure that compassionate quality care has been given. It takes time to facilitate staff development and keep a nursing unit running smoothly. The manager needs to know what is going on in the unit but she need not necessarily have direct involvement with every patient.

A nurse manager can use her time effectively on the nursing unit and administratively in many ways:

1. Acting as a mentor to staff, facilitating and supporting staff to develop to their potential. Time should be spent on employee evaluations and counseling to help define the employees' weaknesses and compliment their strengths.

2. Studying trends and monitoring quality for the nursing unit. Quality is measurable if defined and documented. Issues can be identified and evaluated more effectively by the manager if she is not burdened with a full patient load.

3. Troubleshooting and performing preventive maintenance on clinical issues. Evaluation and problem solving involve the expertise of the manager through past experience and knowledge of new technologies.

4. Handling budget compliance, and prevention and correction of lost charges. Nursing departments are held accountable for lost equipment, supplies, and revenues. Nursing should not be seen as a financial liability, but as implementing effective utilization of resources.

5. Establishing rapport with physicians, other departments, patients, and families. Good relationships with these people result in quicker problem resolution and better avoidance of conflict.

BH DUGGER

◆ HOW DO I MAINTAIN A CONTINUUM OF CARE?

Q What is the role of the nurse manager in creating and maintaining a continuum of care? How do I support the nurse case management roles on the unit and bridge them to the community?

A The traditional role of the hospital continues to change. Currently the transformation of care needs of patients from *only* the acute side of care delivery to other alternatives is quite evident.

As a nurse manager, your role has been and will continue to be the vital link between the global view of health care institutions and their component parts, the unit and patient view.

Nurse managers assume responsibility for translating patient care needs and requirements to both internal and external environments. This view and definition of patient care are taking on new meaning, with care being delivered in a variety of settings; the hospital is just one of many.

The nurse manager, as creator of care standards and outcomes for populations of patients, has generally attended to needs of patients before admission in instances such as preadmission interviews. Nurse managers have been and will continue to be active discharge planners, utilizing appropriate internal and external support systems and referrals.

This component of the ever-changing and expanding role of nurse managers will continue and become more prominent as delivery systems move beyond the walls of the hospital and develop a new model. Some contemporaries and policymakers refer to this as a seamless system of integrated care delivery—a continuum model. Maintenance of old relationships and the development of new ones within the community of the care delivery system can successfully be advanced because they are logical next steps in the work you currently do. The design of a system of case management is a significant undertaking. The same skill, preparation, study, and research utilized when proposing a new system must be employed here—perhaps even more so. Thorough planning is critical to successful implementation.

Case management is an institution-wide system of care delivery that requires clear agendas from the start. Early steps in the planning process would include identification of clear institutional goals, objectives, outcomes, and support. All vital decision makers—administration, nursing, physicians, and other professional disciplines—should plan together, clarify values, determine expected patient outcomes, and consider fiscal implications before implementing systems.

It may be wise to utilize experts in the field to guide your planning and development phase of this system change.

Answers to questions such as the role of the case manager will become more obvious as the system of case management is designed for your specific environment.

LM JOHNSON

M

◆ WHAT CAN I DO TO IMPROVE RELATIONS WITH MY NEW BOSS?

Q My hospital has undergone a corporate reorganization and now has an organizational structure that reflects product lines. As a nurse manager, I now report to a nonnurse who is the product line manager. I find this situation uncomfortable in that my boss evaluates me and my unit from the business aspects of revenues and costs and does not seem to understand quality of care issues. What can I do to change this situation?

A You state that reporting to a nonnurse product line manager is an uncomfortable situation. This is not an unusual feeling for professionals; we tend to resent being evaluated by those outside our discipline. However, there are strategies that can help each of you to be successful while working together toward a common goal.

Get comfortable with the product line concept. A review of the literature will help you gain an appreciation of it and will provide you with ideas so that you can effect positive change in your role as nurse manager. Know that most hospitals are struggling to survive and consequently traditional ways of doing things are being challenged. Look at the restructuring that has occurred in your organization as an opportunity rather than a threat.

You also stated that your boss evaluates you and your unit from the business aspects of revenues and costs and does not seem to understand quality of care issues. Here is where you can have a tremendous effect. Begin by having a formal meeting with your supervisor. Delineate roles and responsibilities to avoid confusion and frustration. Come to agreement about levels of participation and decision making processes. This will be tremendously helpful when discussing financial and patient care issues. Commit to respecting each of these concerns so that they will receive equal attention by both of you. Because product line management has been used to control costs, indicate to your boss your willingness to improve patient outcomes by monitoring and evaluating quality of care issues. Recommend delivery of care models for improved service—after all, patient care services are a product line. In addition, you could "cost out" nursing services, which could ultimately help you focus on quality of care issues. Increased efficiency, better utilization of resources, and reduced duplication of services all can ultimately increase revenue. You therefore have a wonderful opportunity to affect patient care and the bottom line.

There are some other things to consider as you strengthen your working relationship. If you do not have a matrix reporting structure, you may want to give this some thought. Some organizations offer functional supervision for vertical structure. In this way you would be held accountable for nursing concerns by nursing, and you would be accountable to the product line manager for horizontal concerns. These latter ones generally deal with multidisciplinary issues affecting other department managers.

In order to change the situation you need to clearly state what's wrong with the way things are, be willing to collaborate with your supervisor to improve the situation, agree on needed changes, and commit to doing your part. Evaluate your progress regularly. By supporting one another, each of you will be using your organizational and leadership skills to enhance the product line program development, while planning strategically to market your service. Your patients, your staff, and your organization will benefit by this win–win approach.

V MANCINI

◆ HOW CAN I ACQUIRE BETTER BUSINESS SENSE?

Q The role of the manager is changing rapidly from a clinical focus to a business focus. I am having difficulty handling the transition; it seems everything is *my* responsibility. What resources are there to help me be more effective and less stressed during this time?

A It is sometimes during the most stressful periods that we realize the need to reassess what we're doing and how we are doing things. Nurse managers in particular are constantly being asked to accommodate change—often without explanation—so your frustration is understandable.

Balancing during any transition is difficult at best. However, you can alleviate some anxiety by thinking about the following:

1. Ask yourself if you are uncomfortable with the transition because you don't think you have the business skills to be successful. If that's the case, consider taking some courses or asking individuals in the organization to provide workshops. Your education department or your finance department may be willing to conduct classes on business aspects of your role. Remember that you are probably not the only manager in the organization who is struggling. Many of your peers could benefit with this approach.

2. Meet with your supervisor to discuss your feelings. Let that individual know that you are seeking guidance as to how to be more effective. Try to really understand what is expected of you in your role as nurse manager. Then ask yourself, "What is my role? What am I responsible for?" You may need to pull out your job description and review it. If, like most job descriptions, it is vague, get busy rewriting it. You may need clarification from your supervisor or peers, but it will be well worth the time investment.

3. Once there is agreement on the job description, follow through with a criteria-based performance evaluation tool. Each requirement should match item for item. For example, if there is a segment in the job description addressing your fiscal responsibility to the budget, then the performance evaluation tool should contain a segment stating measurable goals for meeting the fiscal responsibility requirement.

4. Review reports that you currently receive to determine how they support your role. You may find that you don't have the right data to make good business decisions. By looking at your job requirements, you can begin to list the tools and reports you need to support your role.

5. Negotiate your yearly goals with your supervisor. As a result of doing this, each of you will know where your energies should be concentrated. Be sure to make these goals clear and measurable. And don't try to accomplish everything in a year; that would just add more unnecessary stress to an already demanding job.

6. Last, relax and have some fun. Don't take yourself too seriously. If you are committed to growing in your role, it will be more easily accomplished with some humor along the way.

V MANCINI

Meetings

♦ HOW CAN I KEEP COMMITTEE MEETINGS FROM TURNING INTO GOSSIP SESSIONS?

Q Whenever the staff tries to get together to communicate about issues on the unit, the discussion regresses into pettiness and gossip. How can I as a manager help to quell the gossip in our sessions?

A Many issues can be resolved in the public forum of a unit staff meeting, but effective meetings don't happen by themselves. Meetings must be artfully constructed by skillful participants. The following points will assist you and your staff in getting the most out of your meeting times.

1. Have a meeting to learn how to have a meeting. Enlist an in-house facilitator if one is available. Include the following:
   ♦ Communication skills for meetings.
   ♦ Scheduling meeting times and items.
   ♦ How to lead and participate.
   ♦ Robert's rules of order.
2. Put together an agenda with staff participation and distribute it in advance. Anticipate the time necessary for dealing with each agenda item.
3. Lead the meeting. Encourage the staff to stick to the agenda. Point out when the discussion strays off course; recognize when the staff have drifted into areas where they may have little or no impact. Be open and direct, and separate personal from professional issues. Some matters may have to be tabled for private meetings between staff.
4. Appoint other staff to compile the agenda, but guide its development. Coach staff to lead their own unit meetings.
5. Use these meetings as an opportunity for team building.

RG HESS

◆ HOW CAN I CHANGE CONSISTENTLY NEGATIVE COMMENTS OF STAFF MEMBERS?

Q Whenever staff meetings are held, one staff member is consistently negative and outspoken, often dominating discussion. What interventions could be used to modify this employee's behavior and facilitate group participation?

A If this behavior is unique to this staff member, it is best to deal with her on a one-to-one basis. The following language is often helpful.

In yesterday's meeting, I felt you had some very good points to make, but I don't think your message was heard by others because of the way it was communicated. It is important that everyone's message be heard and considered. Let's talk about different ways you might convey your message so that it can be heard and so the messages of others are also heard.

Then it is helpful to review the group norms. One norm many groups adopt is the right of each person to speak without interruption for her allotted time and then to respond to questions. (If the group has no norms for communicating and interacting, you may need to help them set these so everyone knows the rules of behavior.)

Discuss very specifically how the staff member could be aware of and work to change phrases and words that trigger a response in others that prevents them from hearing the message. For example, if the staff member uses the term *problems,* she might be counseled to use the word *opportunities.* The phrase *down from management* could be reframed as *from management.* The sentence, "We've tried that before and it doesn't work" could be rephrased as "We've tried that before and the reasons it did not work were . . . However, if we do the following I think it might be successful."

Request that the staff member choose someone who will be honest with her and who can act as a mirror and mentor. This individual would observe the communication and behavior of the staff member and then they would sit down together after a meeting and discuss what was successful and what needs to be changed. The mentor and staff member might also work out an inconspicuous sign language that

the mentor could use to signal when the staff member is using old and ineffective patterns. The mentor can also be helpful when other staff members (who are used to the ineffective communication and behavior) fail to even try to listen to the new communication of the staff member. The mentor can say, "Well, I know I have often tuned Sally out because in the past she was so negative, but I think that what she is saying today is very valuable and I'd like to hear her out." This will help to reposition the staff member with her peers.

Finally, be sure to recognize the staff member when she is more positive and uses effective communication and interpersonal relationships. Even if early steps are small, be sure to recognize them.

JE JENKINS

Mentors

◆ HOW DO I ESTABLISH A MENTOR RELATIONSHIP?

Q I would like to develop a mentored relationship with nurse leaders in our local area. I'm a little uncertain of how to approach this. What would you suggest?

A One of the prerequisites of initiating a search for mentoring relationships is to have a clear sense of the direction you want to take in your career. Spend some time doing a self-inventory of your capabilities and dreams. Develop tentative, realistic goals for a mentoring relationship that are congruent with your dreams. Keep in mind that more than one mentor may be needed to provide the support and guidance you desire.

Following this inventory, make an appointment with the nurse you report to and with the chief nurse executive (CNE) in your organization (if you do not report directly to this person). Ask for guidance in career development in general and in networking with potential mentors specifically. Request input regarding your goals and effective strategies to meet them. In addition to receiving valuable information during this meeting, you will also be marketing yourself as someone who is motivated to take advantage of opportunities that will provide personal and professional development opportunities. As these opportunities become available, nursing administration will be aware of your interest and should facilitate your efforts.

A second avenue to explore is involvement in professional organizations. During your meeting with the nurse administrator(s), ask what professional organizations would provide a good fit with your goals. Have these organizations send information summarizing their purpose, structure, and benefits. Interview the contact people from the organizations to find out what opportunities they offer to become involved and to network with nurse leaders. Once you select which organization(s) to join, volunteer for a committee and attend meetings and educational offerings.

These strategies will provide the opportunity to find a mentor. Some characteristics to look for in choosing a mentor from the leaders you will come in contact with are compatible personality traits and values, high energy level, positive yet practical approach to issues, willingness to provide and receive both positive and improvement feedback, openness to new ideas, willingness to assist you to develop your potential, and belief that a mentor benefits both personally and professionally from the mentoring relationship.

Once you have selected a potential mentor, ask that individual if she would be willing to act in this capacity. Present your career goals and strategies and delineate how you believe this person can help you achieve these. If the person agrees, set up regular times for contact. This contact can be face to face, or by phone, fax, or electronic mail. Assure the potential mentor that you will be very sensitive to time and energy constraints.

Finally, I would recommend that you act as a mentor for a colleague. A number of years ago an article was written that accused the nursing profession of eating its young—the nursing leaders of the future. Nursing must stop patterning itself after the cannibals of the animal world. I propose that we model ourselves after the pride of lionesses and lions that nurture and mentor their young for the survival of the species (or in our case, the profession). If we all view ourselves as mentors, the health care system will hear our roar.

MC HANSEN

Mergers

◆ WHAT WILL HAPPEN TO MY JOB IF MY HOSPITAL MERGES WITH ANOTHER?

Q My employer has announced that the hospital I work for plans to merge with another hospital in the community. What impact will this have on me as a nurse manager?

A It is generally understood that a merger is a strategic business decision whereby resources are combined in order to increase overall efficiency and revenue.

Nurse managers' responsibilities are tied in with those of more than half of all hospital personnel in operations. You are therefore in a very advantageous position to contribute toward a successful merger.

Of primary importance is the decision you must make in terms of compatibility. Learn all you can about the other facility's culture. Try to be open minded and avoid taking on the "fight or flight" attitude. This attitude will only create more personal stress and will get in the way of good judgment. Ask yourself if your management style fits the kind of style needed in the newly formed organization. If it does not, you may need to rethink your continued employment. Throughout this process, stay in touch with other managers—especially those who may have some experience with mergers. While you continue to monitor and assess the changes that occur, your plan to manage your staff should include the following:

- ◆ Keep communication as your top priority. Remember that your staff is experiencing all of the same feelings you are.
- ◆ Learn and communicate any upcoming required changes in titles, benefits, wages, and policy.

M

♦ Role-model positive behaviors, encourage participation and collaboration, and establish positive networks. Think about conducting a joint workshop or research project with the other hospital. These activities not only help promote team spirit but are also great self-preservation strategies.

Remember that mergers generally lower staff morale and therefore lower productivity. In addition, you may see increased absenteeism and turnover in your staff. However, you can minimize stress by encouraging open dialogue. Set up regularly scheduled meetings for the purpose of keeping everyone informed and be sure to ask participants to evaluate each session. Encourage those who can envision the benefits of the merger, and celebrate achievements by hosting a luncheon, by using poster presentations, or through the use of scrapbooks.

Last, avoid surprises. Most of us would rather hear the bad news quickly than agonize over the unfounded gossip.

V MANCINI

M | Motivation and Morale

♦ **HOW DO I PROMOTE SELF-MOTIVATION?**

Q What are effective ways for a nurse manager to create an environment so caregivers choose to motivate themselves?

A The great theories of motivation insist that individuals motivate *themselves*. These theories are generally categorized either as content (Maslow's needs hierarchy, Alderfer's existence-relatedness-growth, and Herzberg's two-factor theories) or process theories (reinforcement, expectancy, and goal-setting theories). They are worthy of your attention because they offer common practical recommendations for managers.

The best managers create and perpetuate a work environment that encourages employees to motivate themselves. Responding to their own unique needs,

people are "aroused" to action by certain cues in the work environment. However, not all individuals respond uniformly to the same cues. Managers must know the people they work with and what those people value in order to customize the workplace for that particular work group:

1. Set clear, realistic work expectations with caregivers in the form of mutually agreed on goals. Then tie valued rewards to these goals. Don't trivialize rewards; for instance, the same raise of a few cents per hour may be more valued in the form of a single one-time bonus.

2. Treat all staff members equitably and fairly in establishing goals and rewards. At the same time, appreciate individual differences. Sensing what rewards are most important to which nurses may be difficult; for example, the recognition provided by prepaid registration at a conference in return for superior work may be more motivating to one nurse than to another who would rather have the extra money. The management trick is to discern these differences in advance.

3. Desired behaviors should be positively reinforced both publicly and privately. This should be done in ways that are meaningful to the individual.

4. Promote risk taking; you must understand which behaviors involve personal risk for individuals. Learn to tolerate mistakes, because the number of failures and mistakes will increase with the number of risk-taking behaviors; support nurses when they fail. Each new risk sets up the likelihood of future risk taking.

RG HESS

♦ **WHAT KINDS OF REWARDS DO STAFF WANT?**

Q What kinds of rewards are proven to be valuable to staff?

A Establishing the proper link between performance and rewards is the single greatest key to improving organizations. Reward people for the right behavior and you get the right results. Consciously work at identifying and acknowledging good behavior; it is too precious to be taken for granted. Seek out your quiet heroes and spend time encouraging and rewarding them. Another reward that will keep your quiet heroes motivated is to take a sincere interest in them, not only as employees but also as human beings. Make people who work for you feel important; if you honor and serve them, they'll honor and serve you. Listen to them. Taking a personal interest in people builds the bond of trust necessary for good teamwork. Other rewards could include:

1. Money. Pay for performance and you get performers.
2. Recognition. Money can be a very powerful incentive; recognition can be even more powerful.
   - Letter for special achievement that goes into the employee's file.
   - Certificates and plaques.
   - Honors, awards, and "Hall of Fame."
   - Changes in job title.
3. Time off. Award time off for improvements in quality teamwork.
4. Favorite work. Give people more of the tasks they enjoy doing as a reward for good performance.
5. Advancement. The traditional way to reward with advancement is to give a promotion up the managerial ladder. But if promotion isn't possible, you can reward an employee with a special assignment or new responsibilities through which the employee can gain valuable experience. An alternative is to create a separate career ladder, complete with titles, pay, and privileges for each level. Great workers can continue to do what they do best and advance without having to become managers.
6. Freedom and autonomy. These can be very effective rewards.
7. Personal growth opportunities. Either give employees new tasks that challenge their creative ability, or give them educational opportunities. Provide continuing education programs and money for nurses to attend programs.

LG VONFROLIO

◆ HOW DO I KEEP MOTIVATION AND ENERGY LEVELS UP?

Q How does one maintain the motivation and energy of staff when working in bureaucratic systems that "move" extremely slowly?

A A common problem for visionaries and changers of the universe is the lag time inherent in helping a larger mass of individuals capture the images of what might be. This is one of the major reasons that bright and creative people leave organizations.

Several issues must be explored when this phenomenon of lag time becomes manifest. It may be due to lack of clarity of the vision, or there may be an incongruence between the vision of the changers and the beliefs and values of those reluctant to change. Each requires a different strategy.

If those committed to change are engaged in action to accomplish the change, their motivation remains high. Therefore it is essential to engage the change agents in addressing these two challenges.

Individuals who cannot capture the vision will often respond to education that enlightens them. A common problem for people who are trying to design a new method is lack of language that accurately captures the essence of the new change. Thus old words are used with new meaning. Individuals will hear the change agent speak, and they will nod in agreement, giving an old definition to a new application of the word. To prevent this phenomenon from occurring, speaking in metaphor helps. It ties a new idea to an older concept that people can understand. Comparing Superman to a "speeding bullet" helped all individuals get a uniform concept of what a super-man is capable of. Without that qualifier, each was left with his or her own definition of the term.

Dealing with resistance because of a difference in values and beliefs is more difficult. We create our belief system through our lived experience. Many people are reluctant to change because they cannot imagine another way of being. Thus creating small changes with big wins is a "safe" way to move forward if there is time for evolutionary change. However, in our current society much change is revolutionary in nature because of the rapid time frame for change. In such a situation, all people should be given support and education to acquire the skills a new way demands. Creating an atmosphere of safety for people to experiment, mourn the loss of old ways without being judged harshly, and celebrate small successes is essential. An environment that nourishes and supports people is the best way to facilitate change in an organization. So if you want to help people maintain their motivation and energy, have

M

them invest it in helping people who lack their gift of vision to move forward to the new frontier that they dream of.

J KOERNER

◆ HOW DO I KEEP MORALE FROM FALTERING?

Q How can staff motivation and morale be kept up when staff nurses are facing such overwhelming changes as decreasing length of stay, fluctuation, and uncertainty in employment?

A This question has dominated the nursing management literature for the past 5 years. Finding an answer has far-reaching implications for the individual employee and the organization as a whole. A motivated staff is critical to organizational survival in the twenty-first century.

The key to organizational and individual vitality can be characterized by the acronym TEEM: trust, enrollment, empowerment, and motivation. Motivation is a direct result of the first three and the driving force behind organizational success.

The first step in creating TEEM is for the administrative team to role-model genuine, open communication in order to build trust. This is done by providing a rationale for decisions. It is also done by being open about mistakes that have been made and stating clearly how the valuable lessons learned from these mistakes will be used to improve future performance. In addition, trust is fostered by timely feedback and continuous follow-up. This will reduce the common problem of fads—management and redesign initiatives that are begun and then disappear without explanation. Small wonder that staff groan when a "new idea" to improve organizational performance is presented.

The second step, enrollment, is facilitated by joint vision statement formulation and strategic planning involving all staff on the unit. To do this, meetings are scheduled with groups of staff members to identify the following:

1. Customers (e.g., patients, peers, physicians, other health professionals, third party payors).
2. Services currently provided and additional services that could be provided.
3. Individual values (e.g., caring, trust, innovation).
4. Common values perceived to be held by all staff on the unit.
5. Perception of the organizational mission.

Following each meeting, the results are summarized and given to all staff. Follow-up meetings are held to develop a consensus statement of the vision. This vision incorporates the agreed upon values into a statement of what the staff believe. It will guide them in day-to-day activities and in planning initiatives for the future.

Using this vision statement, the staff develop goals and strategies for a 1-year period. These strategies must include time tables, lists of who is responsible, and built-in progress reports. An end-of-year report on the success or failure of the strategy is given. Revisions of those strategies that were not completed or not successful can be part of the goal-setting process for the next year.

The third step, empowerment, can be accomplished through a shared governance structure. All decisions are made at the staff level. Managers become consultants, resource seekers, teachers, and supporters.

The final component of this process, motivation, should be the result of the previously described cultural transformation. In order to nurture this motivation, it is important to reward risk-taking. In addition, there must be a climate where all involved view unsuccessful strategies as learning opportunities. Finally, persistence and patience are required. This process is neither linear, easy, nor rapid. This process will, however, provide a structure that will foster the development of the individual and position the team to meet the challenges of the twenty-first century as a team.

MC HANSEN

◆ HOW DO I ENCOURAGE CONTINUING SELF-EDUCATION?

Q How do I motivate staff to continue their learning without depending on the hospital to pay for both attendance and wages, even when we have clinical ladders in place?

A Ask your staff to conduct a personal and professional goals program, or what we call the "Be, Do, Have" exercise. Ask them each to write out what they want to *Have* in their personal and professional lives. This includes material and nonmaterial items, such as houses, cars, vacations, children, time with family, and time for hobbies or volunteer work. Then ask what they would have to *Do* to have these things: make more money, invest money, stop working overtime, manage time better. Last, ask what they would have to *Be* to do these things to get the things they want to have, such as be willing to accept or seek promotions, plan each day, become more educated. In other words, ask them what result they want (Have), what behaviors they would have to exhibit to get it (Do), and what attitude would they have to develop to accomplish it all (Be).

Motivation is internal. *You* can help staff recognize their goals and what it takes to achieve them. Perhaps their goals are different from yours. They may not want to move up the clinical ladder. They may be perfectly content to stay where they are. Or they may not recognize that to truly move up, education is a requirement. They may not understand that their desire to move up must be accompanied by their desire to assume responsibility for their own growth and education. Relying on others places cause in someone else's hands; it removes the source of control. By assuming responsibility for their own education, they control and therefore can create their own destiny. When someone else pays for your education, you owe that person something in return. When you pay for it yourself, you can choose the programs you want and are beholden to no one else. This is freedom! Help them recognize that their investment is in themselves and that this is a characteristic of a truly empowered professional person. Be careful, however, to continue to value the individual who chooses to stay where she is.

Help staff identify what the motivating factor is for self-learning through their goals program. Why will it benefit them? It would be nice if our organizations could pay for wages and attendance at everything, but that's impossible in an era of limited resources, so the options are to pay for oneself or not to attend. Staff will pay and attend only if they see some value to themselves. Help them identify that benefit for their personal and professional future.

RM HADDON

◆ HOW CAN I PROMOTE PEER SUPPORT FOR ACTIVISTS?

Q How can managers encourage peer support of those staff nurses who choose to become actively involved? It appears, at times, that there are too many nurses out there who don't care to get involved, resent the higher expectations, and look at their colleagues' involvement as dumping more of the clinical workload on them. How can we help both groups bridge their gap more successfully?

A The rule of 80/20 applies here: 20% of the staff will arrive early and stay late, 20% will arrive late and leave early, and 60% will follow whomever is winning.

First and foremost, the manager must be supportive of staff involvement. If she only gives lip service and is not supportive, the staff will see through it and respond accordingly. The staff must see daily actions on the part of the manager that support their involvement in activities other than patient care.

1. Use every opportunity to verbalize the importance of staff involvement in the non–patient care work of nursing (e.g., committees, task forces, projects).
2. Schedule coverage for the staff who must be off the unit for longer than an hour. There is no way the other staff can cover a vacancy and do their own work without resentment building up.
3. Explore with your peer managers ways to cover staff.
   - Perhaps sister units could be established. When a staff member needs to leave the unit, a nurse from the sister unit could provide coverage. This could be a reciprocal arrangement and serve to build support among nurses.
   - If you have per diem staff, they can be used to cover partial shifts while a nurse is off for a meeting.
   - The manager herself can assist with patient care periodically to support the staff who are working shorthanded.

In time, the staff will see the value of the work done, provided support is given. It does take time, and the manager's role is pivotal to success.

JM McMAHON

◆ HOW CAN I ENCOURAGE STAFF TO BECOME INVOLVED WITH PROFESSIONAL ISSUES?

Q I've become increasingly frustrated with the staff over the past 6 months when it comes to their getting involved with professional nursing issues. I've tried scheduling issue forums and round table discussions, but nurses never show up because they say they're too busy on the unit. I believe this is just an excuse. How can I deal with this more effectively?

A You need to involve your staff intimately in the planning process. What needs did you identify? What are your goals for development? Don't decide these issues by yourself. Give some leadership to those who will most benefit from the involvement.

Find out what's relevant to their day-to-day practice and which issues hit home with them. Once the staff have identified what topics are important to them, begin to weave in broader issues of concern to the nursing profession. Only then should you establish forums for staff development. Make the forums fun and light-hearted, not arduous and difficult to endure. This can be more difficult and time consuming, but the rewards will be worth it. You can create a working environment that incorporates and reinforces your key messages into everyday practice. You can also show your willingness to support staff development by rewarding employees with compensatory time, research time, or continuing education time for participation in professional nursing meetings.

P MARALDO

◆ HOW DO I GET STAFF TO SUPPORT THE NEED FOR A CONSULTANT?

Q I am a new nurse manager and have taken over a service in which morale and trust among the staff are historically problematic. I have the authority and resources to hire a consultant. How can I get the staff to support bringing a consultant in to help us deal with our issues?

A Low morale on a unit is an "infectious" problem and can be the consequence of many different variables. Low morale can be caused by dissatisfaction with the organization, staffing levels incongruent with the work load, interpersonal conflicts among professionals, stress in the work environment, personal problems outside of work, and feelings of mistrust or conflict with management. Before a consultant is hired, you may want to spend some time talking with each of your staff members to identify the issues that are most troubling to them. Ask them for their help in developing solutions that could be employed to relieve some of the stress. When staff participate in the identification and solution of problems, they take responsibility for changing the morale on the unit themselves. Task forces can be formed to create positive changes on the unit or to investigate ways to improve staff morale.

Just as there are informal leaders among nursing staff who encourage others to constantly progress and perform at high levels, there are also informal leaders who seem to instill a chronic sense of unhappiness on the unit. Negative feelings are infectious and are quickly spread to others. It is often difficult to break the chronicity of unhappiness, but the staff can be encouraged to handle grumbling peers themselves. With peer pressure, the situation can often be dealt with and the grumbling employees will receive less and less positive feedback for their negative behavior.

Once the issues are identified, a consultant who can be motivating and encouraging to the staff can be employed.

JF STICHLER

Negligence

◆ WHAT IS NEGLIGENCE?

Q After having given a bed bath to a patient, one of our staff members left a bowl of hot soapy water on the bedside table. The elderly patient grabbed the table, knocking the water over on herself causing burns to her sensitive skin. Is this an accident or could it be considered negligence? In a case like this, what would constitute staff negligence?

A There is no black-and-white response to the question of negligence in this situation. It is sometimes helpful to consider if it was an act of omission or commission. The latter is an obviously a more serious employee behavior. Before making a judgment regarding this situation, all pertinent information regarding the incident should be gathered, including the employee's perception. In addition, the employee's past performance should be considered. While intent is a subjective process, strictly speaking this in one of the parameters under investigation. The circumstances surrounding the incident should be considered. This is not to suggest that there is a rationale for the incident, but it will assist in determining the possible factors that led to the incident. If this is an isolated occurrence with this employee, as opposed to a pattern of similar incidents, the answer to the question of negligence could be quite different. In some situations it is clearly apparent that negligence occurred. Negligence is the act of endangerment or potential endangerment of a patient by an action or failure to act even though the employee was aware of or should have been knowledgeable of the possible negative outcome. In those situations where negligence is not clear cut, all factors should be carefully evaluated before a judgment is rendered.

SF SMITH

◆ HOW SHOULD I INTERVENE IF I BELIEVE A STAFF MEMBER IS NEGLIGENT?

Q One of the senior nurses on our unit has taken it upon herself to decide which routine care practice she will undertake and which she will not. When asked, she indicates that she is simply setting priorities. I am concerned that she may be approaching negligence. How do I deal with this situation?

A The situation you describe can become a very complex challenge for the nurse manager and the organization. Nurses have long been encouraged to be passive and to follow the rules and dictates or orders as prescribed by the physician or administration. Today's nurses are encouraged to be independent thinkers and to be verbal, active advocates for the patients. How are independent decisions, actions, or judgments evaluated? Are peer review processes in place to measure the quality and outcome of independent nursing actions?

As the nurse manager addressing this situation, you must be clear on whether this individual is exercising

appropriate independent nursing judgment or is simply not completing tasks and, as you suggest, may be approaching negligence.

You should be knowledgeable about organization policies. What do your operational policies or guidelines say about routine nursing care practices? How much independent nursing judgment is allowed in completing routine care? Are the "priorities" being set by this individual consistent with what the nursing care plan describes for the patients?

Remember that your first concern must be the safety and protection of the patients. If after having assessed the actions of this nurse, you conclude that she is not exercising appropriate nursing judgment and is indeed placing patients at risk, you must move decisively to prevent any patient harm.

The situation and the implications are significant enough that, following your assessment of her actions, you should consult with the director of human resources and the chief nurse executive for guidance before proceeding.

GA ADAMS

◆ WHAT CAN I DO ABOUT A MANAGER WHO IGNORES THE NEEDS OF THE OFF SHIFT?

Q What do we do with a manager who appears not to care for the needs of staff on off shifts? The current administrator condones this because she is one of the "good ole girls."

A It is unfortunate when nurse managers see themselves as glorified day charge nurses and, as such, tend to ignore the needs of off shifts. Somewhere, somehow, they've missed the message that they are to be managing a 24-hour process, not just a unit budget.

The advent of managed care will make her behavior stand out as dysfunctional, because achieving decreased lengths of stay while maintaining quality involves all shifts. The "good ole girls" will be tolerated less and less, as *results* rather than sheer "busyness" are evaluated.

For now, there is not much you can do except express very clearly in a letter or a meeting (probably one to one) what needs you want the manager to care about. What behaviors do you want from her that show she is addressing those needs? It might not be as complicated as you, your group, or she thinks.

K ZANDER

Negotiation

◆ DO MEN AND WOMEN NEGOTIATE DIFFERENTLY?

Q Do men negotiate differently than women? I feel like it is always my role to diffuse the male workers' anger. Then, while I'm stewing over the issue much of the day, the men seem to have forgotten about the issue and gone on to other work.

A Studies conducted before the middle 1980s indicated that women did negotiate differently than men. More recent studies on negotiating tactics of women and men, in fact, contradict many pervasive stereotypes about women's weakness in negotiation situations. Many strategies that belied powerlessness have been replaced by more assertive behavior, which reflects the professional and personal progress women have made in the past decade. However, these studies do have mixed results about the communication behavior of women and men.

In Gilkey and Greenbaugh's 1984 study on gender differences in negotiation strategies, it was found that men tended to view bargaining situations as short term and episodic in nature, whereas women tended to view transactions with others as part of a long-term relationship. The women studied adopted more flexible bargaining stances than their male counterparts, which can be partly explained by this attitude toward the length of the relationship. But this difference in negotiating behavior can also be explained by findings in Gilligan's 1979 study describing women's concern for the quality of interpersonal relationships. In West and Zimmerman's 1983 study, it was found that in mixed-sex dyads, men controlled conversations through interruptions and overlaps (when individuals speak simultaneously). Women who are socially conditioned to be polite may experience difficulty in interrupting others.

The attributes of an effective negotiator include clarity, trust, empathy, open-mindedness, confidence, flexibility, fairness, and the ability to listen and present constructive suggestions. If credibility, self-confidence, and assertiveness are requisite communication skills for effective negotiation, then it is incumbent upon women to adopt these skills that will reflect strength and self-assurance.

In Putnam's 1988 study on how men and women negotiate differently, it was found that women report having obtained a good outcome when they feel they have had a pleasant interaction with the other party, even though they have not resolved, or even discussed, the conflict between them. It was also found that women behaved more constructively with men than with women. Men felt they were the more powerful party when negotiating with a woman, and women agreed. Male/female pairs obtained the most good outcomes, female/female pairs the second most, and male/male pairs the fewest.

The results of the study suggest that women need to learn that it is legitimate to say what they want, even if it conflicts with what they think the other person wants. Women also need assistance in seeing that conflicts can be resolved only if they are addressed, and that there are ways of resolving conflicts that maintain, or even improve, the relations between the conflicting parties.

VD LACHMAN

Networking

◆ WHAT IS NETWORKING, AND HOW DO I DO IT?

Q What are some of the basic elements of professional networking and how do I either begin or get connected with a nursing network?

A Networking is probably one of the most under-utilized avenues of support and mentorship for new and developing managers. Networking provides the nurse manager with both professional and personal sources of support. Professional networking requires an investment of time and effort to be meaningful. There are several types of networking that are important for a manager to consider.

1. Internal networking. Professional networking can occur both horizontally and vertically in the organization in which you are employed. Networking in these various "directions" allows you to be exposed to different parts of the organization. Being known in the organization can help you get assigned to new projects and efforts that may be starting up in the organization. You might try having lunch once a week with someone from a different department, or volunteering for hospital activities that would give you exposure to others in the organization. Hospital fund-raising activities are another avenue that might expose you to important people involved in the organization from the governing body or community.

2. External networking. Outside of the organization, networking within the professional nursing community can be a career-enhancing strategy. It also can provide you with some of the support and advice you may not find easily within the organization. Informal mentorship relationships can function well within the nursing community. You can take the following steps for networking in the nursing community.

   ♦ Join at least two nursing organizations: one that represents your clinical area of interest, and one that represents your functional area of interest. These will provide you with access to many people that you "need to know."

   ♦ Get involved in a meaningful way in each organization. Volunteer to be on committees, go to meetings, run for office. Most important, if you make a commitment to do something, do it. Professional nursing organizations depend on reliable volunteers to get their work done. If you deliver, you will be invited to participate again.

   ♦ Volunteer at local nursing schools to teach or be a guest lecturer. This will allow you to get to know the academic community as well.

   ♦ Take the initiative to meet and keep in contact with colleagues that you have met through these valuable associations.

C BRADLEY

♦ CAN I NETWORK WITH STAFF FROM OTHER UNITS?

Q A number of staff in our hospital would like to create a clinical network of support for each other. We are challenged by the fact that we are on different units of service. How do we build a network of support for each other that encourages our growth, development, and professional interaction?

A Relationships can be a nonlocal phenomenon. A traditional definition of relationship is one that occurs in a shared geographic space. With the emergence of telecommunications and the better articulation of shared visions and aspirations, relationships can occur all around the world. However, there are several important ingredients essential to the success of a personal relationship or professional network.

A common foundation of shared vision, values, and beliefs is the unifying framework for a professional network. Creating shared assumptions that make up a shared belief system is essential to development of a group philosophy. Crafting this essential element for the network requires candid and broad dialogue in an environment of trust. This work must be done face to face and over a period of time until clarity and consensus are reached. Some nurses use their lunch hour or meet for breakfast weekly or biweekly until this important piece of work is accomplished.

A second important ingredient is timely, ongoing dialogue. Such dialogue can occur over the phone, in brief meetings in the halls, on shared documents in round-robin fashion, or via a computer modem or fax machine. The key is that the communication contains information that is pertinent to the shared work, and in a time frame that is meaningful to all participants of the network. Thus one of the essential elements that must be identified and planned for by the group in its organizational phase is the type, mode, and frequency of communication expected of group members from each other.

Trust is the glue that holds all relationships together. This is fostered among professionals when ownership of ideas, work, and outcomes is clearly delineated. An important discussion must center around who owns the results of group work. Who will write for publication? Who will speak? Who shares the outcomes with the larger corporation and the nursing community? Establishing group norms for performance and outcomes will enhance the trust level of the group as consensus is reached on how the group process will unfold.

Finally, candid and clear feedback is essential to help the group shape its current and future reality. Through giving and receiving feedback, individuals

N

can better understand their impact on others, as well as others' impact on themselves. This is the key to continued professional development, which is the underlying goal of network building.

J KOERNER

♦ WHAT'S A GOOD WAY TO GET PERSONAL SUPPORT?

Q As a new manager, how can I get personal support in an environment that feels unsafe and untrustworthy?

A A powerful way to develop support is to establish networking relationships with other professionals. Networking uses your abilities to assist others or be assisted by them to obtain your desired outcomes. Using the collaborative relationships of networking enables you to validate data and enhances access to "inside" information.

To develop a networking relationship with others, you must be willing to broaden personal perspectives, explore the various environments for networking, focus on those that are most helpful, attend meetings and conferences that encourage networking relationships, seek out new contacts as well as affirming current ones when the opportunity arises, and support others in a networking relationship.

Gradually, through networking relationships built both internal to the organization and external to it, you can develop the support base needed in your work environment.

J O'MALLEY

New Nurse Managers

♦ HOW CAN I HELP ORIENT A NEW NURSE MANAGER?

Q What should be included in orienting new managers to the manager role? I'm referring to key information, change in socialization at work, and preparing them emotionally for the challenges of hiring, firing, counseling, and loss of buddies at work.

A In the past, to become a nurse manager a nurse had to suffer a rite of passage much like the hazing associated with initiation into a sorority or a fraternity. Candidates were suspect and belittled until they demonstrated the prescribed ability to recite company lines; skills were not shared until the nurses proved that they could survive an initial period of isolation. All the while, these new nurse managers were mourning the loss of old familiar roles and their old staff nurse friends.

Now we've moved on from those times and values. Several provisions can minimize the trauma of role transition and promote a successful promotion:
1. Provide learning sessions to acquire conceptual and technical knowledge essential for carrying out the job. Budgeting, scheduling, and giving performance appraisals are perceived by new managers as frightening and difficult processes to learn. The daily interpersonal skills that managers rely on most, such as assertiveness, coaching, and conflict management, must also be learned.
2. Assign a willing experienced "buddy manager" to act as a role model and coach.
3. Welcome the new manager to the established ranks through formal meetings and frequent informal get-togethers. These are rituals that help managers to feel supported and accepted by their new group.
4. Outline new responsibilities as comprehensively as possible in a written job description. Be explicit about the ambiguities inherent to the managerial role. The new manager has to understand and learn to cope with the ambiguity and conflict that accompany the role.
5. Allow new managers to spend orientation time off of their own units and on units of more experienced managers. Let them observe competent nurse managers in their daily interactions.
6. Arrange for off-unit time to acquire key concepts and core skills of management. Provide opportunities for continuing education sessions afterward.
7. Schedule private time with other managers so that new managers can discuss the application of theoretic bases for management.
8. Phase in the management responsibilities gradually if possible.
9. Keep your office door open to guide and support new managers. Be available, supportive, and nonjudgmental.

RG HESS

◆ WHICH SKILL DEVELOPMENT IS A PRIORITY FOR NEW NURSE MANAGERS?

Q As a very recently hired nurse manager, which skills should I focus on developing now?

A The answer to this question depends on work that you and your supervisor must do together: develop mutually agreed upon performance goals for you. The first step is to review your current job description so that you are clear about what the organization expects from you as a manager. Many health care organizations have widely varying expectations of their nurse managers, and to be successful you need to meet the expectations and requirements that your organization sets forth. For example, common job functions for nurse managers include staff development, personnel management, staffing and scheduling, and budgeting. However, in some organizations nurse managers do not have budget responsibility, but they may be expected to provide direct patient care.

Next, you and your supervisor need to assess the particular needs of your specific area of line responsibility. Perhaps there is currently a high number of new graduates on your unit who require assistance with skill building, coaching, and teaching. Or maybe you have just replaced a very laissez-faire manager who has left a unit with little or no structure in place, and policies, procedures, and standards need to be developed.

Whatever the specific unit issues, you and your supervisor will need to establish priorities and agree on corrective action plans. Each problem may require different skills from you. Finally, you and your supervisor should evaluate your capabilities in relationship to the expected job competencies, and the identified unit priorities, and then agree on those areas of performance in which you will need support, additional training, or periodic coaching. For instance, you may have excellent skills in scheduling, but you never really had to develop or monitor a budget. Or perhaps you feel very comfortable assisting a new nurse in orientation, but you have a unit with very low turnover and few new staff requiring orientation.

Once you know the match between your skills and knowledge and the specific organizational skills and knowledge needed, you and your supervisor can agree on an action plan. This plan should be regularly reassessed with your supervisor and should be changed or modified as the organization, the unit, and you develop.

MC ALDERMAN

◆ HOW DO I PRIORITIZE NURSE MANAGER'S FUNCTIONS?

Q As a new nurse manager, I feel like I am expected to be everything to everyone. How can I prioritize functions and roles so that I can master the most essential skills or roles first?

A One of the first things that any good nurse manager learns is that she can't be everything to everybody without failing at her job. A manager who believes that it is her primary job to run around and put out the fires is out of touch with her real responsibilities. The first and most critical need in this situation is for you to understand your role.

A good nurse manager primarily manages three main areas: human, material, and fiscal resources. She manages these areas by developing processes and systems that will organize these resources and make them available in the appropriate mix and number so that the employees can do the work that is necessary, in our case, provide patient care. Inherent in this role is the need for the manager to develop and implement processes that will work independent of her constant intervention. She must develop systems that work toward empowering her employees. In other words, she should be intervening only when the system fails. Once the initial problem is resolved, her long-term focus should be on how to fix the system or process so that it will work without her intervention next time. No system will be 100% perfect, but over time the number of crises in which the nurse manager needs to intervene should decline. This "focus on the system and process" type style is the best long-term strategy to get the job done today while also planning for the future, when we will all be asked to do more with fewer resources.

CCC LEVENS

◆ HOW CAN I KEEP UP WITH CURRENT AFFAIRS THAT AFFECT HEALTH CARE DELIVERY?

Q How do I as a manager stay abreast of external factors affecting my acute care setting? How do

I lobby the legislature? How do I keep abreast of legisla-tion? How do I keep staff apprised of external forces influencing change?

A One of the best ways to stay involved with external events is by joining a professional nursing organization such as the National League for Nursing, the American Nurses Association, or your specialty nursing organization. Remember, as a nurse manager and leader, it is important to encourage your staff to get involved. Professional nursing affiliations offer many opportunities for involvement in the legislative process and provide you with information on state and federal initiatives.

Through your nursing organization you will have access to information and strategies for successful lobbying. Most organizations hold membership lobbying sessions where you can participate with your colleagues at the state or federal legislatures. Your voice is important. There is strength in numbers, and the nation's two million nurses are a force to be reckoned with.

P MARALDO

◆ WHAT CAN I DO TO RELIEVE TENSION BETWEEN MYSELF AND A FORMER MANAGER WHO NOW WORKS FOR ME?

Q I have recently become the manager of a department in which the previous manager has stepped down and is now a staff member. She has a great deal more knowledge about the department and the institution than I do, and I find that I am tense in her presence. I also notice that she seems tense and sometimes looks quite put off when I announce decisions and new policies. What can I do to ease this situation so we can both be more comfortable?

A Taking over the management of a department is a challenge that demands patience and flexibility. Having the former manager remain in the department does pose an interesting dilemma but must be seen within the broader challenge of role entry and establishing credibility.

As the new manager, you should sit down with your supervisor and develop a plan for orientation

and entry. Within this specific plan, one of the possible barriers to establishing immediate credibility may be the presence of the former manager. You should discuss possible strategies for handling this delicate situation and ask for ideas and feedback from other managers who know and have worked with her in the past. Do not focus exclusively on this situation because other members of the department will begin to see that their needs or talents may not be recognized.

Meeting with this individual and others within the department to establish a relationship will assist in this process. Acknowledging her level of experience and influence within the department and organization is important but should not be seen as a deterrent to assumption of the role. Encourage her to participate in improving the department. Learn more about her as an individual, and ask her about future goals.

Assuming leadership for a department requires patience and skill and an ability to look beyond the approval of others for satisfaction. Use goals of the entry plan to evaluate success in combination with evaluating the atmosphere of the department and general indicators such as productivity and patient care outcomes.

AMT BROOKS

◆ HOW CAN I CRITICIZE FORMER PEERS WITHOUT HURTING OUR RELATIONSHIP?

Q I was recently promoted to nurse manager on the unit where I started out as a new graduate 5 years ago. It's hard for me to give critical feedback to my former peers. What do you suggest?

A By reviewing and identifying the role the unit plays in the hospital's strategic plan, compliance with JCAHO standards, nursing care standards, and policies and procedures, everyone will have a better understanding of the job responsibilities and accountability. Make sure the staff understand your job responsibilities in your new role. Be honest with the staff about your feelings. Once the responsibilities and accountability are defined, you must then determine if the people are qualified to perform according to expectations.

As problems occur, the reason for each problem must be identified. Are additional training and resources needed to support the staff? Otherwise, you must determine the reason for unacceptable performance. As a manager, it becomes your responsibility to deal with issues that interfere with performance and affect patient care. This may be difficult at times. The more clearly the expectations are defined, the more the responsibility is placed on the individual. Although giving critical feedback may not be any easier, you know it is objective and fair to everyone. Gaining trust and respect is vital to the effectiveness of the manager.

SH SMITH

No Code Orders

♦ **HOW DO I APPROACH A PHYSICIAN WHO IS RELUCTANT TO GIVE A NO CODE ORDER?**

Q We have a terrible problem with a physician on our unit who refuses to ever give a no code even though there have been several serious indications for this approach. Patients have been disadvantaged by this refusal. How do we break through and approach this issue?

A I would try to set up a time to talk about it with this physician when she does *not* have a patient on the work area. Talking theory is always easier than talking about people we know. I would meet with the physician alone. Your goal is to talk philosophy. I start here because, whether we like it or not, most of our views are guided by our own beliefs. It is only through dialogue with others that we learn about other views and that it may be acceptable to do something for a patient that we would not do for ourselves or our family. What is important is that we do what the patient wants.

Next, use the ethics committee if you have one in your facility. Ethics committees can help medical and nursing staff open a dialogue about the philosophic issues of no code orders, as well as be consultants for specific cases. Often the issues that arise are communication problems between staff and physicians, between staff and family, or between physicians and patients and/or families. Sometimes patients will tell the nurse that they do not want anything more done, but they never mention this to the physician. Often a conference with the nurse who works most closely with the patient, the patient or a family member, social worker, physician, and a representative from the ethics committee can sort out the communication problems. Each person feels strongly about the "rightness" of his or her own beliefs. The goal in ethics consultations is not to prove who is right but to identify the issues, perspectives, and the patient's preferences.

If you have access to a medical ethicist, she may be helpful in discussion with the physician you spoke of in your question. The approach I have seen ethicists use deals more with identifying issues and views. I have found it to be quite helpful for nurses, physicians, patients, and families.

The Patient Self-Determination Act requires that we ask patients for their preferences regarding a living will and special power of attorney. If patients have expressed a preference, we are required to abide by it. The risk management department of your hospital may be helpful to you in working with the legal requirements of the Self-Determination Act, as well as with physician and staff education about the Act. The American Association for Retired Persons (AARP) may also be a resource for information about this in your community.

Patients and families have rights; they can choose to change providers if the course of action they desire is not adhered to. However, this is not to encourage patients to change physicians. First I would encourage dialogue with all concerned and the use of an ethics committee. If the patient and family are still unhappy, they may chose to change care providers. The problem with this is that a new provider is probably going to be reluctant to come in right away and establish a no code order.

There is one other point: sometimes we think the quality of life of a patient is wretched; we think it would be better to be dead. However, your opinion, mine, and the physician's are of little importance. It is the desire of the patient (and *no one else*) that should prevail. Sometimes the patient is unable to articulate his or her wishes and we rely on the family to tell us what the patient wanted. Sometimes the

N

family has documentation (a living will or special power of attorney), and sometimes they do not but they can make a compelling case for their knowledge of the patient's desire. Our role and the physician's role are to carry out the wishes of the patient. If we do not know or are unsure of the patient's wishes, the current thinking in the United States is that it is better to maintain life.

M PECK

◆ HOW DO I INITIATE DISCUSSION OF THE HOSPITAL'S NO CODE ORDERS?

Q Our nursing staff is uncomfortable with the no code order policy in the organization. They feel that it lacks a communication and interaction between nurses, physicians, and others who have accountability for patient care services. Instead of no code, they would like to establish a mechanism for dialogue regarding patients' needs that reflect varying levels of care. Is this possible? If so, how might we begin such a process?

A End-of-life issues are always emotionally charged. Our society has a difficult time accepting death as a part of the life cycle. We have many more persons living into elderly years of life and much more technology to assist in keeping people alive longer. Only recently have we had "ethics" added to the list of hospital committees to help deal with the complexities associated with such issues.

Patient rights should include a say in the amount of technology employed to sustain life, and yet, those decisions are not always made in advance—despite the work done on living wills.

It is possible to create a structured process that involves dialogue surrounding levels of care for no code orders. Caution needs to be used, however, because there can be much confusion on the part of caregivers who must expedite the wishes of the patients involved. Too many unclear code levels can lead to difficulties in practice. One suggestion is to write a series of "if/then" statements for the patient and family to agree or disagree with in regard to their wishes. This can involve levels of treatment as well as types of technology utilized in code responses.

The best way to begin discussions on the change in this policy is to involve the ethics committee as well as any physician–nurse committees in place within the institution. Key supportive physicians can assist in the process by discussing the idea with other physicians. Within a shared governance system, discussions are helpful within the unit practice councils and large council meetings. The policy change, if and when it is made, needs to be clearly inserviced to all staff before implementation. Ongoing evaluation is necessary.

MT SINNEN

Nurse–Physician Relationships

◆ HOW CAN I DEVELOP PARTNERSHIP WITH PHYSICIANS IF THEY FEEL I DIMINISH THEIR POWER BASE?

Q How can I build true clinical partnership with nurses and physicians for collaborative planning when I am perceived as draining their power base?

A Power is defined as the ability and willingness to effect an outcome. The more one can influence another to change, the more power one is perceived as having. Some basic principles of power that are important to keep in mind as you begin the change process are the following:
1. Power relationships change over time.
2. Power is always limited.
3. The ends of power cannot be separated from the means.

This last principle relates to the importance of remembering that how you manage the process is equally as important as the outcome you desire in achieving the partnership.

Kanter, in her book, *Men and Women of the Corporation,* discusses the four power dimensions of a job. With each of the power dimensions, I will mention behaviors to consider as you work toward your goal of partnership. The first characteristic is visibility, or the extent to which your work is known in the organization. Because of the power of identification, it is important that influential people are aware of your contribution to the organization. If the physician sees you identified with someone of equal or greater power, she will more likely seek to collaborate with you, rather than compete against you. Relevance, or the value of your job to pressing organizational issues, is the second dimension. Take time to identify two to four crucial issues physicians will face in the next 3 years and determine what role nursing can play in addressing them. Another way of partnering is to form a coalition with the physicians to put pressure on a third party for a change benefitting the physicians. The third dimension is autonomy, or the amount of discretion in your job. What decision that could expand your discretionary authority could benefit the physicians? Look for opportunities for nursing to take initiatives that would demonstrate concern for patients and improve the functioning of a systems environment for the physicians.

The last dimension is relationships, or supports and alliances on the job. Examine what contacts you have within and outside the organization that could be of value or benefit to the physicians. Consider how you can use these, or trade on them, to improve patient care or the physician practice climate.

Changing a nurse/physician culture to one of collaboration is a 3- to 5-year process with a lot of backstepping along the way. Measure the cost and benefits before you decide to take the risks necessary to change, but also remember the importance of persuading the physicians that they will benefit and have something better than what they now have. In order to do that, you will have to sell the physicians on the benefit of the changes for them.

VD LACHMAN

◆ HOW CAN I ENCOURAGE COLLEGIAL RELATIONSHIPS BETWEEN PHYSICIANS AND NURSES?

Q Some physicians interact professionally and collegially with the nurses on my unit, while others tend to bully, manipulate, and dominate relation-

ships. What are some specific ways that the "good behavior" can be rewarded and encouraged?

A Physicians are people, no better and no worse than other people. Like most people, they usually respond to adult behavior with adult behavior. An atmosphere of colleagueship is likely to be valued by everyone in it and certainly, in health care, patients benefit from that kind of environment. Physicians not accustomed to adult, collegial relationships with nurses need new experiences. Nurses who remain composed, do not avoid physicians, and actively engage physicians in meaningful consultation about patients are most often responded to in kind. Those few physicians whose behavior is inappropriate should be treated as politely and calmly as possible. Any behavior that is indicative of harassment or negatively affects patients should be documented and reported. In those instances you may be able to at least forge a truce. Keep in mind that changing well-established patterns of communication requires that everyone in the situation—staff and physicians alike—change their behavior.

M MURPHY

◆ HOW DO I RESOLVE DISAGREEMENT BETWEEN PHYSICIANS' AND STAFF'S APPROACH TO PATIENT CARE?

Q How can I improve nurse–physician relationships for myself and the staff I work with in an environment in which physicians are often rude, demanding, and unwilling to communicate regarding patient care issues?

A As with any working environment, it is important that clear boundaries be defined and communicated regarding appropriate conduct on everyone's part. Poor behavior on the part of physicians is often a symptom of other operational issues that they are dissatisfied with, and a permissive climate that has not set limits on this conduct. Physicians' behavior is often *learned* from having issues and concerns responded to only when they become loud and uncooperative.

The first and best preventive measure that you can take as a manager to change physician behavior is to actively solicit and seek out physician input. Physicians should be consulted on aspects of care that affect their patients by the nurse manager and staff. This should not be misinterpreted as having physicians approving nursing practice—related issues. In return, nursing can and should demand behavior that is appropriate to a collegial relationship. Administration and the medical staff governing body must provide support and firm physician discipline if necessary to promote a professional climate of mutual respect and trust. Nursing's contribution to this relationship must be respectful and professional at all times, regardless of physician conduct. I have seen nursing staff who were unified in their efforts significantly overhaul physician behavior through an organized and planned program of "behavior modification." The nurses' single most effective weapon was to reward those physicians who behaved professionally toward the nursing staff.

C BRADLEY

◆ HOW DO I DEAL WITH AN OBNOXIOUS PHYSICIAN?

Q I am a nurse manager of the intensive care unit. The physician in charge of this unit for the past 10 years is egotistical, obnoxious, and verbally abusive to the nurses I supervise. On occasion I have spoken with him about his behavior. He responds with profanity and says he will "get me fired." What should I do?

A Obviously this has been going on for a number of years and I am assuming that you have brought this behavior to the attention of your immediate supervisor and others in authority who should be aware of this problem. That such a situation has been allowed to persist must be difficult for you, especially since the hospital is an employer of professionals and has an obligation to facilitate professional practice, which must be hampered by this behavior.

In this day of litigation regarding workplace harassment, it would seem very important that you begin a paper trail. This means documenting the date, time, place, and people involved when the physician engages in this behavior. You also may need to document the times you have brought this situation to the attention of your supervisor.

However, litigation is not the only, nor the first, route to take. A creative informal approach may provide an effective solution. Approaches have been described by nurses who have put a plan in place to respond to a difficult situation. For example, when staff are aware that the doctor is engaging in this behavior, a prearranged signal is sent out and as many staff as can be made available come and stand around the person being harassed. Such disruptive behavior is a little hard to continue if you have an audience. Another way may be to videotape the encounter when the physician is making a scene and replay it for him at a time that is less confusing. There may be a number of issues that this doctor is dealing with, but there is no excuse for this kind of behavior.

Your concern about his ability to carry out his threat to have you fired is an important issue and one you do need to pay attention to. You will need to assess the willingness of your staff to stand together to bring about changes in his behavior.

You may provide the physician with a copy of a research article that was published on the mortality rates in intensive care units and the relationship to the collaborative nature of the medical and nursing staff. In the article there was a finding of lower mortality rates in those units where the doctors and nurses worked collaboratively than in those in which there was less collaboration. Perhaps a search of the literature would provide some other suggestions, specifically literature related to empowerment strategies.

Ten years is a long time for this type of behavior to exist. The management and human resource literature emphasizes the need to make sure there is a positive working environment, supportive of mutual respect. The foundations of this collaboration need to be established within the educational programs of medicine and nursing where the socialization of the professional has its roots. This is a long-range solution and one we all need to strive to achieve (Cox, 1987, 1991; Pence & Cantrall, 1990).

SR. M FINNICK

◆ HOW CAN I EDUCATE AN OLDER PHYSICIAN WHO PERSISTS IN VIEWING THE NURSE AS THE DOCTOR'S HANDMAIDEN?

Q We have an older, prominent physician who is a major admitter and is from the "old school."

He still expects the nurses to carry his charts and play a subservient role to him. How can I work with him to change his behavior and expectations without offending him?

A In order for you to persuade someone to change his behavior, you have to have two pieces of information. The first is the knowledge of the person's value system. You determine what a person's value system is by watching his behavior and listening to the words that indicate what is important to him. For example, one could conclude from your doctor's behavior and requests that he values subservient nurses. Equally possible is that what he values is being treated with respect, and these "subservient behaviors" are indicative to him of being treated with respect. If he values subservient behavior, then I would search for what else he values. For example, perhaps he values not being bothered for problems that could be taken care of using nursing judgment. If that is the case, I'd point out how protocols, or critical pathways, could enable nurses to take action with guidelines that he and nursing establish. I'd also use every opportunity to tell him of situations in which a nurse's assertiveness solved a problem for his patients. Once you can figure out what he values, and speak to that value, then you are one step closer to persuading him to change.

The second piece of information that you have to obtain is what he sees as the benefits of the change for him, not for nursing. Knowing what his highest values are, you then sell to those values. For example, if he values being respected, then I would take opportunities to treat him with respect in front of his patients, their families, and his peers. By acknowledging his exemplary skills and his contributions to the organization, you show a high regard. The key is to show high regard for what he values.

VD LACHMAN

♦ **HOW SHOULD I RESPOND IF A PHYSICIAN BERATES ME PUBLICLY?**

Q What do I do when a physician berates me in front of other physicians and staff?

A Breathe! There are many ways to address this. It is appropriate to state in a normal tone of voice something like: "It is not acceptable for you to talk to me that way. I am willing to discuss this with you in private." Then walk to a private space to finish the discussion. Another approach is to say: "I will not remain while you make derogatory remarks about me. I am willing to discuss your concerns and would like to do that in private." Most people will stop and listen if your tone is firm, but not out of control. It may help to practice with a colleague who can play your part while you play the physician and vice versa. This technique lets you try both sides without the emotion. Your colleague must be someone who will role-play it seriously with you. If you have consistently negative interactions with a specific individual, you might ask a colleague to observe and then help you role-play a better way to respond.

If you did not address the problem when it happened, or if this is a long-standing problem, you may want to address it with the individual at a time when you are not already involved in a negative interaction. It is just as appropriate to approach the physician at a quiet time, or to make an appointment with the physician, and tell that person that you want to discuss your working relationship. You should have a script, especially if you are nervous about this, so that you say what you want to in objective terminology. For example,

I need to talk to you about our interactions on the unit. When you made rounds on Mrs. Jones you noted that her I&O was not totaled, then said to me, 'What the hell is the matter with you, can't you even add? I wish we had decent nurses on this unit.' I understand why you are frustrated with not having I&O totals; I will address this with the staff and identify the problems. However, I am unwilling to be insulted by you. Yelling and derogatory remarks are not acceptable.

I think you will find most physicians will respond to this statement. You may want to find out what the other issues of concern are for this physician.

If none of this works, your supervisor, the human resources department, and the president of the medical staff are all sources of assistance available to you in dealing with this. These resources can assist you in an objective assessment of the interactions and in seeking common ground that you and the physician can identify in order to work together. Be careful not to "give the problem" to someone else to solve for you. You want to ask others to work *with* you so that the communication problem gets resolved to your satisfaction and to that of the physician involved.

M PECK

N

♦ HOW CAN I IMPROVE NURSE–PHYSICIAN RELATIONSHIPS?

Q We are told that physicians are one of the consumers of our organization and that we must strive to meet their needs. How do you do this and still empower yourself and your staff to assertively deal with situations in which there is disagreement with the physicians' approach to the patient and staff?

A This is probably the most difficult question of all for nurse managers. The answer lies in using two problem-solving approaches. The first approach is the actions to be taken by yourself and your staff. As the manager, you need to do an assessment of both your and your staff's verbal as well as nonverbal communication and assertiveness styles. No person can be empowered who is not ready to accept it, and not all wish to be empowered. If the staff are unevenly balanced between those who wish to engage in professional and assertive behaviors and those who do not, the physician(s) will divide and conquer and nothing much will be achieved. The degree to which the imbalance exists is the degree to which the staff must be worked with in terms of their professional responsibilities to the patient, their job description, and their personal wishes.

Outside educational programs on conflict negotiation, assertiveness, and the professional role are a necessary foundation that must be in place before the physician issues can be successfully addressed. It is very important during this stage that the staff are consistently reminded that the only thing under discussion at this point is learning through discussion and role playing how to increase their comfort level and supportive actions for each other. While learning to increase their own comfort level they should also be aware of the second approach going into effect when the unit is united in its new communication styles.

The second approach relies on using the hospital governance to effect change at the physician level. It is very important for both the medical and nursing staffs to understand that the problem is not nurses in conflict with the medical staff or vice versa but a serious problem with multidisciplinary team effort that ultimately will cause problems with patient care. With this approach in mind, the nurse manager reviews the medical staff bylaws, and the roles and re-

sponsibilities of the various chiefs in ensuring the quality and appropriate ness of care provided by physicians on staff. Using this information, either the vice president of nursing or the manager can approach the chief of staff for suggestions for handling situations in which care is suspect.

The solutions can range from frank and open discussion in the presence of the vice president and chief of staff or the service to a formal complaint, calling the chief of the service when a questionable order is written. If a physician is always on the cutting edge of new trends about which the staff has no knowledge and is therefore uncomfortable, the physician should be asked to provide technical articles and inservice training as a means of ensuring familiarity. The physician should be told in a nonthreatening manner that the nurse must legally question orders about which she is in doubt, and upon not getting appropriate reassurances has been requested by management to call the chief of services for authorization before proceeding. Formal complaints and documentation of any negative incidents should be placed in the physician's file for review when annual privileges are discussed. The hospital administration and lawyer should be kept apprised in serious situations.

S LENKMAN

♦ ARE THERE PROBLEMS INHERENT IN PHYSICIANS' GRADUAL DECREASE IN HOSPITAL CONTROL?

Q As nurses increase in participative ways in the system, it appears that the degree of control doctors have over hospital operations has decreased. Has this balancing or leveling created some problems for staff nurses and nursing managers with the medical staffs?

A There are many individuals who would question whether physicians have, in fact, decreased their degree of control over hospital operations and whether nursing's control has increased. The physician's role as the hospital's primary customer, and therefore the main source of patients and revenue, is vital. The traditional hospital system does not generally encourage or provide opportunities for true col leagueship. However, although the balance of control is not equal, the balance has shifted.

As nurses both demand and exert more professional autonomy, physicians can become defensive and critical. This can certainly create problems for both the nursing staff and the manager. Collaborative practice models that enjoin physicians and nurses in focused discussions regarding roles can be extremely valuable in overcoming resistance. However, they will not alone provide the necessary support to move from the physician-dominated hierarchic model present in most traditional hospitals. In order to truly move forward, a completely different kind of organizational arrangement will be necessary.

C ST CHARLES

◆ HOW DO I HANDLE OBSTRUCTIVE AND NONCOOPERATIVE PHYSICIANS?

Q When working with improving critical thinking on the part of the staff, how do I deal with uncooperative or blatantly obstructive physicians?

A If possible, speak to the physician in private. Explain that you understand she is upset and you want to address the issue. Listen carefully to what is being said. At that point, do not become defensive or offer excuses. Inform her that you will check into the situation and get back her in a specified time period. Use "I" statements rather than "you" statements. If the physician remains uncooperative and obstructive, document and discuss the situation with your director. The medical staff and administration should have a mechanism in place to deal with unacceptable behavior.

Positive relations may be nurtured by addressing issues of interest or concern to the physician. Asking for suggestions and feedback is important. When seeking support for a project or important issue, provide options, with advantages and disadvantages for each option.

SH SMITH

◆ HOW CAN I HELP INVOLVE STAFF IN PHYSICIANS' PROBLEM SOLVING?

Q Some physicians in our hospital feel that when there is a problem on the units, the nurse man-

ager should be the only person that they deal with to solve the problem. Staff feel that the physicians should come to them. The nurse managers have approached the physicians on this topic and they say, "It just takes too much time to deal with all those staff nurses to solve a problem." How can we get physicians to involve the staff in problem solving?

A The nurse manager is key to effective physician–staff communications and dispute resolutions. Before handling a dispute, nurse managers should ensure that the parties involved have exhausted their personal resources. It is not acceptable for physicians to bypass direct communications with individual nurses. Don't let anyone undermine teamwork under any circumstance or for any reason.

However, people generally work best with individuals they feel close to and trust. Again, the nurse manager can make the difference in this situation. With guidance and encouragement from the nurse manager, physicians and staff may begin to problem solve together, feel comfortable with each other, and establish trusting working relationships.

Time and multiple close working contacts will provide the solutions to this problem. Establish joint practice programs, interdisciplinary rounds, and even social mixers to help break down barriers to communication and increase contact between staff and physicians. Also, too often nurses lack confidence to approach physicians and discuss problems with them. Encourage staff by coaching them so they can understand how best to approach their colleagues, and then support them through the process. Give positive reinforcement to both staff and physicians when problem solving first occurs, and reward the positive behavior by using it as an example.

P MARALDO

Organ Donation

◆ HOW CAN I HELP MY STAFF FEEL MORE CONFIDENT WHEN DISCUSSING ORGAN DONATIONS?

Q Some of my staff are uncomfortable about approaching family members regarding organ donation. What can I do to help?

A The question of organ donation is fraught with many personal and social values, beliefs, and religious implications for individuals and their families. Little can be done to eliminate these considerations. However, carefully executed protocols can simplify the process.

Every hospital should have policies that outline the legal and process implications and expectations for organ donation. Following these guidelines ensures that the nurse complies with the law and the organization's strategies for appropriate handling of organ donations. Beyond that, the relationship to the patient and the family becomes critical to the success of obtaining permission for organ donation.

The best approach is to ensure that your state's protocols for organ donation are clear to the donor. Most states have a simple way to give consent for organ donation, usually on the back of the driver's license. Further, as early as possible in the process of admission or in the care relationship with the patient, the caregiver should obtain information regarding willingness to donate organs. Some organizations have these questions as part of the nursing admission assessment process. In their clinical specialties, other organizations have questions regarding specific organs and the patient's willingness to donate them. As much as possible, the nurse should have such supporting protocols available as far in advance of the time of "harvesting" organs as possible.

The most challenging time to try and obtain organ donation is at the time of death or when the patient is in the last stages of life. The emotional issues affecting the key decision makers at the time impede their focus on organ donation. Sometimes the caregiver can appear insensitive when addressing the issue at these critical times. However, a couple of strategies can be suggested:

1. The nurse might communicate with a family member who appears to be supporting, coordinating, or managing the family's legal or functional issues in the hospital. Establishing a relationship with this person early in the patient's hospitalization can offset some of the emotional impact of the request. Your involvement with the attending physician, who should assume key responsibility for this, facilitates appropriate communication regarding organ donation.

2. Often an organ donation can serve to assure the family that the patient lives on in a special way or makes a meaningful contribution to the life of an-

other or others. This message can be especially powerful to family members who want to find meaning and value in the death of their loved one. In the same way the dying person may know that a way exists to continue to contribute after death and leave a powerful personal legacy. This approach brings meaning to the donation and allows a very personal contribution that reflects the value of the dying person's desire to bestow his or her gift to another's life.

Organ donation is a very valuable part of facilitating health and healing. It can be a significant contribution by the donor, which should be the foundation for any discussion with patient or family regarding organ donation. The care team should work in concert to deal sensitively with patient and family regarding the possibility of organ donation. Advanced protocols and processes should be planned by the care team to address this process with expertise and care.

T PORTER-O'GRADY

OSHA Guidelines

◆ **HOW DO I KNOW IF WE ARE IN COMPLIANCE WITH OCCUPATIONAL SAFETY AND HEALTH ADMINISTRATION (OSHA) GUIDELINES FOR BLOOD-BORNE PATHOGENS?**

Q As a nurse manager, what do I need to know to ensure that we are in compliance with the OSHA guidelines for blood-borne pathogens?

A It is increasingly simple to comply with infection control standards, especially those related to blood-borne pathogens. The guidelines from both OSHA and the Centers for Disease Control and Prevention (CDC) are based on the concept of *universal precautions.* These precautions focus specifically on preventing the spread of blood-borne disease and seek to protect both the infected person and the caregiver. These precautions relate to the application of appropriate barriers and insist that such standards be applied universally to protect anyone from the spread of any blood-borne disease.

Because of the spread of life-threatening blood-borne diseases, protective measures are increasingly important. However, such measures should be in keeping with the disease's severity, risk, and nature. For example, the routes of transmission of human immunodeficiency virus (HIV) are clear and specific. When universal precautions and safer sex guidelines are complied with, the disease is virtually impossible to spread. When these precautions are not applied consistently every time contact is established, the risk of transmission is accelerated.

It is important and sometimes difficult to ensure that universal precautions are used faithfully each time contact is established. Although blood-borne diseases may have various characteristics and transmission behaviors, any failure to be continuous and rigorous with regard to universal precautions increases risk of harm to both staff and patient. Managers should access their infection control specialist or risk manager for assistance in the establishment of a policy and practice regarding protection from bacterial and viral blood-borne disease. Education and evaluation of staff compliance are important quality assurance activities and should be incorporated into any quality improvement process.

T PORTER-O'GRADY

Participative Management

◆ WHEN CAN CONSENSUS BE USED TO MAKE MANAGEMENT DECISIONS?

Q In the process of participatory management, at what point does a manager ask for consensus or, instead, simply make a management decision? What is consensus?

A *Consensus* is the agreement on opinion of all or almost all people consulted on a decision. In a work situation, consensus also generally implies that all agree to accept the decision and to work together in its implementation. Making decisions by consensus

has the advantages of disseminating knowledge about and rationale for the decision, engendering commitment to implementation, empowering staff, and communicating the actions to be taken. However, achieving consensus can be an extremely time-consuming process, especially when opinions vary greatly at the onset. Consensus is not necessarily a condition of participative management, since participative management implies that staff are involved in planning, priority setting, and decision making, but the actual decisions may be made by a democratic majority rather than through a consensus process.

This background on consensus demonstrates the essence of the reason for this question. Generally speaking, if the decision to be made has relatively low impact (little risk involved) and little need exists for information concerning the decision, a managerial decision is appropriate. The situation is more complicated when both these conditions are not met. For example, a situation may involve low impact, but everyone needs to be aware of the decision and assist with its implementation (e.g., the bar-coding system for charges is to be changed, thus necessitating a period when two systems are in place, and care must be taken to ensure charges are appropriately accounted for). Alternately, the decision's impact may be widespread, but little assistance is needed with implementation (e.g., the food-service vendor's contract changes, altering the menus available, but actually changing vendors is totally implemented by a few administrative personnel). In these situations the need for consensus must be determined on a case-by-case basis, erring on the side of more rather than less consensus to minimize the potential for lack of cooperation with implementation and for sabotage.

In the final situation, when the risk and impact as well as the need for information are high, every attempt should be made to achieve consensus. In these situations, even the democratic process of the majority may not be sufficient for smooth implementation.

In all these difficult situations, the management decision may still be needed to move the group off center when considerable time has elapsed and no consensus has been reached. Managerial decisions made under these circumstances must be carefully monitored during the implementation phase.

JW ALEXANDER

P

◆ ARE THERE CHANGES THAT CAN BE MADE IN PERFORMANCE EVALUATIONS THAT WILL INCREASE THEIR EFFECTIVENESS?

Q Are there any changes in the future regarding performance evaluations that would make them more effective and meaningful? Right now they seem to accomplish so little of value.

A Almost nothing stirs up as much contention as performance evaluations because there is so much emotional content in the process and so much riding on the outcome in terms of value, contribution, and pay increases. There has been much written on their value and how to make them more effective, yet there still seems to be much uncertainty about them.

Many changes in approaches to performance evaluation will be occurring. Organizations are focusing increasingly on outcome strategies for validating performance rather than performance activities themselves. In the past, performance activities served as the basis for making judgments about a worker's value and contribution. If the worker complied with the activity standards and had a lot of energy and didn't challenge the sensibilities of the manager or the system, she received a good performance review. Research over the years has shown that this really didn't contribute much to the productivity or goals of either the organization or the worker.

Increasingly there has been much doubt cast on the value of process-based performance evaluation activities. As the orientation to work focuses more on outcomes, there is increasing interest in assessing performance in relation to the focus on outcomes. Flexibility in work and roles becomes a key to performance when the emphasis is on outcomes. Therefore defining work process detail on the assumption that it won't change becomes very ineffective. The worker should freely adjust work processes to meet the ever-changing demands reflected in shifting outcomes. Outcome-oriented role expectations and evaluation processes will likely increasingly become the basis for individual performance evaluation. In the context of this process there will be more emphasis on achievement of goals, contribution to the organization, financial impact, and service enhancements.

With the movement to continuous improvement in organizations there is less emphasis on individual performance evaluation. The use of team-based approaches is becoming an important strategy for organizing and performing work. The team becomes the focus of performance and function. Individual roles are viewed in the context of the team's activities and relationships. Performance evaluation, rather than focus on the individual, centers on the performance of the team in relationship to its achievement of predefined outcomes. Individual relationships and team interactions are judged by team members, and issues of compliance, goal achievement, and team member interaction are the obligation of the team to sort out. The role of the manager is directed to assisting the team in evaluating its achievements and outcomes as well as looking at barriers to enhanced functioning and goal achievement. If the team has problems with performance or relationships, the manager assists them in focusing and seeking solutions as well as developing strategies for enhancement of their interaction and achievements. Rather than performance evaluation the manager focuses on team development and effectiveness. This, it is suggested, is a better, more effective way to ensure good relationships and effective performance.

No doubt there will be many innovations in performance measurement and improvement in the next decade. Work redesign, patient-centered care models, and the quality initiative will all work to create more effective ways of defining and measuring work and workers. Continued attention to group process and outcome achievement will form the context for performance for some time. If the manager stays centered on those activities, newer mechanisms for measuring performance and gaining more participation will guide the creation of effective tools for performance evaluation.

T PORTER-O'GRADY

◆ WHAT'S THE BEST WAY FOR ME TO HELP STAFF DEVELOP PROBLEM-SOLVING SKILLS?

Q Should the nurse manager provide structure (issues, problems, focus, meeting times, dates, etc.) for problem solving with staff, or should the staff be asked to do this themselves?

A Timing is everything. The nurse manager's role is to facilitate professional and personal growth and to involve staff in problem solving. This requires that the nurse manager provide opportunities for staff to develop the necessary skills before they are asked to assume responsibility.

Skill building can be a natural part of unit functioning and can enhance the quality of team-building activities. Formal classes can be offered on

- How to run a meeting.
- Role expectations of committee members.
- Decision making in a group.
- Group communication.
- Conflict resolution.

Having staff try out various roles, such as running a meeting, setting up a task force, or heading up a project, requires everyone's commitment to assist in the work and success of these efforts.

Developing a plan with the staff on assuming progressive responsibility for decision making can begin the process of changing the unit's rules and operation. Evaluation of current activities and progress made can become part of the development process.

AMT BROOKS

♦ HOW DO I GET STAFF INVOLVED IN UNIT OPERATION?

Q Our new director of nursing expects the nurse managers to get staff more involved in unit operations, problem solving, decision making, and planning. We are to develop a department-wide plan to begin this process. What is our first step?

A Education is the first step. Concurrently, however, the development of trust is essential. This trust develops only with time as the staff become aware that this level of involvement and empowerment in relation to unit operations is not a ploy to delegate work. Rather, it is a movement toward staff empowerment to improve the quality of patient care and become consistent with the efficiency of current restructuring efforts.

All education stems from the concept that administration's role is to facilitate, coordinate, and integrate the staff's ability to provide excellent patient care. Administration facilitates by ensuring that

mechanisms are in place that free the nursing staff from difficulties and impediments to achieving excellent nursing practice. Coordination occurs when administration uses mechanisms to bring order and harmonious functioning to the nursing staff. Finally, administration uses integration to bring the nursing staff together as a unified whole. Thus the nurse administrator is no longer the person in charge who plans, organizes, directs, and controls. The nurse administrator is now the person who creates the climate and environment in which the professional nurse is allowed to plan, organize, direct, and control the service of the health care organization to deliver quality patient care.

Given this overlay, which requires retooling the philosophy of some nursing administrators but which seems to be the aim of the new director, education can now begin. Assessment of staff's knowledge and skill in such areas as unit operations, budgeting, problem solving, decision making, planning, inventory management, scheduling, counselling, quality improvement, and work load management directs the nature of the educational program. An incremental approach is suggested in which increased staff involvement in one area at a time is encouraged as the assessment and educational efforts determine the staff's readiness to assume responsibility and accountability for that area.

JW ALEXANDER

♦ WHAT DO I DO IF I DISAGREE WITH DECISIONS MY EMPOWERED STAFF HAVE MADE?

P

Q Three months ago the staff on our unit started a clinical practice committee charged with setting and managing the clinical standards of care, practice, and performance for the unit. As manager, I disagree with some decisions they are making. What should I do?

A Review whether the group members are clear about their *terms of reference.* If no terms are established, you may want to assist the committee to develop them. Have you defined for them how the decision-making process will occur and who will implement the decisions? Explore whether ambiguity exists regarding their roles and administration's roles.

For yourself, it might be useful initially to explore why you disagree with their decisions, since this might give you an idea about where to intervene if necessary. Remember that this new committee is only 3 months old and is likely to have growing pains.

Most important, you must determine if the decisions are threatening patient care and safety or violating hospital policy. If so, you need to intervene in the process; however, I suspect this is not the case. You could explore the following possible options.

1. Examine your own needs. Are the decisions different from your own, and do they affect your need to be in charge? It is always difficult to give up the power of decision making, and even when we do, it is unlikely that we will initially feel comfortable. Your role here is to accept your own feelings. Whatever you do, do not get into a power struggle with the staff.

2. Do you disagree because the group's decisions appear naive? We all need to "grow into" decision making; it is a process. We often learn by making mistakes and experimenting with solutions. This group may be doing just that. If you prevent this process from occurring, you may inhibit the group's development; not only may creativity be affected, but you may end up with a group that feels powerless because their decisions are undermined. Your role here would best be teacher, supporter, and role model. Encourage the committee to reexamine their decisions, evaluate them, decide which are the strengths, and develop new plans.

3. Are the group's decisions based on a lack of understanding of management and the system? When a group does not have a grasp of how their decisions affect management practices and other departments and professionals in the system, the members are unable to make informed decisions. They may be making decisions that are beyond their mandate. Your role in this case would be teacher: one who can provide them with additional material on which to base their decisions or one who can assist them to define when they are overstepping the boundaries of their power. The group may also not understand the long-term impact of their decisions. Again, your main role

would be to assist them in looking at the ramifications of their decisions over time.

JB COLTRIN ET AL.

◆ HOW CAN I HELP MY STAFF EXPRESS DISSATISFACTION WITH A NURSING ADMINISTRATOR?

Q Our vice president of nursing is very autocratic and authoritarian. She has been known to anger easily and has fired nurse managers who have disagreed with her views. My staff are very angry at their lack of input and nursing administration's one-way communication style. They want to protest by some quiet demonstration, such as boycotting the annual awards dinner or the National Nurses Week celebration, both of which the vice president perceives as her "personal gift" to the staff. As the nurse manager, how do I support the staff, maintain my status as part of nursing administration, and not get myself fired?

A Your first priority is to assist the staff in understanding their feelings about the situation and identifying appropriate ways to act out these feelings. Once they realize the driving force behind their feelings, they can diffuse the anger and plan actions that will have positive outcomes. Boycotting the awards dinner or National Nurses Week celebration will only serve to increase tension.

Next, the staff need to identify specific areas in which they can improve their input in the nursing administration process. You can facilitate this by empowering your staff with the authority you already have as manager. Once the staff are able to demonstrate their ability to make decisions and produce quality outcomes, they will be able to approach the vice president with suggestions for giving input into nursing administration.

You may need to enlist the assistance of people who work well with the vice president when the staff are ready to take on more responsibility. Building a network of relationships with these workers will help the staff learn the strategies they need to use when they approach the vice president. These relationships will also bridge the gap in trust between the parties concerned. The staff could invite the vice president to nonthreatening discussions and staff meetings so that she can get to know them and build a relationship with them. As this relationship develops, the communication patterns should change, resulting in staff giving input to the vice president.

JG O'LEARY

◆ WHY ARE NURSES NOT CONSULTED WHEN POLICIES AFFECTING PATIENT CARE ARE ESTABLISHED?

Q Why do health care organizations continually make decisions that affect patient care without consulting nurses who are directly responsible for implementing care?

A This question has been pondered by many nurses and managers. The answer centers in the history of women's rights, the past exploitation of nurses, and the traditional bureaucratic structures within America.

Nursing has long been considered a women's job and career. Women throughout history have struggled for equality. As with other oppressed groups, most women remained quiet and subservient even as small groups of women fought hard for equality. Although women have come a long way, much still needs to be accomplished. Just look at the issue of equal pay for equal work or crimes of abuse and rape against women.

In the past, nurses were exploited to work in hospital settings. Nursing students were made to work first or while they were educated, unlike other professionals, who spent time in the university studying. As a profession, nursing has changed dramatically. Pay has increased, as have educational and job opportunities.

Bureaucratic management structures throughout history have been hierarchic. Those "at the top" made the decisions and enforced the policies. Promoted staff fell into the same routine. Little or no regard was given for employees' decision-making skills.

Fortunately, policies are changing. The advent of shared governance, participatory management styles, and continuous quality improvement has brought a new philosophy. The underlying principles include

the belief that the people closest to the work truly understand the work and therefore are in the best position to make decisions about the work. As these novel ideas infiltrate the hospital setting, nursing's voice will become strong, loud, and clear in terms of patient care. This will take time, understanding, and leadership.

MT SINNEN

Patient Advocacy

◆ HOW CAN I ENCOURAGE STAFF TO BE ADVOCATES?

Q As a nurse manager, how can I encourage the staff to be advocates? Whenever they try to do so, physicians object and react strongly, or the administration becomes upset because the nurse identified a problem that may create challenges to the physician or organization. How do we deal with this crisis?

A *Advocacy* is a matter of providing information so that people can make informed decisions. Advocacy is not about identifying problems, but about articulating choices.

Every organization has certain goals and objectives it wants to achieve. No one would be able to object to your advocacy endeavors if you could demonstrate that they are a means to achieving these goals. For example, if you could demonstrate that patient education reduces patient anxiety, which reduces complications and length of stay, and increases adherence to the medical regimen, and if one of the organization's strategic objectives is cost containment, you could link the two together: patients with education and care options tend to use less in-house services and have a shorter length of stay, resulting in a decreased cost per case. No one could argue the benefits of that type of advocacy. However, if you are advocating something that is clearly counter to the organization's goals, objectives, or values, you will not succeed.

P

Relate your advocacy activities to long-term outcomes, not short-term results. Collect and analyze data regarding the benefits of what you are advocating, and present a formal case for the issue. Take each issue as a single case; do not try to do too much at once. Always tie in what you want to do with how it will affect the organization's goals and mission. This is a key to the successful implementation of any activity.

RM HADDON

♦ HOW DO WE ESTABLISH A PATIENT ADVOCACY PROGRAM?

Q We want to establish a patient advocacy approach on our unit that would involve all the clinical providers. Our assumption is that advocacy is a process not specific to any one role. How do we establish an advocacy program that involves the primary clinical providers in patient care?

A The first step in developing such a team, provided you believe support exists for this idea, is to gather some basic information about advocacy in general and about your organization's established mechanisms for ensuring advocacy. You might use documents such as those from the Joint Commission on Accreditation of Healthcare Organizations, the American Nurses Association's Code of Ethics, the American Hospital Association's Patient Bill of Rights, and any state regulations regarding patient rights. This gives you a foundation on which to plan the specific "charge" or charter of your group and to ensure that it reflects the larger organization's and regulatory and licensing requirements.

The next step is to identify all the key stakeholders of your group. This means that you should look both vertically up and down the different levels of your organization and horizontally across different departments to find people who share a common value and interest in this work. These people will assist in smoothing the path for change and provide support for your work.

Next, you should determine the specific purpose of the group meeting, what outcomes you hope to achieve, how often and how long the group should

meet, and where and when they should meet. You also must decide who will lead the group and if the group will need to take attendance or minutes. With this basic plan in mind, you can ask your supervisor to support the use of multiple resources for this purpose, then begin to lobby with the key stakeholders. If you have been clear about the need and expectations for this group, you should find few barriers to starting and continuing it. As with all committees and work groups, periodic evaluation of its purposes and accomplishments is necessary to ensure your patient advocacy program is still contributing to the organization's goals over time.

MC ALDERMAN

Patient Care Delivery Systems

♦ HOW CAN I MAKE INFORMED DECISIONS IN A CHANGING CARE DELIVERY SYSTEM?

Q How can I as a nurse manager make informed decisions in changing care delivery systems, that is, how do I decide between primary nursing, patient-centered models, and others?

A You alone cannot make an informed, effective decision to change the care delivery system. This decision must be a collaborative effort involving input from a variety of constituents and sources. This collaborative decision-making framework promotes the enrollment of these constituents and ensures a good fit between the selected delivery model and the organization.

Before implementation of this decision-making framework, you must be certain that you are willing and able to relinquish the total control, accountability, and responsibility for decision making. It is managerial and organizational suicide to invite participation when the decision is already made or when input will not be used. In addition, it is imperative that you and the organization be committed to this change for the long term versus the short term. Also, setbacks during implementation must be viewed as learning opportunities.

The first step in this process is to solicit volunteers for a working group to collect and analyze the information needed to make this decision. In addition to yourself and staff members, you might consider requesting the participation of a nursing faculty member with expertise in management and health care trends, as well as the medical director for your unit. Critical information that the committee should consider includes:

1. The organization's mission statement.
2. The organization's strategic goals.
3. Projected budget allocations for your unit.
4. Literature review of the structure, costs, and benefits of the different delivery system.
5. Trends in the supply of and demand for health care workers.
6. Patient evaluation of care and the structure of the care environment.
7. Staff evaluation of the current delivery system and suggestions for improvement.
8. Physician evaluation of care and the organizational structure.
9. Profile of the organizational culture.
10. Benefits and problems experienced by other organizations who have implemented the care delivery system being considered.
11. Futurists' predictions regarding the type of care that will be needed.

After analysis of this information, a comparison of the different delivery models should be undertaken using the following format:

1. Major components of the delivery system.
2. Projected cost/benefit analysis in terms of quality, financial aspects, and provider and customer satisfaction.
3. Organizational fit.
4. Flexibility in responding to future changes in the health care environment.

This report serves multiple purposes. It provides the needed decision-making information and the rationale for making the decision. It also serves as a blueprint for the education needed to implement the selected model of care. Finally, the report specifies the framework for evaluation of the selected delivery system's efficiency and efficacy.

MC HANSEN

♦ HOW CAN I HELP STAFF ACCEPT A NEW APPROACH TO PATIENT CARE DELIVERY?

Q We are moving from a staff of all registered nurses (RNs) to a mix of care providers. Most of our nurses are mourning the loss of their all-RN care delivery. This is challenging our ability to be successful in implementing a multilevel system. How can I help them with the mourning process so that we can move past it to constructing a new approach to patient care delivery?

A Many of our nursing staff are understandably confused after being taught, perhaps in their academic classes or by work experience, that total patient care by RNs is the "gold standard" of nursing. They perceive that we are now asking them to revert to a lower-quality approach. Many nurses do not have the opportunity to work in different regions or in many hospitals within their own regions. They are not always aware that many nursing departments were unable to embrace the total-RN care concept but their patient care did not suffer. This lack of awareness and a very real fear of the legal consequences of others' supervision have created a difficult situation for many staff nurses. As these nurses accept the changes dictated by the changing financial situation, they may be depressed and saddened by the perceived loss of a role that gave them the greatest personal and professional satisfaction.

As manager, you must work with your staff to uncover which aspect of care that the staff believed, both collectively and individually, was the most rewarding aspect of nursing care. They should then list those tasks or functions they are no longer able to perform and those aspects they are still doing. To obtain this information, encourage each staff member to write down those items thought to be important, the loss of which is causing sadness. You can then incorporate all the individual responses into a statement for group discussion at a unit meeting. The group should accept all the items listed from the aggregate and either decide to work on one or two items per unit meeting until all items are addressed or form ad hoc groups to address the items.

The work of the groups of staff members falls into two areas. First, with the constraints of the new delivery system, how can they reconfigure the care given to increase the opportunity to expose themselves to those functions that reward them or to increase those that still exist? Second, how can they superimpose on their own needs the ancillary staff's needs for internal and external rewards generated by patient contact? The issue of legacy and stewardship, or the professional nurse's responsibility toward teaching and strengthening others' skills and responsiveness and thus ensuring quality care, in time may recompense or exceed the rewards originally lost. A grieving time of several months should be defined and discussed at the outset. A party should be held to celebrate change and renewal at the end of this period, and everyone should be out of mourning. The unit should adopt a motto or saying to personify their "can-do spirit," with the intent to create the best multilevel system with rewards for all.

S LENKMAN

Patient Classification Systems

◆ HOW DO I DETERMINE THAT MY PATIENT CLASSIFICATION SYSTEM IS NOT WORKING?

Q We have a patient classification system that is not working. We staff our unit with a ratio of one registered nurse to five patients. On some days our patient classification system calls for less staff than the 1:5 ratio, and on other days it calls for more staff. Isn't this evidence that we should develop a new system?

A Although your system may not be right for you, your current problem appears to be that you are not using the system. If you are staffing a ratio of 1:5 regardless of what the classification system calls for, you are using a straight numeric formula. Classification systems generally are based on *acuity* (level of seriousness of the patient's illness or a measure of the patient's resource requirements).

You seem to be using an average staff requirement rather than an acuity system. In budgeting, most of us average or otherwise identify an annual norm from our patient classification system. This number is used to calculate overall staffing needs for the following year. This number gives a manager an average staffing ratio. On a day-to-day basis, however, the staffing needs vary with the patients' level of illness, as evidenced by classification. When you said sometimes your system calls for more or less than the 1:5 ratio, this may indicate your system is fine but you are not using it as intended. If you use it as intended, you might staff 1:5 one day, 1:6 the next, and 1:4 the following; the average is still 1:5. The classification system may have been abandoned because it does not give accurate information for staffing.

I would suggest two approaches. First, talk to whoever is responsible for the hospital's classification system to learn the system's history; she may be able to tell you why it is not being used or may help you make it more useful in your work area. Second, review the literature to obtain more information on classification systems, types, usefulness, and problems. If your system is not useful in your facility, another one may be. Since this could become a major project, I suggest discussing your concerns and plans with your supervisor before embarking on it.

M PECK

◆ IS IT SAFE TO ABANDON PATIENT CLASSIFICATION?

Q Some recent literature suggests abandoning patient classification. If I do what is suggested, I'm afraid I won't meet Joint Commission on Accreditation of Healthcare Organizations (JCAHO) requirements. How can I give up this time-consuming activity and still meet the standards?

A The JCAHO standard's intent is that a plan should exist for nurse staffing in each nursing unit, as determined by a valid system for identifying patients' requirements for nursing care. This does not necessarily require the type of time-consuming, independent, task-focused system that many hospitals have used over the last two decades. The literature suggests that future systems must consider the economic and social environment of health care. Therefore, a system that ties nursing outcomes, staffing requirements, and care costs together so as to demonstrate the value of the service ultimately provides more relevant information to the nurse manager and the hospital.

Integrated, multidimensional systems such as those described in the literature are designed to monitor quality in terms of patient outcomes and the resources (staff, dollars) required to achieve the desired outcomes. These systems eliminate the need to spend designated nursing time classifying patients. Once the system is fully automated, the nursing staffing requirements are automatically generated as the nurse documents the patients' plans of care.

However, an organization needs time to develop and implement the integrated approach, and a prerequisite for these systems is state-of-the-art computer technology. In the interim it is important to define patients' needs for care in a valid, meaningful way that is not overly time consuming or cumbersome to manage. Judgment of a competent professional nurse is a valid means of determining the patient's need for care. Nurses on the unit with the predefined preparation who have been assessed as competent to fulfill this assignment could make this judgment on a day-to-day basis. The nurse manager, selected for the role because of her experience and credentials, certainly is capable of making judgments regarding patient needs and appropriate staffing. Documenting the judgments to provide evidence that patient needs are considered in determining the staffing levels and in assigning nurses to patients is essential in meeting JCAHO standards.

A few simple tools, many of which may already be available, can ensure that your interim approach is systematic and efficient and meets the JCAHO standard.

1. *Staffing standard.* Generally represented in hours per patient day (HPPD), this standard indicates the normal requirement for staff based on the unit's mix of patients. Historical data identifying patient care needs are important to consider when determining the standard.
2. *Master staffing plan.* Developed for each unit, this tool documents the number and mix of professional, technical, and support nursing staff necessary to meet the standard at each census level the unit is likely to experience. With this tool available, nurses who make daily staffing determinations merely need to make adjustments as patient needs change.
3. *Patient needs index.* This tool provides the opportunity to simplify the system until more sophisticated approaches can be implemented. Nurses competent to make this judgment document whether the care requirements for each patient are consistent with or more or less complex than the norm. A symbol or code indicating the index assigned can be documented on the nurse staffing assignment sheet or entered into a computer. The decision to maintain the standard staffing level or to adjust it must also be documented.
4. *Management information report.* This provides the final feedback loop of the simplified system, as well as information to guide the manager in identifying future staffing standards. The report may be prepared manually or generated by a personal computer using simple spreadsheet software. To be meaningful, the report should provide comparative data on volume of patients, patient needs index, staffing requirements based on standard and patient needs, and actual staffing.

In dealing with the issue of patient classification, as with any system, the benefits obtained from the system should exceed the resources expended to operate it. This is reportedly not the case with respect to patient classification in many organizations. Short-term modifications to present systems that enable a unit to meet the objectives of a systematic approach to staffing must be considered. Totally new methods will be available in the future.

SA FINNIGAN

P

♦ HOW CAN I CHANGE OUR PATIENT CLASSIFICATION SYSTEM TO MORE ACCURATELY REFLECT ACUITY LEVEL?

Q Because of reimbursement changes, we are finding on my unit that patients have a shorter length of stay. Although our acuity system usually works, on days that we have 8 to 10 admissions and discharges, resulting in the staff being very busy, our acuity system does not seem to recognize this. How can we change it to reflect the acuity level more accurately?

A The historical measurement of hospital volume based on patient days is becoming increasingly problematic as our delivery of care changes dramatically. Midnight census is no longer relevant to what occurred through the day. This is going to require hospitals to eventually develop a method to calculate work load and volume other than counting patient days or outpatient visits.

Acuity systems often fail to address nursing work load issues that may be more related to volume changes and system issues than those factors that relate directly to the patient. You can deal with this work load issue in the following ways:

1. Work with your finance department to develop an adjusted patient day measurement that would be derived from the work load currently being missed by your system.
2. Work with the vendor of your acuity system to add partial day work load and/or enhanced measurement of intensity on day of admission and day of discharge.
3. Reevaluate how the hospital system is designed to support this turnover of patients. Nonnursing systems often do not keep up with the changing demands of our patient population, thus creating extra work for nursing to fill the gap. For example, could housekeeping be more responsive? Could a discharge lounge or transportation service be established to handle patients who need transportation home?

C BRADLEY

◆ HOW CAN I MOTIVATE STAFF TO USE A PATIENT CLASSIFICATION SYSTEM?

Q How can I get my staff nurses to use the patient classification system? When they do use it, there seem to be many errors or it is incomplete. The data I obtain are meaningless.

A Many nurses have discontinued the activity of classifying patients, which sends an important message to management. Managers should listen to and validate what staff are saying both verbally and through their behavior.

The problem you describe is not unique to your organization. Many nursing units today are facing dissatisfaction and frustration from staff concerning the issue of patient classification. Staff express frustration

with the time required to classify patients and perform reliability audits, since many believe these no longer serve any useful purpose. They often indicate that management does nothing of value with the data, and therefore no meaningful outcome justifies the time spent. Likewise, many managers are also frustrated. Knowing that nurses have learned to use the system to demonstrate a need for additional staff, managers have little confidence in the data. In some situations, acuity levels continue to climb because of the "fudge factor," and the unit budget simply cannot support the increases that would be required.

I recommend that managers give up trying to get nurses to use a system that for all practical purposes has become obsolete. The systems used by an organization must accomplish meaningful objectives. When patient classification systems were developed two decades ago, nursing's goal was to quantitatively demonstrate patients' need for care and thereby "justify" the need for additional nursing staff. In the economic environment today, this is no longer a relevant objective.

Conventional patient classification systems must be replaced by approaches based on more timely values and objectives that match the economic and social environment. Quantifying the time required to accomplish the tasks of nursing must give way to measuring the outcomes of nursing care and the resources, in both time and dollars, required to achieve them. The technology is now available for us to tie our independent systems together to create a multidimensional, outcome-focused management system. Quantifying staffing needs can become an automatic result of documenting a patient plan of care rather than an independent activity of the nurse. More important, the multidimensional approach can assist nursing in demonstrating the relationship between cost of services rendered and outcomes achieved. This can serve not only the nursing profession, but also our patients and health care in general by demonstrating the product's value to those who receive and pay for it.

SA FINNIGAN

◆ WHAT SHOULD I DO IF MY STAFFING FIGURES DISAGREE WITH THOSE OF MY DIRECTOR?

Q I am a nursing manager of a 40-bed mixed medical–surgical unit. I have been informed by my director that I am responsible for calculating my required full-time equivalents (FTEs) for the coming year. She has provided me with the number of patients that have been admitted to my unit this past year, as well as the required hours per patient day. I have a patient classification system that defines my staffing requirements on a daily basis. I believe this classification system is very accurate. Somehow, however, my required staffing numbers for the year don't match those of my director. What is my next step?

A You need to examine several issues here. Are you sure that you have the right calculations for predicting the budgeted FTEs? Whenever a discrepancy in figures exists, it is best to go over them at least twice, then ask someone else to check the figures. If you have done everything right, the actual discrepancy may not be between what you and your director achieve using the same formulas, but rather between what you require by acuity and what your budget allows. You indicate the patient classification system is accurate. How do you know this? Is this a "home-grown" or commercial system? Has a reputable data base of time and motion studies been consistently updated? Are the direct and indirect times calculated separately? Another issue regarding accuracy involves the objectivity of the people using the system. Do you regularly audit the system?

Suppose your answer to all these questions is *yes.* The system is sound and audited regularly, the direct and indirect times are properly calculated, and you strongly believe that safe care is predicated on receiving the staff you show you need. Now what can you do?

With all the facts before you that reflect the answers to the previous questions, sit down and determine your responses to the director when she asks for substantiation. Have another manager act as devil's advocate. Prepare graphs, variance reports, and other materials to support all your points. Calculate the lowest possible FTE allowance that would enable you to feel safe. Are any savings possible by changing the skill mix?

Ask for a meeting with the director to negotiate your budgeted FTE allowance. State your problem with objectivity and levelheadedness, and provide a packet of materials for both of you to demonstrate your conclusions. Be prepared to negotiate, with patient outcomes as the goal. After your request is considered, if the ruling is that the original budget must

stand, ask for assistance with work redesign to enable the nurses to better handle the existing work load.

S LENKMAN

Patient Rights

◆ CAN WE INCLUDE PATIENT RIGHTS AS PART OF THE ORIENTATION TO OUR UNIT?

Q We believe in the patient bill of rights on our nursing unit and want to establish a patient rights process as a part of our nursing care. Is it possible to include issues regarding patient rights in the assessment or to involve patients in understanding their rights as a part of their orientation to the unit? Are there liabilities connected with doing this?

A Increasingly in our society, people expect to be informed and to understand what is expected of them and what they may expect from others and organizations. Large institutions such as hospitals can and do appear very intimidating and somewhat hostile to patients. The patient's bill of rights informs patients about aspects of care to which they can hold the organization and its caregivers accountable.

Most patients are unfamiliar with hospital protocol. A hospital is a complex, foreign place, and medical care is often frightening to patients. Whether a patient is admitted voluntarily under a physician's care or as an emergency, hospital staff and nurses alike have a primary responsibility to inform patients as soon as possible in the process of their rights and, equally important, of what the institution and its caregivers expect of them.

Some institutions communicate patient's rights in the admissions department; others do this in the nursing unit. Regardless of where this occurs, the nursing assessment and orientation process should (1) reinforce any information received by the patient in the admitting office and (2) cover both the patient's rights and the institution's expectations. This should be done with tact, care, clarity, and patience.

Because we operate in an increasingly litigious environment, and based on the organization's policies and procedures and on the patient's plan of care,

P

nurses need to communicate rights and expectations fully, carefully, and with good judgment. In addition, both need to be legibly and accurately documented in the patient's record.

Nurses need not be concerned about liability in informing a patient of various rights; however, errors of omission may present definite liabilities to both the organization and the nurse. When patients are not fully informed of their plan of care, the unit's or organization's rules, or whatever may be required of them (no matter how minor or inconsequential it may seem at the time), problems may arise.

Therefore I recommend that patient rights and institutional and caregiver expectations be included in the unit orientation process. Liabilities exist, but by exercising care, thoroughness, and good judgment and by documenting and witnessing as appropriate, the potential for future litigation can be greatly reduced, if not eliminated.

GA ADAMS

◆ WHAT IS THE BEST WAY TO MAINTAIN A BALANCE BETWEEN PATIENT RIGHTS AND STAFF RIGHTS?

Q How do we balance patient rights with staff rights so that both are not violated, abused, or harmed? In our unit, a thin line often exists between patients' acting out and violating the staff and the staff's reaction to this aggression. How do I as a nurse manager balance these two concerns?

A A growing concern for assaulted staff has been reflected in the literature over the past decade. Curtin and Flaherty (1982) state that:

although the primary focus of ethical concern in any clinical decision ought to be the welfare of the individual and, although the patient has an integral if not central role in decision making, the patient has no more right to coerce the professional than the professional has to coerce the patient.

Nurses must not be subjected to patient behaviors that cause harm, abuse, or violence. Proactive measures should be instituted to protect staff and others from violent patients. These include the provision of adequate security support, education of staff in the prevention and management of aggressive and assaultive behavior, and ensuring that adequate professional and ancillary staff are available to meet patient care needs routinely, especially in high-profile areas such as hospital emergency departments and waiting rooms.

Early, expert triage should be initiated to identify patients at risk for violent behavior so that they are placed in the appropriate clinical setting as soon as possible. Clinical managers must maintain an environment for patients and staff that serves as a safe haven based on knowledge, security, and awareness, yet supports the individual who may have experienced physical assault. Ongoing education and the development of alternative strategies to avoid future attacks are key factors in assisting the staff. Caring and support to cope with feelings of anger, anxiety, fear, and shock related to incidents of abuse also convey to staff a sense of genuine concern from nurse managers and help to ease a difficult experience (Lipscomb and Lone, 1992).

J TROFINO

◆ WHAT SHOULD I DO ABOUT A COLLEAGUE WHO TALKS ABOUT PATIENTS AWAY FROM THE UNIT?

Q A fellow nurse always talks about patients outside the nursing unit. She is never discreet about what she says. What can and should I do?

A You must intervene immediately. Patients have a right to strict confidentiality regarding their health care information and to be protected from unnecessary dissemination of that data. Confidentiality is a fundamental part of our professional code of ethics and a legal obligation of your organization. Your organization probably has a policy on confidentiality, or you may refer to the Joint Commission on Accreditation of Healthcare Organizations manual, or the American Nurses Association Code of Ethics. As soon as possible, you must schedule a meeting with this employee and discuss this issue with her. You must clearly state the standards of confidentiality that you expect and specifically describe the times you have observed her violating those standards. Although it is important for you to hear what the employee has to say regarding your observations, you must make it clear that NO acceptable reasons exist to violate this standard and that failure to comply with these professional behaviors will result in immediate disciplinary action. A new or inexperienced nurse may not know the organization's policy on confidentiality, but a nurse cannot be totally unfamiliar with the professional standards of confidentiality. Once you have stated the expected standard and the required behavior change, you must monitor this employee to ensure that the change is consistently enacted. A follow-up meeting in several weeks to praise new behaviors will assist in maintaining this change by reinforcing your commitment to this critical performance standard.

MC ALDERMAN

Patient Safety

♦ **HOW SHOULD I RESPOND TO STAFF WHO HAVE VOICED COMPLAINTS ABOUT PATIENT SAFETY TO THE JOINT COMMISSION ON ACCREDITATION OF HEALTHCARE ORGANIZATIONS (JCAHO) AND LEGISLATORS?**

Q I am a nurse manager at a 250-bed acute care facility. I have just received a copy of a letter directed to the administrator, board chairperson, JCAHO, and legislator for the area. It outlines a long list of complaints expressed by the nurses in our facility, some of which relate to patient safety. What course of action should I take?

A Given the scenario described, I would surmise that the staff are using this avenue of communication because they believe previous concerns and issues have gone unheeded or unresolved. Although this may or may not be the case, this action most likely will elicit a definite organizational response.

First, you must accept the staff's perceptions of these issues and determine what staff need and expect as a form of resolution. You should delineate

which issues are within the staff's control to resolve and which are not.

As a staff advocate, you should carefully evaluate the identified issues and assess what are real versus perceptual issues. Patient safety issues should be dealt with first. It may be helpful to provide a variety of open communication channels so that all staff can contribute to the discussion of the issues.

Preparing a response is important to both staff and those interested parties who will undoubtedly question the complaints. Proactively contacting all recipients of the letter immediately helps alleviate any concerns or doubts it may have generated. You must reassure all parties that these issues will be taken seriously and resolved. Timely follow-up is critical, and using staff to provide written resolution can sometimes be a constructive way to involve those who initiated the complaint. It also helps them understand the serious nature of communicating concerns outside the organization in this manner.

After the issues are addressed, follow-up with staff should eventually include a discussion about internal channels and how staff might present issues and concerns in the future to ensure resolution without placing the organization at risk.

C BRADLEY

♦ **WHAT SHOULD I DO IF I HAVE INSUFFICIENT EQUIPMENT AND SUPPLIES?**

Q How do I deal with situations in which equipment or services are not available when hospital policy clearly states that for safety reasons they *must* be available?

A First, you should call for the necessary equipment or service. Follow hospital policy and procedure to document the missing equipment or service. This may require completing an incident report or quality assurance reports.

Second, begin checking for the equipment or service before it is needed. Whenever an item is missing, call and document the follow-up. Identify the negative consequences that do or could result from the missing item.

If this activity fails to produce the needed equipment, request the development of a task force to review the policies and procedures regarding the safety issues. Then work out a plan to achieve policy outcomes.

J O'MALLEY

◆ WHAT SHOULD I DO IF STAFF ABUSE PATIENTS?

Q As a nurse manager, I have been informed that one of the staff has verbally and even possibly physically abused a patient. I have not validated the claim but suspect it is true. The accused staff member denies it, and the patients cannot confirm it. What should I do?

A This situation is always of great importance but difficult to deal with. The collection of valid information is a primary consideration. As a manager, your job will be made much easier if you have the necessary "evidence" to effectively discipline or remove the employee. Your human resource department *must* be consulted in this matter.

Evaluate carefully the degree to which you believe your patients are at risk. This should guide your actions and your time frame. Unless you have sufficient evidence to deal with the employee immediately, it is best not to inform the employee of your suspicions. This allows you more latitude in conducting an investigation. From the question, however, it appears that this staff member has been informed that you have concerns.

You should include several other considerations as you make a plan to deal with this employee:

1. Carefully interview the source of your original information to determine how much evidence you have at this time. Is this employee willing to document the information?
2. Is timing of this investigation critical based on the end of a probationary period or upcoming evaluation period?
3. What shift does this employee work, and to what degree is this employee normally supervised?
4. If the employee is licensed, have any complaints ever been made against her license? Call the state licensing agency.

5. Recheck any references and previous employers to determine if previous problems of this nature occurred. Speak with former immediate supervisors if at all possible.
6. Follow up with previous patients cared for by this individual. Ask questions in a manner that does not lead patients.

Depending on your level of concern and evidence that this patient abuse is a valid issue, you should ensure that competent supervision is available for this employee and the supervisor is well informed of your suspicions. A written memo reinforcing any relevant nursing or hospital policy or procedure should be given to the employee. If valid evidence is obtained, you should work closely with your human resources representative to act expeditiously.

Such situations serve as a good reminder to review with other staff how you expect patients to be treated and what employee responsibilities are in ensuring patient safety and reporting any inappropriate care.

C BRADLEY

Patient Satisfaction

◆ WHAT ARE THE BASIC ELEMENTS IN A PATIENT SATISFACTION PROGRAM?

Q We are interested in focusing more on patient satisfaction. What should be some critical elements in a patient satisfaction program at the unit level?

A The most critical element in a patient satisfaction program is the commitment of top management. These programs have become popular as a marketing tool. The hope is that satisfied "customers" will return when further care is needed and that their word-of-mouth publicity will be positive. However, unless the institution as a whole possesses patient satisfaction as a core value, the program will suffer from its cosmetic nature. Staff and patients alike will identify the counterfeit nature of the intent.

An authentic patient satisfaction program is backed by the resources for staff development so that employees understand the importance of their role and receive training in the specific behaviors that convey caring. When all employees fully understand their role as patient advocates and feel supported in behaving in a caring way and in protecting the patient from the institutional system when needed, patient satisfaction increases.

Some specific behaviors are:

1. Call the patient by his or her preferred name or title. Treat each patient as a person, not an object.
2. Make eye contact.
3. Ask open-ended questions. Listen for the answers.
4. Gently touch, when you sense this is permissible.
5. Allay fears as best as you realistically can.
6. Provide information at the level of the patient's understanding and tolerance.
7. Respond to needs in a timely way and follow up.
8. Utilize effective pain control methods and medications.
9. Provide comfort measures.
10. Function as the patient's agent for protection during vulnerable times.

Do your best to preserve the dignity of each person. Laugh and cry with the patient. Remember that what is routine to you is not routine to the patient. Finally, nurture yourself regularly so that you have the stamina to care for others without hurting yourself.

J HIXON

◆ WHAT CAN I DO IF STAFF IGNORE A PATIENT'S COMPLAINTS?

Q Our unit has been receiving several complaints from patients and their families about the care provided. I have repeatedly brought this to the attention of the staff and given them specific performance expectations to change this. They say they will work on them, but I find they are not accountable and do not follow through. How can I get them to improve on this serious situation?

A Sharing patient and family feedback about care with staff members is an important step to increase awareness about how patients perceive the care. First, discuss with your staff that the patient's and family's perceptions are "reality" for them, regardless of how factual the perceptions are. Second, be sure staff know that ensuring *quality* in patient care is everyone's responsibility. Although performance expectations have been set with the staff, they might not know how to make substantive changes that will improve patient care. To facilitate staff accountability in improving the quality of care, you may want to assist them in forming a council or committee to identify and review quality indicators, including a review of patient satisfaction forms. The committee can develop specific alternatives that would help prevent the complaints from recurring. The members should be selected by the staff and should represent each shift. Once the committee is functioning, its members should discuss patient and family complaints and the resultant suggestions for improvement with other staff members in staff meetings, rather than the manager doing so, to reinforce that improvement of patient care is the staff's responsibility.

If the staff committee identifies specific trends that negatively affect patient care, the committee must develop specific action steps to reverse these trends. They may need management's assistance if one or more nurses are implicated in several patient complaints, although it is extremely worthwhile when the staff committee talks with the offending staff member on a peer-to-peer basis. Some newly formed staff committees may need some education and training on how to manage breaches in quality care with their peers in a manner that coaches rather than disciplines the staff member.

By including the staff in the identification of quality issues and in the possible alternatives for solving them, they will accept accountability for making the changes necessary to ensure quality for patients and their families. As a manager, you may want to ask yourself if the proper administrative supports are in place for the staff to be successful in improving patient care. The manager is responsible for ensuring that:

1. Appropriate staffing is available for the level of care to be provided and the volume of patients served on the unit.

P

2. Necessary supplies are immediately available and accessible so that unnecessary energy is not expended securing needed supplies and equipment to care for patients.
3. The work environment supports the professional practice of nursing.

JF STICHLER

Patient Transfer

◆ HOW CAN WE IMPROVE THE TRANSFER FLOW OF PATIENTS FROM THE CRITICAL CARE UNIT (CCU)?

Q One of the significant problems in our CCU is a transfer of patients to other units of service. Often, more patients are ready for admission than our discharges allow. What are some actions we can take to balance the rate of admissions to CCU from surgery with the slower rate of discharge to other units in the hospital?

A The best solution to this situation is to use a good patient acuity system that allows for prospective work load management. Using this type of system helps you to predict the work load 6 to 8 hours in advance. Thus time is available to make adjustments. The nature of the adjustments varies depending on the shortfall: is it caused by lack of beds or lack of staff?

If the situation involves lack of beds, you need to be able to prepare patients for discharge to an intermediary care unit. Relationships and trust must be established with the physician groups so that they are willing to move the "least ill" patients to a "regular" unit. Establishing these relationships with physicians should be facilitated because the same surgeons you ask to "move out" a patient one day will be the ones that you are "making a bed for" another day. If your institution has implemented managed care, the nurse case manager should be invaluable in making these adjustments.

Collaboration also needs to the established with the intermediary care unit ("regular" unit) staff to accept these patients. This task may also require some cross-training of these unit nursing staffs to care for more critically ill patients. A mechanism must be in place that allows these regular units to obtain more staff if their work load becomes greater than their scheduled resources. All these relationships are feasible in an institution that has an environment of cooperation and integration to provide quality patient care for all.

With the advance planning, establishment of relationships, and cross-training completed, 6 to 8 hours should be adequate to make the necessary adjustments when the rate of discharges and admissions is out of balance. In a surgical intensive care unit, of course, emergencies lead to unplanned admissions in shorter periods. If the mechanisms previously described are in place, however, they can be implemented in a much shorter time frame because everyone is familiar with the process.

JW ALEXANDER

◆ WHAT CAN I DO IF MY UNIT RECEIVES TOO MANY PATIENTS AT ONE TIME?

Q Our unit receives admissions daily from the admitting office, day surgery, labor and delivery, and emergency room. I have met with the managers of these various areas and explained the difficulty in receiving too many patients to our unit within a short time. Although they seem to understand my dilemma, they state that they have to transfer their patients to make room for incoming patients. What steps can I take to handle this problem?

A A common cause for the perennial problems between departments is the lack of a broader *systems perspective.* Individual units see their work and issues in isolation from the other departments that they interface with on an ongoing basis. A possible solution to such situations is the development of an *interface agreement.* Such a process, when adopted by the entire system, gives managers a way to create a win–win situation when unit needs are in conflict.

To initiate an interface agreement, a meeting of the major stakeholders is called. Staff and management from the units involved meet to identify the issues inherent within the problem. Often the list of stakeholders may include people from supporting departments such as housekeeping, who are responsible for cleaning rooms to allow a timely transfer. A candid, considerate discussion is essential so that all issues can be expressed. If the units have disagreed for a long period, it may be helpful to invite a facilitator to keep the discussion focused on the issues rather than personalities.

Once the problem has been thoroughly investigated, a list of solutions is generated. In this brainstorming part of the meeting, no idea is too insignificant to list. Once all possible solutions are listed, a reasoned approach is crafted by all parties present. Then each unit makes a commitment to which strategies and behaviors their unit members will be held accountable for. This is put together in a document that lists stakeholders, problem, steps to resolving the problem, and each unit member's accountability. The document is signed by the managers from each unit, demonstrating the unit's level of commitment.

The interface agreement document is then shared with the staff on each unit. It is posted in a position of prominence so that all may refer to it as need arises. This document becomes part of the continuous quality improvement (CQI) process. If a member of one unit is not supporting the document's contents, this is reported and proper action is taken. The document may be revised by the group of stakeholders whenever the need arises. It may be removed when the problem has been completely resolved.

J KOERNER

Peer Relations

♦ HOW DO I IMPLEMENT A PEER REVIEW SYSTEM FOR STAFF?

Q As a nurse manager and a professional, I believe that nurses should provide feedback to one another on practice in a peer relations format. With the diversity in terms of education, years of experience, and personalities, how can I make this happen? Can you give me some idea of the major barriers I will need to plan for?

A Successfully implementing a peer review system depends less on the diversity in terms of education and experience than on the level of staff maturity. By maturity I do not mean age. I mean the level of psychologic and professional maturity as described in the situational leadership model. In a mature work group, a healthy balance of emphasis exists between relationship and task. The staff can successfully work together through the stages of group development to achieve a high level of trust and an ability to explore issues, including practicing constructive resolution of the conflict that arises in every effective group.

Some barriers to achieving sufficient maturity in a work group are lack of trust, insecurity (personally or institutionally), and "turf" and competition issues. To move past some of these barriers, enough group members must have a healthy self-esteem to reach out and begin the process. Even then, some work groups are simply not ready to handle the delicacy of the peer review process and agree on the competencies on which they will be evaluated.

The current move toward competency-based evaluation does help as a motivator. However, remember that it can be a serious error to attempt to implement peer review in a group that is not ready. Don't fool yourself about the level of staff maturity. If necessary, bring in a consultant to assist with that assessment. If you base your planning on a realistic, objective assessment, the project has a good chance of succeeding.

The steps in establishing a peer review system follow.

1. Clarify these questions for yourself:
   ♦ Exactly what do I want to accomplish?
   ♦ Who will have the power to reward and punish?
   ♦ Who will control the substance of the competencies on which staff are rated?
2. Establish a temporary planning committee with the power to structure the peer review system. This committee may appoint subcommittees. The committee identifies core values, adopts standards and criteria, and constructs operating procedures. When this work is accomplished, a peer review committee is formed according to the approved criteria of the planning committee. Members of the committee may be appointed or elected by the staff. The staff on the committee must possess clinical competence similar to that of the employees who will be rated, as well as integrity, profes-

P

sional commitment, ability to make decisions, and interpersonal skills. Considerable resources may be needed for development of the group.

You and your staff can obtain valuable information from a substantial body of literature on the peer review process (e.g., American Nurses Association, 1988).

J HIXON

♦ WHAT SHOULD I DO IF MY STAFF IS DYSFUNCTIONAL?

Q I've been reading that some work groups have difficulty getting the work done in a quality way because they are more or less dysfunctional. How can I determine whether department staff are demonstrating dysfunctional behaviors to a degree that affects the work, and what can I do about it?

A By definition, *dysfunctional* means impaired or incomplete functioning and can therefore only be described as a deviation from a group's normal functioning. A healthy, mature group effectively and efficiently accomplishes the tasks to achieve prescribed goals and standards. Also, positive interpersonal relationships are marked by collaborative problem solving, mutual support, and a sense of camaraderie.

In the initial developmental stages of testing (I) and infighting (II), normal behaviors for these stages could be labeled as dysfunctional. For example, in stage I, *testing*, individuals may act fearful or evasive as they constantly monitor verbal and nonverbal messages of other group members to determine what is acceptable and unacceptable behavior in the group. Each person proceeds with personal, conventional ways of becoming involved, such as staying in the background and observing or actively participating with good humor. Two examples of dysfunctional behaviors at this stage include the following:

1. Not drawing out silent members.
2. Certain people consistently not showing up or being late for meetings.

A manager can prevent a group from being stuck in this stage by establishing an effective welcoming structure and by facilitating the group's getting to know one another. The manager who helps the team

establish ground rules early within the group can avoid problems in this stage and in stage II. By brainstorming the potential task and relationship problems, the group has a list to convert to ground rules. These ground rules begin with "We will," followed by a positive statement of the acceptable behavior. Two ground rules to change the identified dysfunctional behaviors are:

♦ "We will attend at least 80% of the required meetings, and habitual tardiness and absenteeism will be confronted by peers and/or the chairperson."
♦ "We will ask for comments from silent group members."

In stage II, *infighting*, individuals sort out personal relationships of power and influence. Some behaviors that indicate dysfunctional behavior in this stage follow:

1. Disruptive, aggressive, and passive/aggressive behavior exists, and individuals are not confronted.
2. Members often restrain their critical remarks to avoid "rocking the boat."
3. People do not follow through with decisions made by the group.

A manager in this stage needs to help members by modeling effective conflict resolution skills and by allowing disagreements to surface and be worked through. If power and control issues are not faced and resolved, the group will remain in stage II and therefore become dysfunctional. An example of a ground rule relevant to this stage is "We will support the majority decision, even if we disagree with it, by following through with the decision."

You must remember that most problems in groups result from dynamics in the group, not individuals. Therefore it is crucial for you to confront ineffective group norms (group habits) by establishing ground rules, as well as facilitating group development.

VD LACHMAN

♦ HOW CAN I INSTITUTE CHANGES WITHOUT ALIENATING COLLEAGUES WHO PREFER THE STATUS QUO?

Q I have begun to involve the staff in more and more aspects of unit management, such as hiring, financial management, decision making, and program development. The head nurse colleagues are putting subtle pressure on me to stop this practice because they believe "Everything is just fine the way it is." How can I continue on the path that I believe in but at the same time not alienate my management colleagues?

A This is a difficult situation because many different issues may be contributing to it. The primary concern about the relationship between colleagues should be confronted head-on. You must let your colleagues know that you take your responsibility as a manager seriously, as do they, and therefore you promote policies and practices that you believe enhance patient care and staff satisfaction *on your unit*. Units or departments develop their own character or personality and thus cannot and will not operate exactly the same way. What works on one unit will not necessarily work on the next without some modifications. It may be useful for you to note alterations or practices that are unique and appropriate for colleagues' units but that would not work on your unit. If your colleagues' motivation for criticism is envy or fear, all you can do is clarify your own motives, share your rationale for change with anyone who asks, and continue to do what you think best.

M MURPHY

♦ IF A COLLEAGUE SHIRKS DUTY AND HER MANAGER WON'T DO ANYTHING, WHAT CAN I DO?

Q I have made complaints to the manager about an employee who shirks her duties, but nothing happens. What can I do now?

A As a first step, staff members should provide direct feedback to each other regarding performance. Although uncomfortable for staff members, this process is very beneficial to professional growth. This process can be facilitated by consulting a clinical nurse specialist or other available resources.

If this intervention is unsuccessful, the staff member should meet with the manager to share her concerns. If the manager agrees that a problem exists, she generally will take the following steps:
1. Discuss with the person the expected behavior and job competencies.

2. Identify the deficiencies in behavior and that behavior's impact on expected outcomes, such as safe patient care.
3. If necessary, set up with the employee an educational plan and a behavioral plan that identifies expected behaviors, and review dates to document changes in behaviors.

J O'MALLEY

♦ HOW DO I GAIN CREDIBILITY WITH NONNURSING MANAGERS?

Q How can I gain credibility most quickly and effectively from other nonnursing department head peers who do not consider a nurse manager their peer?

A Credibility is gained by the outcomes individuals are able to achieve. Managers often wrongly assume their title automatically gains them instant credibility and respect. Credibility and respect have to be earned; they are not simply handed to people. Nurse managers sometimes set themselves up for failure by bemoaning that they "get no respect." This, unfortunately, taints all nursing because nursing as a whole is viewed as "complainers versus doers." A nurse manager is very much a peer to other department managers outside nursing. Because there have always been multiple nursing managers in an organization, administrators have often been unwilling to give them the same recognition as other managers. In addition, nursing has traditionally had directors between them and the vice-president, which has further distanced them from being recognized on the same level with other managers.

Nursing managers need to recognize the unique strength they bring to hospital operations. Patients come to the hospital for nursing care. Physicians choose a hospital because of the quality of nursing care. Nursing managers are in a key position to help achieve the success of the hospital. As a result, nursing needs to ensure the care provided is based on highly held standards of care. This care is not only nursing care, but *all* care provided. The nursing manager must take a proactive role in all issues related to patient care. Nursing managers must participate actively and positively on committees and pursue inno-

P

vative approaches to patient care. They must actively advocate for patients, ensuring that activities within the institution are carried out for enhanced patient care delivery. How nursing accomplishes this will determine the perceived credibility of the nursing manager. If this is done in a whining, defensive manner, laced with complaining about having not enough staff and too many high-acuity patients, credibility is lost and nursing is tuned out. If the nurse manager can do this in a positive, enthusiastic, outcome-oriented way and bring solutions to the table, colleagues' respect for her and nursing will be greatly enhanced.

The nurse manager is in a pivotal role to recognize and advocate for the changes needed to enhance the delivery of patient care. Nursing has always been at the end point of the service that is provided by everyone in the institution and should be in the middle of redesigning and restructuring how that care is delivered. It is unfortunate, but nursing's traditional role has been more that of a martyr than a crusader for change. Nursing has been widely recognized for the ability to succinctly and clearly recite failings rather than solutions to problems within the institution. Nursing has not been perceived as being able to do anything to solve problems.

The nurse manager must be seen as the initiator of change. She must be seen as actively seeking, negotiating, and selling her ideas of change to others. The nurse manager must look outside nursing and become familiar with the work of other disciplines. She should spend time with other disciplines learning about their work, their issues, their ideas, and how these relate to or correspond with overall patient care.

The nurse manager must be able to talk in terms of what the patient wants and needs, not what nursing wants and needs. She should also develop collaborative relationships with managers of other disciplines, seeking their advice or thoughts on issues she is experiencing. Another good strategy is to invite a manager outside nursing to have lunch or just stop by to do some joint problem solving. This results in face-to-face contact rather than communicating only by phone; adds a personal, collegial dimension to the relationship; and provides an excellent opportunity for the nonnursing manager to see nursing in another way. The nurse manager should be seen as an advocate for teamwork and collaboration and actively role-model the behavior. Nursing management then becomes the leader in beginning to integrate all disciplines to address patient care issues collectively.

Finally, the nurse manager needs to expand her knowledge beyond patient care (clinical knowledge). Understanding the budget and how it is developed and monitored, coupled with an ability to discuss finances, whether productivity, cost per unit of service, cost per day, return on expenses, managed care, per diem, capitation, census, or operating margin, will be critical. She should be well versed in how the hospital is doing financially and why it is above or below budget. She should know whether her unit is on budget not only from a staffing and salary perspective, but also on the census projections. She should have a plan to address the budget variance and inform all the appropriate people who can agree with or assist with her plan.

The nurse manager needs to understand and articulate what an integrated delivery system is and how the hospital fits into that integrated system. Understanding the payor makeup of her patient population, length of stay, costs per discharge, and clinical outcomes serves to enhance her credibility. Developing strong, collaborative relationships with the medical staff in monitoring outcomes of critical pathways and providing high-quality, cost-effective care helps the nurse manager gain respect and credibility with her colleagues.

The nurse manager is an equal peer with counterparts in other departments; however, the old paradigm of unequal status has evolved from past behaviors and thinking. Nursing has adapted to that mentality and must now change that image by changing how nurses have traditionally viewed themselves and behaved. The nurse manager needs to demonstrate her ability to create and seek new ways of doing things by involving all the disciplines that interact with the patient. Also, she must be able to talk in a well-rounded, articulate manner relating clinical, business, and financial issues at the same time.

J TORNABENI

◆ WHAT IS THE BEST WAY TO ESTABLISH PROFESSIONAL RESPECT FOR NURSING?

Q What is the most effective strategy, plan, or process to establish professional respect for nursing within the health care structure?

A Effective strategies, plans, and processes to overcome the lack of professional respect in any setting depend on nurses themselves. From my experience, I believe nurses should consider two views on respect. First, as with trust, respect is earned or is afforded to everyone until someone gives you reason not to respect or trust. Consistent demonstration of clinical competencies in the delivery of care to patients plants a firm foundation from which mutual respect will grow.

Second, nursing's uniqueness must be emphasized. What is it we really do? The answer can be provided in short, practical, respectable terms and even shared with the patient at the bedside. Knowing who we are and what we do and broadly communicating it provide additional role clarity to our colleagues.

The three "R"s suggest initiatives that we as nurses might employ to further our attainment of mutual respect:

1. *Redefine.* We must redefine the needs to be addressed by ourselves and our organization.
2. *Reassess.* We must reassess our inherent strengths, which may have been overshadowed in the past.
3. *Reinvent.* We must reinvent our structure to respond to realities.

LM JOHNSON

Performance Evaluation

♦ HOW DO I MANAGE STAFF THROUGH EVALUATION USING THE PERFORMANCE MANAGEMENT PROCESS?

Q How does one manage a staff through evaluation under the performance management concept?

A To manage a staff through evaluation under the performance management concept, it is helpful first to understand the terminology and methodology involved. Webster has defined the term *evaluate* as "the process of finding the value or amount or determining the worth of; to appraise." Traditional methods of evaluation involve a yearly meeting between the boss and the employee during which the employee is given feedback on performance throughout the previous year. Most often this one-way process involves a paperwork shuffle and may include goals for the upcoming year. The evaluation feedback frequently centers on how the work has been done and the staff member's performance and productivity within that context. Minimal emphasis is given to individuals and their aspirations, creativity, or self-actualization.

Evaluations for professional staff sometimes have centered on the process of peer relations, or peer review. In this method professionals complete a self-evaluation in which they critique their own work process and request feedback from other professionals. All comments are taken into account when the evaluation is completed, most often by the manager.

With the advent of continuous quality improvement (CQI) or total quality management (TQM), many institutions are taking a second look at their evaluation process. In this philosophy, evaluation focuses on the work process rather than the individual. Teamwork is stressed. Monetary rewards are structured differently as well. Merit raises change to pay for performance or incentive pay; money is not provided merely for years on the job.

Each facility will structure the performance management process and techniques differently. However, some central issues can assist the manager in preparing for and encouraging staff toward this new method of evaluation.

1. Educate staff regarding organizational mission and values. These concepts permeate performance management methods.
2. Increase employee participation in the evaluation process. Employee and manager together must understand the process, tools, and structure.
3. Learn to coach and advise employees. The manager's role shifts to these skills within the performance management concept.
4. Emphasize evaluation as a part of the normal work flow, not a separate, formal process.
5. Stress innovation within the work environment. Creative ways to continually improve communications between manager and staff are the focal points in the process.

MT SINNEN

P

◆ HOW DO I EVALUATE STAFF WHOM I RARELY SEE?

Q Our performance evaluation system requires that I review every nurse's performance annually. I rarely see the night or evening staff, and I really don't think I can review their performance. Isn't there a better way to evaluate these people?

A Yes, but it will take some ingenuity on your part. First, most organizations require the nurse manager to do these evaluations because they are a means to encourage the development of employees who will meet the organization's objectives. From the organization's point of view, productive employees are desired, and the nurse manager often seems to be the best person to ensure such employees exist.

In this case, however, I would recommend a *peer review process* similar to a performance appraisal, except the evaluation is done by persons of equal status. A peer can give a critical, yet empathic evaluation of one's work. A spirit of trust must exist for this process to be successful; your facilitating skills are needed in this area. The person can perform a self-evaluation according to a predetermined set of criteria, then name two peers to do a similar evaluation. They should then meet and discuss the evaluation. In the beginning these sessions could be done with you as observer or facilitator, but as skill in this type of evaluation grows, the process should be left to the peers.

If this peer evaluation is unacceptable, another method is for you to plan a certain number of times during the year to spend some time on those shifts. This would have several advantages, such as giving you a better appreciation of what these shifts accomplish and perhaps allowing you a different perspective on which to make administrative decisions. It would also provide you with some anecdotal information on the specific people you are evaluating. This would not necessitate working complete shifts but may entail overlapping two shifts. For example, you could work from 8 PM to 3 AM once or twice a month for several months over a year.

A more common practice is to have the evaluation done by the charge nurse on those shifts. However, this option excludes your input and ignores your requirement to review every nurse's performance.

SR. M FINNICK

◆ WHAT SHOULD I DO WHEN STAFF DISAGREE WITH MY INTERPRETATION OF STANDARDS?

Q When I evaluate some employees, we disagree regarding the content and interpretation of the standards. How can I prevent this?

A Nursing standards should be written in a clear understandable way, established by authority, and consistent with the nurse practice act in your state. Standards are created to define the best nursing care, decrease complications, and ensure timely, appropriate interventions. Standards should be measurable and attainable according to the nursing staff's knowledge level.

Communication is the key to good employee relationships. Here are a few suggestions to avoid misunderstanding and to communicate effectively with the employee:

1. Define terms clearly. For example, "clean" to one person may mean clearing a path from the door to the bed. "Clean" to another person may mean having everything put away in its assigned place, the floor cleared and vacuumed, and the furniture dusted.
2. Avoid making personal comments when evaluating the individual's performance. If nurses are slow in accomplishing their work load, one should not infer that the reason is "obesity" or "laziness." Focus on specific examples of behaviors. Suggestions for improvement are generally better accepted and appreciated.
3. State criticism as positively as possible, and make sure comments are constructive.
4. Let employees explain their perception of the standard, then you provide feedback. They may have a knowledge or educational deficit that prohibits them from adhering to the standard. This provides you an opportunity to discuss your differences in interpretation.
5. Allow employees to have input into determining the standards of practice by which they work. The nurse at the bedside often is better able to decide what will and will not work in actual practice.

BH DUGGER

◆ HOW SHOULD I CONDUCT AN EVALUATION MEETING WITH AN EMPLOYEE WHOSE WORK IS UNSATISFACTORY?

Q Recently during a performance evaluation, the staff member's performance was rated "does not meet standard" in most categories. These issues were clearly documented by peer and manager observations. I have documented each previous discussion with this employee and have them on file. However, the staff member had rated herself "far exceeds" in most categories. How should I handle the evaluation meeting? How can I evaluate her in a positive way yet remain reality based?

A This is a unique situation whereby you seem to be dealing with both types of employee problems, performance and conduct. Let's deal with the performance issue first. Apparently, previous conversations between you and your staff member have not produced positive results. This may be caused by lack of understanding of expected outcomes, inability to meet those outcomes because of lack of skills, unwillingness to change because of no previous consequences, and so on. Whatever the reason, you must formalize the disciplinary process so that either performance improves or the staff member is terminated. After all, you do not want to continue to support the employment of a staff person whose performance "does not meet standard" in most categories.

When meeting with this individual, you must focus on specific behaviors rather than the person. Ask yourself, "What strengths does this employee have that can help in modifying the unproductive behavior?" Also, think about what additional resources might be needed in terms of enhancing her knowledge or skills. When you meet with the employee, examine each standard within the category and compare it with the actual work performance. Offer specific examples that clearly point out why the performance was substandard, and state what the employee could have done differently to meet the standard. Ask your employee to comment, and allow her to express opinions. Avoid placing blame by remaining focused. Be especially attuned to nonverbal cues or long silences; do not be afraid to say, "I was hoping we could discuss this today, and I'm wondering what your silence means."

Outline each problem behavior by priority: patient care–related issues first, followed by inappropriate interactions with families and relatives, to poor work habits with peers or physicians, and so forth. Once this list is agreed on, write a plan of action that is specific in terms of behavior relative to who, what, where, how, and when. Be prepared to discuss alternatives; what you may have planned for this individual may not be agreeable. A workable action plan must be your goal, so be prepared to be somewhat flexible.

Follow-up is extremely important with this particular problem. Considering that this has been an ongoing issue for you, it is imperative that you provide frequent feedback. I suggest you meet with this individual weekly to review performance. This tight supervision will help you in dealing not only with performance but with conduct issues as well. Stay focused on the issues, and don't get sidetracked with unrelated topics. Again, be specific with your feedback and provide encouragement when you see good work. Finally, do not be surprised if this individual really doesn't "get it." Remember that in the end, if you have done all you can to help preserve her self-esteem, perhaps the best you can offer this employee is to counsel her into a different position.

V MANCINI

◆ ARE PERFORMANCE STANDARDS THE ONLY CRITERIA FOR EVALUATING PARAPROFESSIONALS?

Q Is performance standards review the only way to hold paraprofessionals accountable for their patient care activities? Is a better process available?

A Standards developed by the organization are the umbrella for a multifaceted, integrated performance appraisal system. This system requires ongoing and collaborative evaluation processes. It also requires an organizational culture that promotes accountability, self-appraisal, and lifelong learning. Two examples of innovative evaluation strategies congruent with this culture are care partner review and

P

competency assessment. Both strategies assume interactive evaluation processes between nurses and paraprofessionals.

Care partner review involves collaborative evaluation of patient care activities by a team composed of two nurses and two paraprofessionals who have worked together. Evaluation conferences, lasting approximately ½ hour, are conducted at least once a month. Additional conferences may be scheduled by either the paraprofessionals or the nurses. The purpose is to celebrate successes collaboratively and problem solve areas needing improvement.

During the conferences, cases selected by the nurses and the paraprofessionals are critiqued. Suggested criteria for case selection include exceptionally effective care activities, ineffective care activities, problematic communication between the care partners or other health team members, a question regarding the rationale for care activities, and indicators of quality below expectations. In addition to case critiques, previously developed strategies for improving performance are reviewed and revised, and new strategies are formulated as indicated by the current case review.

The results of these conferences are documented and used for the annual performance appraisal of the nurses and paraprofessionals. The individual being evaluated uses the documentation in self-appraisal of performance; the evaluator uses the data to improve the validity of the evaluation process. In addition, these reports are used to document the unit's accomplishments, develop future goals, and guide budget development.

The second evaluation strategy, *competency assessment,* involves evaluation in three performance areas: cognitive, psychomotor, and affective. Measurement of cognitive abilities may include paper and pencil testing, computer simulation and testing, and oral responses to questions. All strategies should focus on critical thinking abilities.

Psychomotor and affective skills can be evaluated using a "skills fair" format. The participants demonstrate all critical psychomotor skills annually through return demonstration. Critical affective skills such as caring and respect for all individuals can be evaluated using vignettes and role playing. In addition to the critical skills, those psychomotor and affective skills identified as needing improvement during the care partner conferences are reviewed and evaluated.

It is important to remember that all evaluation strategies must be anchored in the organization's performance standards. Also, the purpose, benefits, tools, and methods of effective performance appraisal must be clearly explained. In addition, all team members should be asked to evaluate the process and offer suggestions for improvement. This is the hallmark of a culture that embraces accountability and lifelong learning.

MC HANSEN

◆ CAN PATIENT SATISFACTION BE INCLUDED IN THE INDIVIDUAL STAFF PERFORMANCE EVALUATION?

Q If we incorporate patient satisfaction in our evaluation of performance, would it be possible to include patient satisfaction in the individual staff performance evaluation?

A Organizations should be designed to achieve their goals. It is especially appropriate that patient satisfaction with health care interventions be evaluated. If this dimension is part of your performance evaluation, you can incorporate it into individual staff performance evaluations. However, criteria must be developed against which each individual can be evaluated.

As in any other standard that is part of the evaluation process, an adequate, representative sample of responses must be available from the patients the nurse has cared for during the evaluation's time frame. Consumer input is essential to ensuring quality of care. If this becomes part of your evaluation, the primary factor is to ensure that the measurement is valid and reliable. Care must be taken to evaluate usual behavior with patients and avoid magnifying isolated situations. Those involved should also know that this item has been added to the usual performance appraisal, and the nurse should have the evaluation form to review before the evaluation.

The nurse manager may be called on to obtain this information. Ways to achieve this feedback include mailed surveys and postdischarge patient interviews (see Lebov, 1988).

SR. M FINNICK

♦ WHAT ARE BASIC ELEMENTS OF A GOOD PEER REVIEW PROCESS?

Q I need guidelines to follow and actions to take in developing a peer review process on my unit. What are some of the basic elements I need to know to ensure good peer evaluation?

A Peer review is a universally accepted benchmark of a profession and is generally seen as a method of ensuring accountability to one's colleagues and to society. Unfortunately, the traditional top-down management review of staff performance is still the most frequently used form of evaluation in nursing.

Starting a peer review program can be difficult. Fortunately, we can refer to several nursing resources in beginning the process. From a national perspective, the American Nurses Association (ANA) provides published standards for all areas of practice. In addition, many of our specialty organizations provide information on the formulation, implementation, and evaluation of standards of practice.

In general, peer review can be a means of implementing accountability-based practice. The review should be based on preestablished, universally accepted standards and should be conducted as a formal process by staff. The elements of the peer review process follow:

1. Staff are educated on the peer review process and have ample opportunity for input into the system and process.
2. Objectives of the program are clear and uniformly applied at all levels of nursing practice.
3. Criteria for measuring performance are valid and reliable.
4. The role of staff and supervisors and their interaction must be clearly outlined in the process.
5. An agreed-on method for collecting performance data must be developed.
6. Where and how performance data are collected must be documented and agreed on.
7. It is paramount that management and staff agree on whether peer reviews will be used in personnel decisions.
8. It also is helpful to emphasize communication and conflict resolution skills in the initial training for peer review.

Within the peer review process, management has the roles of facilitator and coach. The nursing manager ensures that staff are well versed in the process and assists in the program's evaluation. Staff accountability can be facilitated by peer review and can become a powerful tool for motivation in the workplace.

GL CROW

♦ HOW CAN I DEVELOP GOOD PEER REVIEW?

Q The nursing staff on my unit is struggling with their role in peer review of work performance. How can I facilitate effective peer review and dialogue?

A Peer review is considered one of the most problematic types of evaluation but is always listed as a strategy for staff development. The problem with peer review is the fear that less-than-perfect evaluation feedback will jeopardize annual evaluations and merit raises and lead to hard feelings among the participants. The value of peer review is that, when done honestly, it is one of the most effective tools for improving performance. In addition, it promotes effective interpersonal communication and acknowledges others' perspectives of caring.

My first recommendation is to not use the phrase peer review but rather *peer development evaluation.* This changes the focus from a hit-or-miss isolated effort to an integrated, collaborative one.

As nurse manager, your first step is to identify the purposes of the peer development evaluation. Possible purposes are to identify educational needs, enhance insight into areas needing improvement, provide data for performance appraisals, and promote accountability for work team outcomes.

The second step is to delegate process development to a committee of volunteers. The committee should have access to current literature describing peer development evaluation. The tasks of the committee include:

1. Developing evaluation criteria that are derived from performance and professional standards of care.

P

2. Designing evaluation tools.
3. Determining the procedure for implementation of peer development evaluation.

When determining the implementation procedure, the committee should consider the following:

1. Review should be done by individuals at the same level or a higher level of expertise.
2. A variety of data should be examined (e.g., care activities, documentation, contribution to unit and organizational goals, self-development activities).
3. Evaluation should be conducted at least twice a year.
4. Feedback should be written, specific, and immediate.
5. A meeting should be held to discuss the written feedback and develop specific strategies with time frames to improve performance. Both parties are responsible for monitoring outcomes of the strategies.
6. All staff should evaluate and be evaluated.
7. Evaluators are randomly assigned.

The next step is to present the committee outcomes to the staff and teach them how to effectively evaluate *and* be evaluated. Then a pilot project should be undertaken for 1 year to fine-tune the process. During this time the peer development results would not be used for annual performance appraisals.

After the pilot project, participation in peer development should be added to the performance standards for all employees. This demonstrates its importance and reinforces the joint accountability of the reviewer and reviewee to make it a development process for both.

The key to effective peer development evaluation is trust: trust in one's peers, trust in administration, and trust in the process. This changes the perception of the peer evaluation from distrust to mutual advocacy, where all involved share the responsibility and accountability for peer development.

MC HANSEN

♦ **HOW CAN I ENCOURAGE STAFF TO WORK AS A TEAM?**

Q How can I structure the evaluation process to encourage staff members to become "team players" rather than "every person for herself"?

A Most generally agree that a major purpose of the appraisal process is to evaluate what employees have done well and to develop a plan for them to do it even better during the next appraisal period. Other purposes are to identify employees for promotion and identify education, training, and development needs as a basis for rewards such as merit increases and other benefits. If not handled or structured properly and fairly, the appraisal process can deteriorate into a negative experience for all and become a demotivating factor in the workplace.

Today's employees are rightfully demanding more input into the systems and processes that shape the work environment. Therefore, consider undertaking the following activities to structure the appraisal process to engender greater cooperation:

1. Ensure that the objectives and criteria to measure performance are clearly written. Ensure that both ends (outcomes) and means (processes) are part of the evaluation criteria.
2. Next, decide who will do the evaluating. Although still not widely used, peer evaluations can be a very motivating factor in the workplace. Peers have the most contact with each other and therefore have the best opportunity to evaluate both ends (outcomes) and means (processes). One hallmark of a profession is that its practitioners are accountable to their peers, as well as to society and the agencies where they work. The move to an accountability-based practice system may be facilitated by peer review and can inspire increased cooperation.
3. Provide educational and developmental activities to educate the staff on the benefits of peer review. Staff must participate in the development of the program in order for them to "buy in" and have a sense of ownership and accountability.
4. Begin the process of peer review slowly. Often we decide on a course of action and proceed too rapidly, not allowing staff the time to assimilate what the changes specifically mean to them. Leaders must accept the level at which staff are operating and work from there. Wanting things to be different and acting on that desire without staff involvement will only lead to frustration and could ultimately destroy your staff's chances of developing into a team.
5. Have staff and management jointly monitor and evaluate the effectiveness of the education, train-

ing, and appraisal processes. Allow for modification in your program; reimplement; and evaluate.

When management and staff work cooperatively to develop an appraisal program, it has a greater chance for success and can be a motivating part of the workplace. Accountability for the program is facilitated by participation and can increase cooperation between management and staff.

GL CROW

Policies and Procedures

◆ HOW DO WE REPLACE OUTDATED POLICY AND PROCEDURE MANUALS?

Q We find that our policy and procedure manuals are not used, are inadequate, and describe nursing care in very functional ways. We would like to replace these manuals with some more viable mechanism for articulating nursing care. Is it possible to replace them? If so, what can we replace them with, and how should we proceed?

A The trend in the past few years has been toward a decrease in the number of policies and procedures. A popular misconception is that policies and procedures are required. Actually, the number of policies and procedures required by regulatory agencies is very limited (less than a dozen). Thus, determining the number and types of policies is an organizational decision.

As the profession of nursing has progressed toward a more autonomous self-directed role, the need for rigid detailed policies and procedures has lessened. Some believe a detailed step-by-step outline of tasks is necessary for new employees or graduates. However, making reference materials available can be accomplished by other means. Those tasks that new employees are expected to perform should be part of a basic competency and orientation program. For ongoing reference, many texts are available that succinctly outline the major principles and steps. It is recommended that the nursing division evaluate and standardize a basic text for each department as reference.

The next step in revising the manual is to identify policies and procedures required by regulatory agencies. Some organizations still find that they need to retain some policies and procedures. These should be limited to those that are unique and specific and require uniform performance of a task. While reviewing the policies, the nursing division could eliminate those that are routine task or basic nursing knowledge. Those retained should also be streamlined, with detailed basic steps eliminated.

The move away from policies has been replaced with a move toward standards. *Standards of practice* outline the care delivered to a group of patients. They should be outcome based and reflect quality care. Again, many good references could be used as a base from which to build the nursing division standards. These standards can be incorporated into quality assurance and improvement programs as well as documentation systems.

SF SMITH

◆ HOW CAN I IMPLEMENT A POLICY I DO NOT AGREE WITH?

Q How can I go about implementing a hospital policy that I don't support?

A I believe this is the most difficult burden of management and at times can make you question why you are in management. Try to remember that you are a teacher, not a cult leader, so you can explain and enforce policy without total belief, as long as the policy does not conflict with your ethics.

In the prepolicy phase, you should:

1. Bring up your disagreements in meetings, along with suggestions: "I agree we don't want families in our ICU 24 hours a day, but 5 minutes an hour is too short because . . ."
2. Tell your boss about your concerns.
3. Clarify "what if" questions so everyone gets a clear picture of the implications of the policy if it were to be enforced.
4. Set up a research plan, with your unit becoming the control group.
5. Agree with policy makers on goals of the policy, and see if you can get a time-limited exemption.

P

6. Request a 6-month review of policy by an objective task force if you cannot get the policy changed.

After the policy announcement:

1. Make sure you thoroughly understand the policy and how to manage it.
2. Let staff voice their disagreements. Write them in staff meeting minutes. Encourage them to work with you to cite ways the policy can be carried out.
3. Invite administration to come to your staff meeting and hear concerns directly from your staff.

K ZANDER

Power

♦ HOW CAN WE ENSURE THAT NURSING DEPARTMENT HEADS ARE PAID COMPARABLY WITH OTHER DEPARTMENT HEADS?

Q Nurse managers in our organization are continually told that they are department head personnel. However, when compared with other departments, such as pharmacy, laboratory, x-ray, and cardiac services, they are not identified comparably. Also, when salaries and wages are reviewed, the nursing department head is paid significantly less than other department heads in the hospital. Is this typical and appropriate, and if not, what strategies should we undertake to correct it?

A Without discussing the long history of social injustice in hospitals, it is sufficient to say that most hospital executives today recognize that a mistake was made years ago in not fully recognizing the importance of nurse managers to their success and the need to integrate them into the formal department head ranks.

Let's separate the issues of designation, pay, and benefits for a department head from the greater struggle the system faces in this change process: a resocialization and realignment of the informal power structure that has existed in the hospital for years. This change is a major cultural transformation process. The social issues of integration of a new group of managers into a fairly bureaucratic, stagnant power structure are significant enough that one could expect such a change, if actively pursued, to take at least 2 to 3 years. So don't expect change overnight. This is the type of process that requires careful planning. It must be customized for your institution and must involve all levels of management.

First, you need the support and encouragement of your nurse executive. She needs to lead the effort for the nursing division. She must help you raise consciousness of the problem that exists and help educate her colleagues as to why they must pursue change. Education is an important strategy in this type of project. You can never overeducate people regarding what they are trying to accomplish and why it is important. The change cannot be viewed as a power struggle. It must be viewed as a restructure and redesign effort necessary for us to be able to adapt to the changes being forced on us externally because of health care reform. The nurse executive must be educated, as well as the nurse managers, on the importance of presentation and communication of the issue. Once the issue is identified, a diversified task force of managers and executives should be suggested as a method to map out specific plans to help accomplish the task at hand. This group can examine possible structure redesigns, educational efforts, resocialization strategies, and so on, all of which will be needed to effect this change. Nursing cannot do it alone. We can, however, lead the efforts to create a collegial atmosphere inside our institutions.

Remember that you are dealing with a major transformation effort here, and it needs to be carefully planned and evaluated.

CCC LEVENS

♦ MUST I ALWAYS OBTAIN MY SUPERVISOR'S APPROVAL FOR CHANGES I WANT TO MAKE?

Q I am coordinating a very important program that has definite impact, but I have no power to effect change without going through my supervisor (director of nursing) before the change can be initiated. Isn't this an example of power without authority?

A Each individual has the power to effect change. The roles within an organization provide structure to promote positive, sustained outcomes consistent with an organization's mission and philosophy. The coordination of a very important program requires planning, organization, and support from multiple levels within the organization. Change is difficult and presents many challenges to both individuals and the organization. The participative change cycle is initiated as new knowledge is introduced in hopes that it will be accepted with commitment toward the change. At that point in the cycle an effective strategy would be to identify those respected individuals who can use their power to support the process. Change continues as other people pattern their behavior along with those whom they perceive as leaders (Hersey & Blanchard, 1988).

Authority is one type of power that is vested in an individual as a direct result of the position one maintains within an organization. *Power,* however, can be defined in the following ways: "The resource that enables a leader to gain commitment from others" (Hersey & Blanchard, 1988), "the potential for influence" (Rogers, 1973), or "the production of intended efforts" (Russell, 1938).

Personal power is defined by Hersey and Blanchard (1988) as "the extent to which leaders join the confidence and trust of those people that they're attempting to influence." Your role in effectuating this important program is to establish good lines of communication with your supervisor by using your personal power as well as information power, in addition to employing the participative change cycle strategy. According to Hersey and Blanchard (1988), you are in the position of "selling up" by attempting to influence based on personal power and rapport to establish an effective relationship. An understanding of the impact of power and how to use it effectively, as well as a thorough knowledge of the change process, will produce the desired outcomes. Authority is only one type of power, and although important, the use of authoritative power is not the only way to accomplish a positive outcome.

J TROFINO

◆ HOW CAN I REGAIN STAFF SUPPORT?

Q I am a new manager selected from my unit with input from my staff. As a new manager, I implemented a number of changes we (staff and I) always talked about wanting. The staff are not reacting as I expected; they are angry with the changes I made and say I am now "power hungry." How might I approach this group to redefine my relationship with them and to get the unit back on track with our goals? What might I have done differently after first accepting the position?

A You chose the words, "*I* implemented a number of changes" and "staff are angry with the changes *I* made." That is where the problem lies. You want to be able to say, "The changes *we* have implemented and made." You had the best intentions and learned a very valuable lesson: the importance of collaboration in decision making.

Two issues are involved here: the implementation of change without staff collaboration in the decision-making process and the defense mechanism of projection by your staff nurses. When people are bombarded by a change outside their control, the impact is likely to be felt in many different ways. You must remember that individuals' reactions will always be personal before ever being focused on organizational concern. When people are faced with a new situation, they have emotional reactions that relate to their self-interest. Also, employees are culturally programmed not to trust their bosses.

Remember to have your staff collaborate on important issues; seek each other's opinions and expertise. Make decisions by consensus. The implementation of changes within a unit has an enormous impact on how your staff thinks and feels. When people have been left out of the decision-making process, they often feel powerless and unneeded. They become dependent on others, anxious about their value to the organization, cynical in their dealings, and understandably resistant to well-intentioned efforts to "empower" people. Those who provide the service have essential information necessary for improving quality and making sound decisions. People who have some say in decisions that affect them are much more likely to carry out those decisions with enthusiasm and ef-

P

fectiveness. Unclear or misunderstood decision making causes mistrust, confusion, miscommunication, and a sense of powerlessness.

Projection is a frequently used defense mechanism employed by those individuals who want to maintain their dependent stance. They may find the thought of independent action too threatening to consider but are unable to admit this to themselves. They fear failure in taking risks with new behaviors and fear the rejection of those whom they depend on and whose approval they seek. They protect this fragile area of their ego by blaming others for their circumstances; they become victims. They bemoan their situation with a pathetic helplessness or a righteous anger over what others have done or are doing to them.

Meet with your staff and be frank about your perceptions and the decisions you have made. Admit your error and move forward. Be open to feedback. You need to be able to accept sensitive feedback about your own communication and leadership style. In fact, you should be on a continuous hunt to track down feedback about how you come across. Willingness to accept personal feedback is a critical element that will enable you to grow as a leader. Be open to adjust personal behavior as a result of feedback. Facilitate, rather than direct, discussions and meetings. Be a catalyst for others' discussion and reflection. Communicate in ways that encourage others to offer their views.

Remember that the process of change is helped when the persons affected can participate in the decision-making process and in the planning for change. The greater the participation, the more assurance people have of being able to influence the direction and impact of change and consequently to identify and resolve their personal resistance.

The following guidelines are useful for the prospective change maker:

- ◆ To aggressively pursue committed members who want to be involved in decision making.
- ◆ To be more aggressive in seeking ideas and suggestions from committed members and to ensure that prompt feedback regarding use of these ideas and suggestions is provided.
- ◆ To establish joint problem-solving sessions so that all nurses on the unit share and better understand each other's problems.

LG VONFROLIO

◆ HOW CAN I MAINTAIN INDEPENDENCE AND NOT OFFEND COLLEAGUES?

Q How can I keep from mindlessly accepting my boss' or colleagues' priorities and values as my own without alienating those I work with?

A Nothing has as great an impact on a work team's ability to achieve seemingly unbelievable accomplishments as the creation of a shared vision. Too often it is assumed that the values, priorities, and objectives of management differ greatly from those of the caregivers on the "front lines" of giving life to the organization's mission. More often than not, the reality is that the information we operate from, and our consequent perspectives of the issues we face, differ more than our fundamental values.

As a nurse manager you are in a very pivotal position as it relates to the development of a vision shared by managers and clinicians alike. You have a good understanding of the clinical issues and can speak about them knowledgeably in management deliberations. This is not, however, a substitute for having clinical experts represent their own perspectives in managerial decision making. You also have managerial expertise and an understanding of the resource realities that impact clinical practice. It is your responsibility to facilitate a broadening of your staff's perspectives to include health care reform initiatives at the federal, state, and local level that are going to affect their lives; information about your hospital's financial health; strategic initiatives and priorities; and any other information you have access to that would assist them in developing a "big picture" mentality. Implement any creative strategies you can think of to share information. Some possibilities include regular discussions at staff meetings, special housewide staff meetings, incorporation into your current committee or council structure, brown bag lunches, or nursing grand rounds. Essential to all of the discussions is identifying what quality patient care means to us, the essential aspects of our mission, the realities of our changing health care environment, and coming to terms with the reality that we do not have the option of increasing the cost of care.

It is a critical time in health care. Nurses will be greatly disadvantaged if they cannot merge their clinical and managerial skill to design new approaches to care delivery. The best way to mobilize our resources is to work together to find that common ground in which excellent patient care and resource realities are balanced. As a nurse manager, you can take the lead in implementing these discussions. Invite your vice-president to participate. Challenge your staff to creatively grapple with how we will deliver care differently in the year 2000. You'll be pleasantly surprised to find the chasm between the values of staff and management was only as wide as the information gap.

JE BEGLINGER

Preceptors

♦ **WHAT ELEMENTS ARE ESSENTIAL FOR A SUCCESSFUL PRECEPTOR PROGRAM?**

Q In defining and planning a preceptorship program for both new graduate nurses and veteran nurses, what elements are essential to ensure successful outcomes?

A Essential elements of a successful preceptor program involve the following actions:

1. Clarify expectations of all involved (learner, preceptor, educator, manager).
2. Select preceptors for their clinical expertise, communication skills, and ability to coach, support, and advise.
3. Provide preceptor development and support. Many institutions have a 2-day staff development program for new preceptors.
4. Place learners on shifts and in situations as close as possible to those in which they will be expected to function. This increases not only their competence, but also their development of confidence. Preceptorship is first and foremost a *clinical* teaching situation, so guard against too much time spent in classrooms.
5. Ensure a positive learning environment. The learner should feel welcome, liked, and supported.
6. Assess the competence level of each learner. Use the principles of adult learning.

7. Rotate preceptors. Overusing even the best preceptor can lead to burnout.

These pointers apply to both veteran and new graduate nurses. However, new graduate nurses have some special needs. They are frightened about entering the clinical situation. They are acutely aware that their competencies are not sufficiently developed to enable them to practice safely with independence. They also need friendly nonjudgmental support during the role transition from student to practicing nurse. Support during this time has been well documented as a tool for increased competence, earlier independence, recruitment, and retention.

J HIXON

Productivity

♦ **WHAT CAN I DO TO HELP STAFF BE MORE EFFICIENT?**

Q How can I help staff to set patient care priorities and to better use their time?

A One of the first approaches would be to assess how the nurses on your unit are approaching their patients:

♦ Do they use the nursing process, and do you have a nursing model in place? Many nurses have not been taught the nursing process and models, and a good place to start would be educating them in these areas.
♦ Once this is in place, begin by helping them to look at how they assign patients for care; have them assign their patients by need, not by numbers. Help them to set assignments globally for the whole unit in a way that is a learning experience for them.
♦ Work with them to identify low-priority activities that don't always need to be accomplished, such as routine tasks that may not need to be done and care that could be done by the patients themselves or their families or delegated to another professional. Have your nurses ask themselves, "Why do we do this?"

P

♦ Foster the idea of research-based care that helps to identify ritualistic practice and unnecessary repetition. Look for ways to disseminate research that relates to practice.

♦ Examine relationships with other health care professionals in a systems fashion. Plan care with other disciplines, and work together with them to coordinate care. See that their schedules and those of the unit fit compatibly. Make changes where time can be saved.

Don't forget to use the strengths you already have and to use the staff who are skilled in setting priorities and who efficiently use their time as mentors and role models for those who are not as skilled.

JB COLTRIN ET AL.

♦ HOW DO I MANAGE NONPRODUCTIVE TIME?

Q I'm having a tremendous challenge as a manager with nonproductive time. What is nonproductive time, and how do I best manage it?

A *Productive time* is time paid that is worked. *Nonproductive time* is time not worked on the unit that is paid for out of your budget. It usually includes vacation, sick, overtime, orientation, on-call, bereavement, education, and severance time. For example, if a staff nurse works Monday through Friday, 40 hours, day shift, she is paid her salary per hour times 40 hours. If she works overtime at time-and-a-half pay for an additional 2 hours on Tuesday, she now has used up an additional 3 hours (2 hours at 1.5 times pay) of your budget, even though you only received 2 hours more of productive time. Other productive costs that "eat up" your budget include incentive pay, such as weekends and shift differentials and charge nurse differentials.

The best way to control nonproductive time is to try to "flatten it out" during the year. This includes spreading vacations and orientations throughout the year when possible. Alternately, you may budget for fluctuation if you know when it will occur. Some hospitals are controlling nonproductive time by limiting paid jury duty time or bereavement leave. Other hospitals have implemented modified work programs to move some nonproductive time into a different budget during recuperation.

The difficulty in understanding nonproductive time is that it varies unit to unit and month to month. Keep a daily or weekly log of nonproductive use of time if your finance department does not have this type of report available to you, so that you can remember who was on jury duty, bereavement, modified work, and so on. Also, be sure to check with your finance department so that you clearly understand how productive versus nonproductive time is defined in your organization.

D SHERIDAN

♦ WHAT IS THE BEST WAY TO MEASURE NURSING PRODUCTIVITY STANDARDS?

Q Much discussion surrounds nursing productivity standards. What are the advantages and disadvantages of "cost per unit of service" versus "hours per patient day" as a nursing productivity standard?

A Productivity is often defined as the measurement of the ratio of resources consumed to the yield or output of an enterprise. The formula used is Input ÷ Output × 100 = % Productivity. Accurately measuring the productivity requires clearly defining the end product. A unit of service can be considered a hospital's end product; it is why the patient comes to the hospital. In other words, a unit of service is what a hospital sells to those who either consume or pay for the service.

When payors purchased care on a per-day basis, a patient day was a fairly accurate unit of service indicator. Thus labor hours per patient day was a meaningful statistic. Today, as more payors contract for care on the same basis as Medicare, the diagnosis-related group (DRG), the unit of service has changed. It might be a chest radiograph, a tonsillectomy, or any other combination of services. Conventional nursing productivity systems have measured only one resource element, labor hours, when in reality several resources contribute to the end product. As more payors contract for a fixed payment for a unit of service, knowing the cost of providing the service becomes increasingly important. Since nursing continues to represent a major component of a hospital's inpatient services, the ability to identify and control the total cost per unit of service effectively, both from a pricing and an operational standpoint, has become a matter of survival.

The goal, however, is not to try to find the one perfect productivity measurement, but rather to use several measurements to gain insight. Cost per unit of service is useful in providing broad information representing a number of variables, including labor hours and salary rates, accumulated in terms of the hospital's end product. It is a useful statistic for comparison of cost per unit of service with revenue per unit of service. If the cost per unit of service exceeds the standard, examining hours per patient day can help in determining the cause. Hours per patient day is a narrower statistic and is beneficial for analyzing labor productivity alone. It will continue to be valuable for developing the full-time equivalent (FTE) budget.

Productivity can be a difficult concept to manage, but it is central to management effectiveness. Without productivity objectives (standards), an organization does not have direction. Without productivity measurements, it does not have control. It is therefore necessary to establish various productivity standards and monitoring systems as tools for meeting the challenge of operating successfully in today's and tomorrow's environment.

SA FINNIGAN

◆ HOW CAN I HAVE ACCEPTABLE PRODUCTIVITY FIGURES IF MY STAFF IS UNABLE TO KEEP PACE?

Q The work load on my unit is getting increasingly heavy, and some of my employees are getting older and less able to keep up with their previous pace. They have been loyal over the years, but I must meet my productivity figures. What can I do?

A The first area the manager should examine is the work load, using objective data and resource requirements. Although productivity is an important indicator to monitor, it does not give the entire picture, particularly if changes or increases in patient population have occurred. The manager needs real data to know if it is the employees who cannot keep pace or if the work load has exceeded the resources. If the resources match the work load and some employees are unable to meet expecta-

tions, the manager needs to address this on an individual basis. Following are some strategies to consider:

1. Assess each individual and assist her in examining the details of her work. Counsel her regarding performance.
2. Assess the care delivery system and consider reallocation of duties to increase efficiency and effectiveness, better matching abilities to tasks.
3. Investigate with the human resources department, if appropriate, possible early retirement plans.
4. Career counsel employees and assist them with considering other job options within the institution that would better match their capabilities. Explore their perception of work and their ability to perform tasks.

It is important to know the organization's culture in relation to tenure of these employees. Different cultures handle long-tenure employees in different ways.

SF SMITH

◆ CAN A COMMUNITY-BASED MANAGER MEASURE PRODUCTIVITY WORK LOADS?

Q Are any measures of productivity of work load appropriate to community-based managers?

A Traditional measures of work load units cannot be used for community-based nursing case management, since time is spent with patients establishing rapport that will improve quality and fiscal outcomes. Instead, results can be evaluated by comparing the case management group with health maintenance organizations (HMOs), measuring number of emergency room visits, length of stay, critical care days, and patient days per 1000 enrollees. Results also can be evaluated by using quality indicators that include symptom management, patient satisfaction, facilitation of decisions regarding quality of life issues, and other expected outcomes as perceived by the patient. Nursing case management is a process that depends on the patient's needs, so to measure work load units such as home health (per visit) may not produce the cost-efficient outcomes of a continuum of care.

DD GILES

◆ WHAT IS THE BEST WAY TO MEASURE PRODUCTIVITY OUTCOMES OF STAFF DEVELOPMENT ACTIVITIES?

Q What is a reasonable method for determining the productivity outcomes of various activities involving staff development?

A Staff development activities include educational programs, management training, and departmental problem solving. These programs may result in outcomes such as clinical advancement, reward opportunities, or perceived autonomy. Staff development activities can be costly because the staff is pulled away from patient care and replacement caregiver costs are incurred. The benefits generally outweigh the cost, however, because the staff reaches higher levels of professional function and expertise.

Productivity of the nursing staff can be measured in terms of time, cost, or patient and quality outcomes. Time spent on developing staff nurses to reach their potential in leadership and organizational skills can prevent employee vacancies and turnover and enhance recruitment for the department. Costs to prevent problems and solve potential issues result in less time spent than waiting for small problems to become major ones. Quality and better patient outcomes result from well-run departments that can focus on patient care rather than staff problems and complaints.

Staff productivity outcomes as a result of staff development activities can be determined in several ways:

1. *Patient satisfaction surveys.* Data should be collected from patients on an ongoing basis to evaluate the level of care received. Meeting patients' needs clinically and for comfort indicate positive staff attitudes, commitment, and interest. A baseline level of acceptable performance should be decided and used as a measure of quality. Trends in variances should be determined according to department and monitored closely.

2. *Nursing satisfaction surveys.* Periodic questionnaires are helpful in determining perceived nursing productivity and autonomy, degrees of institutional loyalty, and satisfaction with management, administration, and hospital structure. Frustration is often the result of underutilized skills or a pressured environment. A 2-year interval between surveys usually allows for reaction to change and corrective interventions to be effective.

3. *Low nursing turnover and vacancy rates.* Bedside nurses need to be the most skilled clinically. Longevity and high educational achievement should be rewarded so that the most experienced and skilled nurses can stay at the staff level. Enhanced autonomy and expanded accountability are provided by staff development investments. Productivity is increased by keeping and using existing staff.

4. *Decreased infection rates.* Additional education and empowerment of staff in the overall quality of patient care result in development and participation in techniques that result in decreased length of patient stay and reduced mortality. Staff members who are aware of the causes and signs of infection are more apt to practice correct techniques of universal precautions and develop improved methods of patient care.

BH DUGGER

Public Speaking

◆ ARE THERE SKILLS THAT WILL HELP ME TO BE MORE AT EASE WHEN SPEAKING PUBLICLY?

Q I have had many opportunities to speak before various groups; however, whenever I begin to think about doing so, I freeze up and become very uncomfortable. Are there some skills that I can apply to make me look comfortable at public speaking?

A Often when we speak before groups, we worry about all the things that can go wrong. It is more helpful to prepare for the talk and think of all the things that can go right. Athletes have done this for years, as have successful speakers. Successful speakers usually admit that they experience some anxiety before any public presentations. So how do they do it?

1. Know what point(s) you want to make. Keep it simple; that is, don't have more than three major

points you wish to make. More will confuse your audience.

2. Think of all the questions people might have about your topic. Select those that are pertinent to your points, and be sure to answer them in your presentation.

3. Think of images that illustrate your point(s). Talk with colleagues to gather examples or receive feedback regarding your examples.

4. Outline your points to organize your thoughts. Use a mind map such as the one in the figure to see your talk as a whole. This uses the right side of your brain and permits you to see your presentation holistically.

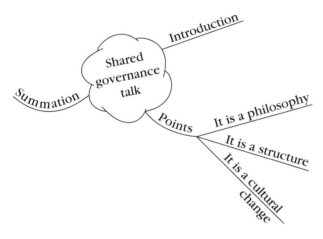

5. Practice giving your talk to the mirror with a tape recorder. Listen to how you sound: your tone of voice, pacing of speech, volume, inflection, and diction. Make changes and practice several times again. Ask a friend or two whom you trust to listen and critique you.

6. Each day for a week before your presentation, in a quiet place, sit and close your eyes. Visualize yourself giving the presentation successfully. Imagine you are backstage calmly standing or sitting by yourself. You have your eyes closed, and you are breathing slowly and deliberately, thinking about your favorite place where you can be most relaxed. You hear yourself introduced, and the audience responds with enthusiasm. Imagine yourself calmly walking to the podium and arranging your notes. You smile at the audience, take a slow deep breath, and let it out slowly. You hear yourself begin to speak from your diaphragm clearly and slowly so the person in the back row can hear you. As you scan the audience, notice everyone

intently listening to you. They are responding with laughter to your humor and thoughtfulness to your serious points. You look at different individuals and speak directly to them. They respond to you. A little later you start to feel nervous, and you picture each person in the audience as your best friend or in some humorous way, such as your pet dog who listens intently to you or wearing a ridiculous clown outfit. You pause. Take a deep, slow breath, letting it out slowly, and continue. Then picture yourself concluding your presentation and the audience applauding in appreciation. Watch yourself give them a big smile and walk confidently off the stage. You did it!

7. Now do it for real and enjoy it. Remember, they came to hear you because you know something they don't and they want to hear it.

JE JENKINS

◆ HOW CAN I FIND OUT ABOUT SPEAKING OPPORTUNITIES?

Q I have been told by other management colleagues that I am a very good speaker, am poised, and present myself well. I like having the opportunities to speak before groups and to challenge myself in a speaking role. Are there opportunities for nurse managers in speaking? Are there nurse speakers that I can be connected with to help expand my abilities and increase my opportunities to speak?

A *What* you have to say is at least as important as how you say it. Developing a repertoire of topics or issues that you have the expertise to speak about is the first step. Assuming you have done this, many opportunities exist to speak in the nursing world. Many state nursing associations have speaker's bureaus, and they are often looking for volunteers. Your state undoubtedly hosts various annual meetings. Watch for the "call for papers" for these meetings and respond. The first step is to broaden and expand your audiences. Once people have heard you and like you, your name will be mentioned when program planners are developing the agendas for conventions and meetings, and you will be asked to present more and more often.

P

Feedback regarding your presentations can be received by asking for it. You can ask someone whose speaking skills you admire to come to a presentation and provide critique. This is often more valuable than program evaluations. In the end, many opportunities exist in your nursing and broader community. Volunteer, and the rest will come.

M MURPHY

Quality Improvement

◆ HOW CAN I DIFFERENTIATE BETWEEN QI AND QA?

Q What should I emphasize if I want to clarify the difference between QI and QA?

A QA is *quality assurance,* which was designed as a program to ensure that patients receive quality care. Important aspects of care are identified and thresholds determined. Once thresholds are met, a new aspect of care is identified.

QI is *quality improvement,* which is an ongoing program to ensure that patients receive quality care. Important aspects of care are identified and monitored on a continuous basis. The thresholds must be met for 3 consecutive months, then quarterly. This ensures that the important aspect of care is continuously monitored to maintain quality.

K KERFOOT

◆ IS CQI JUST ANOTHER FAD?

Q What is continuous quality improvement? Is it the "wave of the future" or just another fad?

A *Continuous quality improvement* (CQI) is seen by the regulatory bodies in health care as the next step in the logical progression in quality improvement. The purpose of CQI is to prospectively identify opportunities to improve the quality of a product or service. In health care, CQI is based on the belief that all professionals working in a health care agency have a responsibility to monitor and improve their performance. Also, the CQI approach views patient care as composed of structures, processes, and outcomes, as provided both individually and collectively.

Rather than view CQI as the "wave of the future," it is better viewed as an evolutionary step along the way of demonstrating to consumers that health care providers are seriously engaged in monitoring and evaluating the care they are providing. The concept of assessing and improving nursing care has been pervasive since the days of Florence Nightingale. Evaluating nursing care has evolved from performing audits, to monitoring individuals, to naming and claiming specific nursing outcomes, which is the present focus. This evolution will and should continue. What can be considered transitory or faddish is the name attached to the process. It is the *process* that is important, not the label.

SR. M FINNICK

◆ IS THERE A DIFFERENCE AMONG TQM, QA, QC, AND CQI?

Q I sometimes get confused when discussing the following terms with the nurses on my unit. What differences can be pointed out among total quality management, quality assurance, quality control, and continuous quality improvement?

A *Quality assurance* (QA) is a systematic approach to ensure desired patient outcomes. QA programs are based on structure, process, and outcomes. The system identifies a deficiency, evaluates the data collected, and solves the problem. The process usually originates from a suspected problem. Individual performance and improvement concerning high-volume and high-risk procedures are usually areas that departments specifically target. Employees are expected to collect data to determine the nature and extent of the problem.

Employees are more readily inclined to participate in data collection when they believe that the data will be used for specific action to improve the environment or solve the problem. For example, the number of intravenous restarts has increased. The number of restarts versus the number of new starts this year was compared with numbers from last year. A monitoring tool is developed to investigate the reasons for the frequency of the restarts. Is phlebitis or infiltration the problem? If phlebitis, is it mechanical, bacterial, or chemical? Employees are more apt to take the time to do data collection if they know that the goal is not just to count restarts, but that restarts and work load can be reduced by identifying the specific antibiotics that need to be further diluted or administered over a longer time, or that the intravenous catheter that was recently introduced is causing a greater incidence of phlebitis and should be replaced.

Continuous quality improvement (CQI) is a continual process to improve performance. It is multidisciplinary and focuses on the process, not the individual. It is based on resource effectiveness, expected outcomes, credentialing, safety, and patient satisfaction. It examines appropriateness of care proactively, problem prevention, and cost reduction. Quality improvements are designed to eliminate waste, duplication, and rework. Responsibility belongs to employees at all levels, from administration to environmental services. Some examples are patient falls, medication errors, skin integrity, and pain management. Performance improvement examples focus on high-risk areas to reduce length of patient stay, deaths, returns to surgery, and readmissions.

Total quality management (TQM) resulted in concepts adapted by quality experts J.M. Juran and W. Edwards Deming, who introduced TQM to the Japanese in the 1950s. Dr. Juran began working with American industry in the 1970s to increase customer satisfaction, empower employees, increase revenues, and reduce cost. To achieve this, he included quality planning, control, and improvement. *Quality control* (QC) is defined as implementation of a monitor or method to maintain a positive result for all quality improvements. QC denotes constant record keeping and determining trends from data collection. TQM is a business process that integrates departmental quality assurance, customer relations, and marketing programs into one process.

BH DUGGER

♦ HOW DO I IMPLEMENT CQI?

Q Can you detail "how to" steps on the best way to implement continuous quality improvement?

A Continuous quality improvement (CQI) is a culture change determined by management philosophy. Implementing this process successfully takes time, and it must be viewed as replacing what exists, not as an add-on program. The steps are complex because you are asking people to change their thinking paradigms, to accept a different philosophy of managing, to value individuals for the value they add to their daily work, and to focus on process, customer, and outcomes based on strategic objectives.

- Step 1: *strategic planning, vision, and mission goals.* The organization must know where it is going and *if* CQI is the way to get there.
- Step 2: *administrative commitment.* Administration must be willing to do whatever it takes to make the process work. Commitment versus compliance is key, and the reason for using CQI must be to achieve the strategic objectives.
- Step 3: *education, which eventually becomes ongoing.* All staff must understand the direction of the organization, be familiar with the new vocabulary, and have a common framework from which to proceed.
- Step 4: *process improvement.* Processes are identified by staff as obstacles to achieving the strategic goals and are refined and simplified by task forces made up primarily of staff. At this step the entire organizational structure begins to change because now business is conducted differently and decisions are based on data and strategic goals.
- Step 5: *ongoing measurement and evaluation.* Continuous data collection and measuring incremental improvements in processes replace committee meetings and emotional disagreements.
- Step 6: *rewards and recognition.* Human resources changes policies and procedures to reflect a new working environment that moves from policing to rewarding *group* behaviors.
- Step 7: *feedback.* All processes and plans must be continually updated and revised, which begins the entire sequence over again.

Detailing these steps would take more than the allotted space. Look for these steps, however, in any implementation process.

The implementation takes 5 to 10 years according to successful organizations. The importance of the strategic plan and the educational component cannot be underestimated. The educational process must be-

Q

gin with management development so that management can allow change. Management is cause and all else is effect; therefore, managers must be ready and prepared to empower staff to create a new structure and future. The education must also include business planning so that everyone in the organization understands their role in achieving the mission. Basic skills such as communication, team building, goal setting, delegating, and time management must be stressed as much as statistical tools and task force training.

A very important step in implementing CQI is that the process must be designed to fit your organization's climate and culture. Do not become a slave to a model or a particular proponent such as Deming or Juran. Design what will work best for you, borrowing from all the models and proponents. Keep it flexible, and don't be afraid to seek help. Successful organizations frequently use the assistance of consultants for some or all aspects of planning and implementation. Outside sources bring new perspectives and are not hampered by the organization's baggage and history. They can often move an organization more quickly because good consultants know which questions to ask, which will free staff of the mental paralysis caused by tradition and past events.

RM HADDON

◆ HOW CAN I ENCOURAGE ADOPTION OF CQI?

Q What are some practical approaches to stimulate nursing and medical staff to accept continuous quality improvement and become more involved?

A As in any major transition, there are four main strategies to increase commitment and participation in continuous quality improvement (CQI) programs for all disciplines.
1. *Carefully examine attitudinal and educational needs.* People do not use their discretionary energy on activities that are confusing, meaningless to their work, or unconnected to their professional values. There is nothing worse than a CQI inservice to staff that laboriously goes through the minutiae of fish bone diagrams. Why is the orga-

nization pursuing this initiative? How will it help me in my work? How will I be helped to prepare for my participation? What really is expected of me? Providing case examples tied to the professional's area of interest, with demonstrated improvements, is a strong way to increase commitment.

In addition, the competence of those facilitating the CQI program must be unquestionable. People do not follow leaders who are unprepared or who possess only superficial knowledge. Be careful to not fall into the trap of assigning the CQI coordinator role to the wrong person. Sometimes we err when we give it to someone who wants to get out of patient care or, even worse, to someone we do not know where else to place.

2. *Provide adequate staffing and adequate time to do the work well.* CQI takes the dedication of adequate resources. Evaluate staffing variables before implementing the program, and make adjustments as necessary. Inadequate time will prevent action teams from engaging in the appropriate amount of planning, critical thinking, assessment, and strategy implementation. In its place will be "quick fix" solutions to complex system obstacles, which will be designed to meet criteria rather than to create real change. In addition, failure to fund adequate time and resources for CQI work will result in burned out pioneers, who will communicate their disappointment to the rest of the organization.

3. *Build in reward systems.* Professionals who assume increased responsibility should be compensated adequately. In addition, organization recognition programs should reflect the real struggles encountered by CQI teams. Consider, for example, a recognition reward for the team with the "most persistence in communicating needed change."

4. *Ensure involvement of staff from all levels of the organization.* Our quality assurance legacy reminds us, in the definition and the assessment of quality, of the authority of the individual performing the work. The organization's senior management must continually look for opportunities to recognize the contributions of the individual to the quality of the whole. Organizations do not produce quality care; people do.

CK WILSON

◆ TO WHOM SHOULD THE NURSING QUALITY IMPROVEMENT COORDINATOR REPORT?

Q In hospital organizations, to what person or persons should the nursing quality improvement coordinator report? Who is directly responsible for nursing quality improvements?

A *Nursing quality improvement* is a broad term that can be defined as any improvement activity, either clinical or operational, in which a standard is set and monitored and corrective action is taken, if necessary, to meet or exceed a defined standard. Involvement in some aspect of quality improvement should be the responsibility of every member of the nursing department. Some institutions may identify a specific individual for overseeing and coordinating nursing quality improvement. Others may use a committee with representatives from the various nursing areas. Regardless of the structure in your specific institution, nursing quality improvement is the direct responsibility of the nurse executive, and the reporting relationship should support that responsibility. It is also important, however, that nursing interfaces and is part of the overall hospital quality improvement effort and is represented in any hospital-wide committee or activity.

C ST CHARLES

◆ WHY DO STAFF HAVE TO DO DATA COLLECTING?

Q Why do staff have to perform data collection for the QA monitoring and evaluation program? Shouldn't that be the job of the QA department?

A Quality assurance (QA) is undergoing dramatic change. However, this question implies that past thinking related to QA is still in place and in need of change. Continuous quality improvement (CQI) requires new thinking and approaches related to the role of all staff members to improve all operations. In the past the involvement of staff in QA activities included data collection.

CQI provides an opportunity to redesign systems in both structure and process because of desired outcomes. Although the collection and monitoring of data are achieved in a variety of ways, the use of data offers clinicians, administrators, and all hospital staff different opportunities for decision making by using the data to provide the basis for analysis, discussion, consensus building, and action. CQI works when there is a clear commitment to everyone involving themselves in improving the system. This will take time for the learning and changes in behavior to occur, but the spirit and performance of the staff will reflect their understanding and willingness to make a difference in improving patient care.

AMT BROOKS

◆ HOW CAN I GET MANAGEMENT TO COMMIT TO CQI?

Q I need some advice on encouraging top management to write a specific plan to implement continuous quality improvement instead of merely giving it lip service.

A Many top management and administrative people are simply giving lip service to continuous quality improvement (CQI) because they are not sure what it is. Although top management in most institutions generally value the need for "quality" in our hospitals, we continue to struggle with trying to define what that is and how to achieve it. How do we balance CQI with available resources? Quality assurance (QA) was the accepted strategy for years until we realized it was only addressing the "outlier" issues. While recognizing that those were important to deal with, those of us inside the system knew that we needed to dig deeper. The problems that we face every day are more system problems than people problems. With this slow recognition came CQI efforts. Its value as a process is beginning to be seen as critical to our long-term success as an industry, especially under the cost constraints that currently face us. However, CQI was marketed initially as a total quality management (TQM) packaged program that was the answer to all our problems, and intelligent executives rightfully questioned the value of that type of approach. Initially, therefore, CQI ran into

Q

some commitment problems by more than just a few executives. That cloud is starting to lift, and the time is right to start really pursuing the value of this process for all our systems.

Keeping history in mind, several possible strategies exist for starting or redesigning CQI in your facility. Organizing educational efforts about CQI is one possibility. The Joint Commission on Accreditation of Healthcare Organizations (JCAHO) requires education by all managers and executives to meet JCAHO standards. Inviting top management to attend with you in order to see what value this process may have for your institution is a good strategy. Participating in the updating of your CQI plan, previously called the QA plan, is another strategy. During those efforts you could identify other supporters of the concept and talk with them about how you could spread the word and educate others on the value of the process. Separating *service* CQI efforts from *clinical* CQI efforts can be another effective strategy in some organizations. Clinical CQI efforts may be more readily acceptable to clinicians and may be viewed as more of a grass-roots effort truly focused on improved quality, in other words, less suspect than service CQI efforts, traditionally viewed as more marketing oriented. Effective clinical CQI efforts bring quick results and allow the true value of the process to be more visible to top management, especially if you use a multidisciplinary approach to the analysis. Don't sit back and wait for top management to get on board; be the spokesperson for the efforts. Middle management can lead that effort and through progress and education can lead top management forward.

CCC LEVENS

◆ ARE THERE TOOLS TO MEASURE CQI?

Q I need basic tools to measure QA initiatives other than compliance versus noncompliance. Are there any good tools to measure success in continuous quality improvement?

A CQI is very different from quality assurance (QA). QA looks for compliance to a given standard and whether staff are operating according to that standard. CQI does not measure behavior, but rather outcomes of the process. Therefore, measure-

ment tools are designed to measure the results of the *process,* not the behavior of the persons involved in the process. A good CQI process does not measure by quotas such as 80% or 100%, but rather looks for incremental improvement along a continuum. The goal is continuous improvement of the *process.* For example, if you were interested in measuring the number of patient falls from bed within the QA framework, you would simply count the number of patient falls and look for trends in time of day, shift, staffing patterns, and so on. Within a CQI philosophy, you would measure the assessment process used by nurses and others to determine need for medications, restraints, or side rails. In other words, you would be interested in knowing *why* patients fall out of bed, not just how many do. The purpose then would be to design structures or procedures within the organization that would decrease the number of falls. Your interest is in the "root cause" of the falls. Root cause is determined through data collection. Once this is known, you would then continually revise practices and continually monitor the results until the outcome is achieved.

The processes you select to measure should always be tied to your strategic goals; therefore, as you measure your processes, you determine the organization's goal and mission achievement. If, for example, a strategic goal is cost reduction, you would determine the cost savings involved in preventing patient falls, so the actual measurement tools of this QI initiative would be dollars saved each month as a result of the decreased number of falls. Your measurement tool in this case would be a cost-accounting one.

There is no mystery to QI measurement, and it requires no special tools. Simply decide where you are now, and incrementally measure your improvement status toward overall goal achievement. If you want to know what tools are available, you may want to purchase a book from JCAHO entitled *Using Quality Improvement Tools in a Health Care Setting.*

RM HADDON

◆ HOW DO I GENERATE MY BOSS' INTEREST IN CQI?

Q How can I motivate a boss who is neither committed to continuous quality improvement nor interested in quality assurance and improvement (QA&I) without alienating her?

A Motivation is a complex issue that, in this case, is made even more complex because we are talking about the boss. The crux of the issue is to how to create a change that is win–win. To do this, you must be able to demonstrate the payoff for the other person.

Often our inability to accept change results from our inability to see how the change will benefit us personally. Therefore, persuasion will become your most powerful tool. It is suggested that you follow these steps:

1. Enter the negotiation process from the perspective of win–win. To do this, you must have knowledge of what motivates your boss to keep things the way they are and what might motivate her to change.
2. Establish that you are a credible source of information for why CQI or QA&I will benefit the boss and the agency. Do your homework on the pros and cons of these processes. Be specific and avoid generalizations.
3. Make your presentation clear and concise. You may want to present an executive summary with follow-up of a more in-depth analysis in writing. In your presentation (orally and in writing) ensure that you present convincing evidence for why the change is needed.
4. Know the target well. Ensure that you tailor your presentation to your boss' needs. If patient satisfaction is most important to her, then highlight how these processes will improve patient satisfaction.
5. Be logical. Present your argument logically, and ensure that your presentation is internally consistent and clear.
6. Be aware of the environment and timing. Do not make your presentation at the end of a busy day, late on Friday, or the day of a JCAHO visit.
7. Finally, be enthusiastic about this endeavor. If you do not act like you are sold on the idea, the boss will not be enthused either.

Change is a very threatening event. Often we fail because we are unable to convince others of the need for change. The ability to persuade others is a developed skill that improves with practice and a belief in the benefits of change.

GL CROW

◆ HOW CAN I UNITE MANAGEMENT TO SUPPORT CQI?

Q How can CQI be implemented to address multisystemed problems when there is only lip service from the vice-president of the organization? The chief executive officer (CEO), on the other hand, is supportive of CQI.

A CQI is the responsibility of all persons in the organization. It is a philosophy of shared values and goals by which all employees must be educated and assigned responsibility. The process is based on utilization of appropriate resources and identification of costs, causes, and trends. Corrective actions should be based on research and solutions rewarded and celebrated. Communication should be multidisciplinary and organized.

Top-level administration should make sure that all levels of employees have the necessary education about the QI process and incorporate the success and effectiveness of CQI into all job descriptions and performance reviews. All employees should be empowered to be involved in the process. This process does not occur quickly, and results are often drawn out. Time lines should be established and selected problems should be prioritized and realistic.

The nurse manager should focus on departmental quality assessment and, through the larger goals of quality improvement, identify specific problem issues without finger pointing at other departments. Even if the problem is one person's responsibility, the issue should be stated as a system problem rather than an individual downfall. It will eventually become apparent that other areas need to become more deeply involved in the QI effort.

BH DUGGER

◆ HOW DO I UNITE STAFF TO SUPPORT CQI?

Q How can I get the entire staff involved in QI activities?

A There are two critical and fundamental requirements of staff involvement and participation in QI activities: the manager's belief that QI is an important and valuable method to improve clinical care and systems and an expectation by the manager and/or the institution that staff will participate.

In addition, the manager must

♦ Provide education regarding QI skills and tools.
♦ Commit to work on real issues that have meaning and value to the staff.
♦ Create an environment in which staff can work in groups across traditional organizational boundaries.
♦ Recognize staff's efforts.
♦ Reinforce efforts.
♦ Celebrate successes.

C ST CHARLES

♦ HOW CAN I MOTIVATE STAFF TO PARTICIPATE IN CQI?

Q In the institution where I am a nurse manager, we have implemented a program of CQI and each unit has a CQI committee. I have been able to find only a few nurses who are willing to participate on the committee. Those who are not willing or will not participate complain about the decisions that are made and in some cases sabotage new programs that the CQI committee has suggested. What can I do?

A The nurse manager is the formal leader of the clinical nursing staff, and according to Deming, "Leaders play a key role in fostering quality improvement." Also, "The job of management is not supervision, but leadership. To lead in quality improvement, the responsible individuals must have knowledge about and be actively involved in quality" (JCAHO, 1991).

The leader is responsible for finding the right people for the right jobs. The leader will need to "influence" others' behavior to accomplish tasks and achieve goals. In an attempt to do this, the leader must have a sound understanding of the process for planning and implementing change. A knowledge of the problem begins with a "diagnosis" and includes an attempt by the leader to define (1) what is actually happening, (2) what is likely to happen if change is not introduced, (3) what people would like ideally to happen, and (4) what barriers or blocks are stopping

movement to the ideal outcome. "Implementation" is the stage of the change process that translates data gathered during the diagnosis stage into change, goals, plans, and strategies (Hersey & Blanchard, 1988).

The nurse manager needs to evaluate the motivation or lack of motivation of the resistant staff nurses. According to Hersey and Blanchard (1988), "The motivation of people depends on the strength of their motives. Motives are sometimes defined as needs, wants, drives, or impulses within the individual. Motives are directed toward goals, which may be conscious or subconscious."

A major component of successful change is the need to educate staff nurses regarding the process and the effects the change will have on them and their practice.

Nurses have a need to know why the change is occurring, how it will benefit the patient and the staff, who will assist them in the change, and when it will take place. The most important aspect of the educational component is to maintain open lines of communication. Staff nurses must have encouragement and support regarding suggestions about new programs. Although all suggestions cannot or will not be implemented, they must be given merit and acknowledged. Encourage those staff members who make complaints about the decisions to continue to voice their opinion; however, with each complaint, an alternate solution must be presented. This excludes the solution of returning to the past system. The complaints must also be supported with concrete information and rationale of how the proposed solution does not support QI. This will allow the nurse to express her views but change the negative energy into positive. A more positive environment will be fostered, and the nurse may be rewarded for her input. This will in turn generate a more positive attitude regarding CQI (Arnold, 1993; Wakefield & Wakefield, 1993).

The nurse needs to know that QI is everyone's responsibility, not only that of the unit representative. The Joint Commission concurs,

A top-level commitment to quality, a nonpunitive environment, education in quality improvement techniques, attention to opportunities to improve systems, and commitment of resources to carry out ongoing improvement all can result in improved understanding of quality, desire to improve quality, and actual quality improvement (JCAHO, 1991).

The CQI committee must make the program inviting for even cynical people. The program must possess the characteristics of open communication and the overarching goal of seeking quality outcomes.

QI is still a relatively new concept. It focuses on outcomes and has a unit-based decentralized structure. Every unit should have its own QI program, identifying its most important issues and suggesting the most feasible means of dealing with them. Rather than using set standards as many quality assurance programs do, this innovation calls on nurses to exercise professional discretion. By taking this approach, the emphasis is on accountability and responsibility by providers of care, with nurse leaders supporting staff nurses in their increased decision-making role. "QI challenges nurses to maximize the care and services they provide, and the very nature of the program necessitates that they take active, participative roles in carrying out procedures" (Calder, 1991).

J TROFINO

◆ HOW DO I ENCOURAGE HOSPITAL EXECUTIVES TO PARTICIPATE IN CQI?

Q What are some methods to use to encourage hospital executive staff to not only "talk the talk" but "walk the walk" of CQI changes? It seems staff always change but administration does not.

A CQI, by anyone's definition, is the "scientific method" applied at a group or organizational level, that is, plan, do, check, and act. As such, it is relatively new for administrators who have not had experience in problem solving as clinicians. When implemented at its fullest by knowledgeable administrators or those willing to learn, CQI can create major cultural changes in not only the processes of an organization, but the morale and actual behaviors of the people in the immediate environment. After several years of using CQI, a growing consensus among staff, managers, administrators, and consultants is that its possible benefits are sustained only if administrators *do* "walk the walk."

Some ideas for managers entering into a CQI endeavor with administrators revolve around making sure you know where your authority lies. Authority is a negotiated entity that has to do with power. Don't accept a committee assignment or new project until you are sure about the nature of support you will receive to enable you to do the job you've been asked to do. Specific resources to be negotiated are

1. Time commitments (estimated) of you, groups, and the manager of the particular aspect of CQI you are considering.
2. Reporting structure (verbal).
3. Typing, statistics, data, and computer expertise available to you.
4. Budget for phone, field trips, seminars, consultations, and so on.
5. Confidentiality.

As you get deeply into the CQI process, keep administration involved and intrigued. Besides issuing brief but interesting reports that always give credit to responsible groups and individuals, you might try

1. Inviting key administrators to CQI meetings to hear the process firsthand.
2. Holding an annual forum so that everyone can hear about the successes. Ask the administrators to speak.
3. Being clear what specific behaviors you need from them rather than vague "support." Put support in behavioral terms, such as "Please facilitate purchasing a fax machine for this unit" or "Our group needs legal counsel about this issue. Please give us suggestions by our next meeting as to how to proceed."
4. Practicing "walking the walk" yourself. It may be contagious.

K ZANDER

◆ IS IT POSSIBLE TO MEASURE THE IMPACT OF CHANGE ON QUALITY OF CARE?

Q Our ultimate and final goal in hospitals is to provide quality outcomes for our patients. We all struggle with restructuring and empowerment issues. Are there any ways to track the impact of these changes on quality of care and clinical outcomes?

A To track changes in quality of care and clinical outcomes, you need to have a baseline with which to compare information. How are you measuring quality of care now? What are important elements in evaluating clinical outcomes? Once you decide what those are, you need to structure sampling times to follow changes that may be occurring in your indicators.

Evaluation research provides a framework for you to look at many changes over time. You may want to contact your local school of nursing to invite a faculty member to help you design such a plan. Once you have developed your plan, ongoing monitoring is necessary to adjust your structure in the direction that will continue to provide quality patient outcomes.

CE LOVERIDGE

◆ **WHEN NURSES WORK AUTONOMOUSLY, HOW CAN I IMPLEMENT CQI?**

Q In my agency, we are moving toward implementation of theory-based practice in which it is assumed that a professional registered nurse is expected to function as an autonomous and independent practitioner whenever this is appropriate. How can I, as a nurse manager, identify and apply the criteria for CQI in this setting?

A Theory-based practice and CQI are congruent. Practice that is theory based must be continually evolving as patients' needs change over time. CQI is the continual enhancement of work focused around the patients' needs and desires as defined by the patient. It requires careful and consistent data collection and observation. Assessing the impact of theory-based practice can occur though chart review, data collection, case reviews, or satisfaction surveys of patients, physicians, and nurses. Data demonstrating patient outcomes with similar diagnosis can be clearly accumulated through consistently applying theory-based practice and principles.

The focus of quality is outcome. Outcomes are largely determined by the quality of the processes that produce them; therefore quality efforts should center on process.

One of the primary attributes of CQI is that the people doing the work have the information on how to improve it and should be making decisions about how to improve it. Teams composed of people who

clearly understand the job should work together to improve the work process and systems that support the work needing to be done. Knowledgeable staff are needed to analyze the processes and to look at more efficient, effective ways to get the work done. In CQI it is recognized that, for the most part, it is not the people, but rather the inadequate systems, that create barriers and get in the way of getting the job done.

Empowered staff who can function independently and autonomously and who use theory-based practice are capable of using data to examine how work is done and how to effect change. Empowerment of the professional nurse leads to a willingness to challenge and ask questions about the way care is delivered and how it can be improved. The manager must create an environment in which staff feel the initiative and support to challenge the way things have been done.

In organizations that are appropriately decentralized and "right sized," it clearly cannot be an expectation of the manager to identify where all the areas for improvement exist. The manager can play a role in establishing and supporting team goals and encouraging groups to set goals but cannot possibly know all the processes and potential areas for improvement. The manager's role must be to provide information, support, resources, and consultation for the practitioner.

Autonomy and independence go hand in hand for CQI to succeed. Autonomous teams of staff using theory-based practice understand their clinical responsibilities and can manage their own practice if trust and respect for the practitioner truly exist. The manager's role is to create an environment for staff that uses their clinical expertise, supports their decisions, supports conflict, and pushes for change that makes sense. Autonomous people must feel the support and reward for taking risks when trying to fix a process that is inefficient or not working.

The manager must understand the theory-based practice the staff is using and must be well educated in the concepts and principles of CQI. She must be articulate in her understanding of the tools and principles and able to help advise the staff, support their data collection, and help them interpret the data and facilitate action necessary to respond to what needs to be done.

So how does the manager get this all started? She should first select a representative sample of the staff who have a good understanding of the theory-based practice being used. She should then provide them with instruction concerning the tools and principles of CQI and with a facilitator's course. This ensures thorough integration of the two and ownership of both theory and CQI by the staff. Management must be willing to develop staff in the same way management is educated to function in a CQI environment. Management often falls short in recognizing and ensuring that staff are given the same amount of training and support management is given to understand and feel comfortable with the changes being made.

J TORNABENI

could discuss the candidate and come to a mutual decision on hiring.

4. Once mastery of skills and a track record of success are established, HR might be willing to turn over the hiring decision to nursing and feel comfortable backing out of the process.
5. Keep a record of the before, during, and after progress of nurses hired and their success in performance to document the outcome of the change.

JM McMAHON

Recruitment

◆ HOW CAN I GET MORE CONTROL OF STAFF RECRUITMENT?

Q In our hospital, recruitment is exclusively a personnel service function. The nurse manager cannot make specific choices with regard to candidates. She can only recommend to the personnel department those candidates she believes are appropriate. This is not working well for our organization. What can we do to address this serious problem in the recruitment of staff?

A Since this issue is a policy issue, administration must be involved. The vice president for nursing and the vice president for human resources (HR) ultimately must discuss the conflict and compromise on alternatives. It is possible that HR is not comfortable with nursing's ability to choose candidates, or it could be that control of hiring decisions is the real issue.

1. Ascertain HR's comfort level with nursing interviewing and hiring skills.
2. Have HR present a program on these skills if they are lacking. Classroom methods, role-playing, and videotaping mock interviews are tools that could be used.
3. Establish a matrix structure for decision making on hiring. The nurse manager and the HR recruiter

◆ HOW DO I BEGIN THE RECRUITMENT PROCESS?

Q The centralized recruitment process of our hospital is no longer funded. Many recruitment activities now belong to each unit of service. I am unfamiliar with some of the dynamics of recruitment but need to recruit additional nursing staff to my unit. Since we have no centralized recruitment process, how should I approach recruitment of new staff?

A The most immediate and reasonably effective resource available is your current staff using "word of mouth." Use the informal network. Promote and sell the differentiating characteristics of the patient care area informally as well.

More formalized approaches might include the traditional postings, media, and other advertising methods employed jointly with other areas within the system to minimize the fiscal impact.

Develop alliances with educational facilities in the area. Clinical rotation opportunities for student nurses and other allied health professionals give you immediate access to potential new employees. Seek opportunities to become a voluntary clinical faculty for the various schools, increasing your and your institution's visibility.

Enhance your learning curve in HR management (recruitment) through workshops and peer networking and with other HR departments that have demonstrated successful recruitment efforts.

Develop a plan that begins with getting the word out and defining the need. Allocate time to this important aspect of your job. With good preparation up front, you will alleviate nonproductive interviewing.

R

A good description of the patient care area that you can promote or sell would include sincere and honest responses to questions of interest to applicants. Questions generally posed would include nurse/patient ratios; rotation frequencies; straight shift opportunities; turnover rates; average daily census; self-scheduling; management and patient care philosophies; relationships with physicians, staff, and others; opportunities for advancement; modality of patient care delivery; and, of course, mention of salary and benefits.

A strategy of shared interviewing, in which the applicant receives firsthand information from actual staff associates, has merit and is worth exploring.

LM JOHNSON

♦ **WHAT IS A "HEADHUNTER," AND HOW CAN THIS PERSON HELP ME?**

Q I was recently called on the nursing unit by a "headhunter" who was recommending me for a position in another organization. Was it appropriate for me to discuss those matters over the telephone on my work unit? What exactly does a headhunter do in the recruitment process? How can I best use such services for my own career advancement?

A It would be appropriate to have only a limited discussion with a headhunter over the telephone on the work unit. You could express interest in a particular position and, if interested, provide the headhunter with information on how to contact you at home or on off-time. It is a matter of professional responsibility to not disrupt your work in this regard, and one would expect a headhunter to respect this position.

A headhunter is in business to make money by providing recruitment services. Generally these individuals seek out people who may have qualifications and interests for positions being recruited for by individuals or institutions. Usually a headhunter attempts to find people to apply who match those requirements. Headhunters are not typically in the position to screen candidates to identify the most qualified; they function more to obtain phone numbers of potential candidates and, in the process, potentially market a position to generate interest. A headhunter may also be used by an individual seeking a particular position in order to create this type of match. In this regard the headhunter often functions as a point of contact between recruiters and people looking for new opportunities. Most often, headhunters are used in filling positions that are difficult to fill or when individuals or institutions may be seeking more focused recruitment or job identification with discretion.

A headhunter's services can best be used for your own career advancement when you are looking for specific types of job opportunities. To assist the headhunter in identifying possible jobs, you should know personal strengths and what you are seeking in a job opportunity. If the positions being sought are clearly identified, a headhunter could be helpful in connecting you with those who are recruiting for positions of interest to you. Headhunters often can provide a more global picture of opportunities available.

You would best be served professionally by ensuring that the headhunter you are using is reputable. Provide this person with an accurate, concise set of information on your résumé.

J O'MALLEY

Research

♦ **HOW CAN I STIMULATE INTEREST IN NURSING RESEARCH?**

Q How can I help staff nurses become interested and involved in clinical research at the unit level and use research to direct their practice?

A Nursing practice is the essential component in the circle of nursing research, theory, and practice. As a nurse researcher, I am concerned that nurses in practice have often been criticized for lack of interest in research when in fact they are justified in calling for research that is truly useful to inform nursing practitioners. Such criticism is not helpful to nursing staff or to the development of nursing knowledge to update practice. It would be helpful if nursing researchers and theorists would give more attention to questions and methods of inquiry that have meaning to nursing practice.

Much research reported in the literature does not fit nurses' ways of thinking about and doing clinical nursing. For example, many nurses in practice know that the unique, whole persons they nurse are not represented by particular attributes, statistics, and outcomes of standard research methods. These nurses ask that researchers' questions involve real nursing and that researchers' methods be useful in working with real nursing practice problems. Some methods of research unique to nursing are now being developed. At the same time, nursing staff are often unclear on the meaning of nursing research to their practice.

Some questions to help nursing staff prepare to use nursing research are:

♦ What concept of nursing guides the practice of nurses on this unit?

♦ What questions, issues, or problems are faced by these nurses in their daily practice?

♦ How can the staff find and work with research that is consistent with values and beliefs guiding practice on this unit?

♦ How can research about the particular problems be located and evaluated?

♦ What are particular strengths and areas for learning concerning use of research for each nurse on the unit?

One example of involving nursing staff in nursing research occurred over a 2-year period in an acute care community hospital and addressed questions raised by nursing staff (Parker, Gordon, and Brannon, 1992). Nurses, with genuine support of administration and nursing researchers, formulated research questions congruent with their values and unique clinical settings. Nursing staff participated fully in learning and doing nursing research. Success of the research depended on all participants' willingness to engage in the project.

ME PARKER

♦ **HOW CAN I GET STAFF TO READ NURSING RESEARCH LITERATURE?**

Q I circulate one nursing research article each month to the nursing staff to use in their practice, but it never seems to make much difference.

They say they don't have time to read. How can I get them to apply literature to their own practice?

A To apply research to practice, the user must be familiar with research methods and must be critical of the innovations that research suggests. I know that nurses prepared at the baccalaureate level have some exposure to critical reading of research, but it is limited and usually occurred before they started working in the hospital setting.

I have found two approaches that help. The first is to require research-based policies and procedures. For staff nurses to use research, they need to see its use in a way that supports them. Staff will research a policy, looking for one or two articles, often with the goal of validating their own opinion. Once they begin to review the literature, they find support for or opposition to their views and are motivated to keep searching. I have never required extensive research support, but one to three articles with at least one being research, encourages critical thinking and the use of research in practice.

The second tool I am familiar with is the use of journal or study groups for specific problems or issues. For instance, our facility was still using in-line intravenous filters after others had stopped. Many strongly believed that the in-line filters prevented infection. A group of staff nurses, with a clinical specialist leading and our director for nursing research assisting, formed a study group that reviewed the literature and research on in-line filtration and found that the evidence did not support the use of in-line filters. The infection rate did not increase, and the cost savings were significant.

Lack of a hospital-based nurse researcher should not be a problem, but you need someone with experience in critical use of research. A clinical specialist, master's-prepared manager, or a faculty person from your local college are options to help staff start to use research in practice.

M PECK

R

♦ **HOW CAN I INCREASE STAFF AWARENESS AND USE OF NURSING RESEARCH?**

Q In my BSN program, I became excited about using nursing research findings to improve quality of patient care. In my community hospital, no research is done, and to my chagrin, I see no use of nursing literature to help improve nursing practice. Most of my staff are licensed practical nurses (LPNs) and associate degree nurses (ADNs). Is there anything I can do to increase their awareness and use of nursing literature and research?

A Several reasons exist why nurses do not use nursing research in their practice. Many are not prepared educationally to understand research methodology or to interpret the findings from the statistical results. Research terminology may be intimidating to some nurses, who may not have been exposed to concepts such as theoretical framework, conceptual models, or other research terms. Some nursing studies may not have direct applicability to practice but may be important studies for knowledge development.

Exposure to research involving practice or your specific specialty is one easy way to enhance nurses' understanding and appreciation of research. One hospital Xeroxed short research articles or a summary of the research findings and posted the articles in the nursing lounge, communication book, nursing station, and bathroom-stall door. A short summary of the research with comments on how the findings apply to a particular specialty is helpful to nurses without much exposure to research.

Research is reported in many styles according to the journal publishing the article. For nurses not experienced in reading research, you may want to search journals that publish research findings in a narrative format rather than in the usual research reporting style. Journals other than nursing publications also include research applicable to nursing practice and should be scanned for information to be shared with nursing colleagues.

One of the best ways to begin to appreciate nursing research is to participate in a study. If no resources are available in your hospital setting to develop a research project, you may want to contact the nearest school of nursing to discuss developing a joint project appropriate for your nursing specialty. Enlist the help of some nurses on your unit to participate in data collection, observations, interviews, or other methods used in your study. Participating in the study increases their awareness of research methodologies and how findings are generated.

Quantitative studies are often more intimidating to nurses who do not understand research. By sharing the summarized findings of such studies and how they are applicable to your setting, the nurses can be exposed to research without struggling with the interpretation. Qualitative methodologies are often more easily understood by inexperienced nurses, and you may want to share some of these studies or enlist their participation in a qualitative study appropriate for your unit.

Planning an inservice program or a series of programs on research at the basic level could also be helpful. It is important to keep the programs short and focus on one small aspect of research to avoid overwhelming the nurses with too much information at a level that exceeds their ability to understand and appreciate.

Once the nurses begin to demonstrate more interest in research, consider developing a research council to review articles and choose some to share with the staff in a discussion round table, staff conference, or inservice meeting. The committee could also serve as a support group for those who want to embark on a small study or enhance their research skills. Establishing a research committee extends staff involvement in promoting research on their own unit.

JF STICHLER

Retention

◆ WHAT CAN I DO TO PREVENT RAPID TURNOVER?

Q What actions can I take as a nurse manager at the unit level to prevent high levels of turnover? We have a high-stress unit and a challenging patient population.

A A nurse manager is responsible for maintaining a positive environment for staff. Many opportunities arise in a day to recognize hard-working staff. Thanking staff for a job well done, pitching in to help when someone appears frazzled, occasionally buying a pizza, starting an exercise group, and having a party for no reason are just a few ways that relieve stress. Always put yourself in their shoes and remember that laughter goes a long way. Many relaxation techniques can be helpful for staff. Also, providing staff with the opportunity to give presentations of difficult clinical cases can enhance learning while recognizing expertise. Contact your staff development department for further suggestions.

JG O'LEARY

Retirement

♦ **WHAT PLANS SHOULD I DEVELOP FOR RETIREMENT?**

Q I am a nurse manager and have been with this organization for 20 years. I am looking ahead to retirement, although I have about another 15 years of active management practice. What plans should I be making? Where can I turn to assess whether I will be adequately financially prepared for retirement, and what activities should I undertake *now* to make sure that I am?

A Three major areas come to mind when discussing future retirement: your finances, health, and remaining years of work.

A good financial advisor is important. Although a good one may be hard to find, ask friends, family, and retirees. Attend seminars and workshops in your city (many brokerage firms and trust companies offer them free of charge), and take courses in relevant subjects at your local college. You may decide that you want to start investing in a house if you haven't already bought one, and you may want to begin a retirement savings fund. Remember that these last 15 years will likely provide you with your greatest earning potential.

In the event that you move or are moved from your present position, you must prepare yourself for other opportunities. Keep yourself current in your field and in management practices. Be prepared to diversify your skills to accept a lateral transfer. If your position is eliminated, be prepared to assume other roles. Always be aware that nursing is changing, and stay on top of those changes.

Your health is an important factor in your existing life and your retirement. Establish an exercise, eating, and healthy life-style program for yourself now. You want to enjoy your retirement, not spend it sick. You should also make certain that you have enough insurance in case you take ill or become injured on the job. Long-term illness can interfere significantly with your savings and retirement plans.

Ask yourself, what type of retirement will I want, and what will I be satisfied with? Establish your goals and begin to work toward them. You are already ahead of most people who don't think about retirement or plan for it until it is upon them.

JB COLTRIN ET AL.

Rumors

♦ **HOW SHOULD I DEAL WITH AN EMPLOYEE WHO SPREADS RUMORS?**

Q A staff nurse on the unit has been spreading rumors about me with unit staff and other employees. What should I do?

A Usually, this type of behavior is an attempt by the employee to meet her power or belonging needs. This person may not feel valued or recognized or may have reasons to try to diminish your power and influence with staff. Staff are usually able to sort out the truth through their own direct contact and experiences with you. If you have accurate information regarding the content of the rumors, it is appropriate to discuss this with the individual. It is important that this type of behavior be directly confronted in a calm, objective manner. As a manager, you also must explicitly define your expectations for behavior to this employee, as well as the consequences if the behavior does not change. It may be helpful to use a facilitator to discuss this topic if it is a pervasive problem or has significantly interfered with your relationship with staff.

C BRADLEY

R

Salaries

◆ HOW CAN I RELATE NURSES' SALARIES TO PRODUCTIVITY?

Q How can we link salaries with productivity so that a better connection exists between what nurses do and what they are paid?

A Centuries ago, Justinian postulated, "Justice is the firm and continuous desire to render to everyone that which is his due." Unless there is a clear understanding of what is expected, however, it is difficult to connect the reward to the expectation. A nurse manager often has difficulty assessing productivity in nursing. Can we put a monetary value on having compassion for the dying, teaching the living, and tempering the machinery that sustains the critically ill? Can we put a value on the other myriad tasks and the talents, art, and science that our staffs possess?

We can tie salaries to this "productivity" only if we have a clear idea of our institution's overall strategic plan, mission, and philosophy and reward the players who help us move toward those goals. To accomplish this, we must start first with the "big picture."

1. Be familiar and knowledgeable with the strategic plan for your organization. Be a player, and align yourself on any of the subgroups, product lines, or interests that affect your unit. For instance, if yours is an orthopedic unit, be involved in the planning for outpatient screening, sports medicine interests, and community outreach programs for rehabilitation.
2. Involve your staff in the planning process so that they understand what part your unit or area plays in the greater scheme.
3. Establish the standards for performance that will be rewarded. On an individual basis, these performance standards must be stated in terms of specific outcomes and behaviors that can be documented and measured.
4. Communicate to the staff what these expectations are, and advise them in understanding how this fits into organizational productivity, goals, and missions.
5. Identify the rewards, whether they are recognitive, monetary, or both.

6. Align any gain sharing or profit sharing with the institutional goals. In most environments, the first benchmark for this reward is patient satisfaction. Others often used for employee rewards are related to attendance, cost containment, decreased lost charges, decreased patient days, new programs, or reduced turnover.

We all need to see and understand how our actions fit into the greater plan, but we also need to understand how we will be rewarded monetarily for that participation. As managers, we must ensure the reward is sufficient; too little is not an incentive for productivity.

MA SORENSEN

◆ HOW CAN I REWARD EMPLOYEES WHO ARE "TOPPED OUT"?

Q Most organizations have a number of "topped-out" employees who receive no monetary compensatory reward each year. As a manager, what can I do to reward them?

A Provide incentives for topped-out employees to attain higher levels of education. Nursing has an unusual number of advanced educational opportunities, and you should encourage your staff to take advantage of them. This may seem costly at first, but when you consider the mobility nurses have between health care settings, offering opportunities that enlarge their professional perspective clearly will enrich your own setting multifold.

Provide topped-out employees with nonmonetary opportunities within the organization, and help them explore monetary opportunities outside the organization. Most professionals have many opportunities to receive compensation for speaking engagements, consultation, or writing, which reflects well on your organization and helps the employee grow.

P MARALDO

◆ WHAT ARE SOME ALTERNATIVE WAYS TO COMPENSATE?

Q Are there ways to reward extra effort and energy by staff nurses other than paying hourly rates, overtime, and similar benefits?

Many creative ways are available to reward nurses through compensation and benefit programs specifically designed to meet their needs. First, before a compensation and benefit program is developed, you should find out exactly what your nursing staff wants. Some nursing groups prefer certain types of benefits over others, and therefore it is necessary to have a more flexible benefits program. Other nurses may prefer the independence of having a professional salary program in which they are paid an annual salary and expected to operate like other exempt salaried employees in an organization. Also, hospitals have implemented creative incentive bonus programs that emphasize quality improvement and other rewarded goals, since the hospital reaps the benefit and efficiencies that the nurses help promote.

Hospitals have been extremely traditional in their approach to compensation and benefits for nurses. It is time for human resource departments to break away from traditional models developed for work forces of the 1950s and develop progressive, innovative models that meet the needs of today's nurse. One must realize that the average nurse today is 41 years old, female, and married, and she is looking for scheduling flexibility. Many compensation and benefit programs, however, focus on an hourly mentality and benefits that are not very meaningful to the nurses. Nursing managers can play a role in providing this vision and leadership for an organization. Research the various creative models discussed in the literature and used at other hospitals. Lead the effort to break away from the stereotypic hourly mentality that exists in nursing pay practices. Be creative!

KJ McDONAGH

♦ **WHAT ARE SOME INNOVATIVE WAYS TO REWARD STAFF?**

Q What ways are available for rewarding staff differently from simply hourly wages?

A We are often reminded that most of us did not choose nursing as a way to get rich. Although we expect to earn a decent income, we realize that we stay in nursing for more than just the salary. I have found that, as managers, we try to answer the question about rewarding staff by ourselves or try to look to what others have done. The best way to learn what nurses want and how they would like to be rewarded is to ask the nurses. The manager who takes this fairly unusual step must not do so lightly. The manager must be truly open, honest, and fair and must be ready to hear whatever is brought forward. An atmosphere supportive of creative ideas is essential, and the manager must be willing to offer information to help nurses create realistic alternatives.

We sometimes apologize for what is called "nurses' idealism" when we would do well to pay attention to the ideals held by nurses and build reward systems accordingly. Exploring questions about what originally brought us into nursing and what has kept us in nursing can lead to illuminating and essential internal rewards. Caring, compassion, wanting to help, a desire to be competent, and increasing growth in an excellent practice are usually cited as answers to these questions. Realizing respect of the self and others for these values can empower nurses.

Exploring ways these values are or can be incorporated in practice is encouraging and will lead to increased creativity and a sense of owning and prizing one's practice. Genuine honesty and fairness from managers and staff are essential in exploring values and creating practice settings that recognize and support ideals guiding our commitments.

ME PARKER

♦ **HOW CAN WE MAKE A SMOOTH TRANSITION FROM HOURLY TO SALARIED PAY?**

Q I'm a manager in a fairly progressive hospital environment. We are trying to shift the mindset of our nurses away from the "hourly pay" mentality toward a "salaried" program. With all the complexities woven into nursing compensation structures over the years, we are finding it an extremely difficult and burdensome task. Do you think this is still a critical factor in future compensation? If so, can you give us some advice so that we may see some light at the end of the tunnel?

A Before we can have the pleasure of seeing the "light at the end of the tunnel," it may be helpful to examine why we are going through the tunnel in the first place. The idea of a "salaried" versus "hourly" mentality has much broader implications than how a nurse is compensated for her work.

S

We have often heard that when nurses stop punching time clocks, they will magically become more professional. Consequently, many institutions changed from time clocks to hand-written time cards. I believe the effect of this isolated practice did not have a significant impact on our journey from blue-collar to professional status.

The salaried nurse, by virtue of the method of payment, is no more professional than the hourly nurse. The movement to professionalism is much more complex, and compensation methods are only one component of that journey.

Although I believe all nurses should be salaried and free to negotiate their wages and working conditions, this is not the panacea for the journey to professionalism. I agree that the complex pay rules enforced by union contracts and state and federal labor laws do pose a threat to this process. However, I also believe that if we, as a body of 2.2 million nurses in the United States, wanted this changed, we could accomplish it.

At present, I suspect that this move would be seen by staff and the union solely as a means to get increased work out of the staff without paying for it. This is precisely why I suggest that although it is a noble goal and a hallmark of professionalism, we have some basic workplace-related issues to conquer first:

1. Move all patient care decisions to the staff level.
2. Increase staff input into budget formulation and control.
3. Institute a peer review process that is designed, implemented, and evaluated by staff and management.
4. Move to accountability-based practice.
5. Realize that the relationships between union and management must improve so that the previous four points can occur.
6. Insist that our institutions of higher learning build into the curriculum the expectation and skills to become an entrepreneur and the skills to negotiate individual compensation packages.

The way nurses are compensated is an important issue. However, compensation levels are also important. It will do nurses little good to be salaried if our salaries are below those of other professionals who provide comparable services to society. Rather than work on this singular issue, it would be much more effective for us to work on the entire issue of compensation and its relation to professionalism.

GL CROW

Scheduling

◆ HOW CAN I HELP QUARRELLING STAFF TO RESOLVE SCHEDULING PROBLEMS?

Q There has been a continuing conflict between one vocal staff nurse and several less vocal staff regarding holiday time off. The less vocal staff have come to me to make a decision that will be fair to everyone. Our policy has been to encourage staff to resolve their own conflicts, but I see intimidation as a part of this situation. What should I do?

A This situation provides you with a unique opportunity to coach staff in problem-solving skills. It is important that each participant in this discussion understand what the others want and need to have a successful resolution. I would recommend that you act as facilitator for this discussion with the staff. You should not attempt to solve the problem but should continue to provide coaching by clarifying what is being said, asking questions, and redirecting. You also should ensure that no one person dominates the discussion or interferes with the consensus-building process. Each participant should be asked for her opinion of the process and her level of satisfaction once the issue is resolved. Your involvement as a facilitator does not diminish or conflict with your philosophy to let staff solve their own problems. This is an important role to play in developing staff.

C BRADLEY

◆ WHAT CAN I DO TO IMPROVE COMMUNICATIONS AND BUILD A TEAM?

Q How can I increase communication and build a team with all the flexibility we now offer with staffing plans? Eight-, 10-, and 12-hour shifts, weekday and weekend plans, plus PRN and part-time schedules make it difficult.

A The growth of flexible shifts has increased staff options and satisfaction. It has also challenged management to manage communication and patient care continuity. When all staff worked 8 hours, we could get by with one staff meeting. Today, we must schedule multiple meetings covering the same material. You need to schedule five or six staff meetings 1 week a month, covering all shifts twice. This gives all staff the opportunity to attend. The attendance will be lower at each meeting, which can foster dialogue and team building. Collective minutes of the issues presented and discussed should be posted, with all staff required to read and initial the minutes each month.

JM McMAHON

♦ HOW CAN OVERTIME BE MANAGED FAIRLY?

Q Occasionally the staff is faced with mandatory overtime in the operating room (OR). We presently have a roster and rotate the mandatory overtime among all staff. Is this a fair way to handle overtime?

A The fact that you ask the question indicates that there may be some staff in your OR who believe your rotation roster is not altogether fair. Staff satisfaction with the method is as important to its success as an external evaluation of fairness. Literature suggests that some aspect of personal time management contributes to nurses' perceived autonomy and that a direct correlation exists between feelings of autonomy and overall job satisfaction. Therefore, although the mandatory method you describe may not be unfair, it might need reconsideration to create a sense of ownership of the plan by staff.

Generally, a method that considers the staff's individual needs and desires, while accomplishing the unit's objectives, has greater potential for support by both management and staff. Consider developing a roster of staff who are interested in working the overtime. Then rotate the available overtime among those on the "interested" list first. If none of the interested roster staff is available for a particular need, the general roster could be used.

Another approach would be to have a few flexible part-time (PRN) staff available to use when the schedule runs behind or a higher volume of cases increases the demand for staff. PRN staff could fill some of the demand without the added expense of costly overtime.

Again, although these approaches may be workable and fair, staff ownership of the method is most important. To accomplish this, your OR unit could appoint a representative group of staff, including a manager, and charge the group with developing the guidelines for handling unscheduled staffing needs. They are likely to design a method better than either you or I could create alone, and it will meet your OR and your OR staff's needs.

SA FINNIGAN

Self-Managed Work Teams

♦ WHAT PROBLEMS ARISE WHEN DEVELOPING SELF-MANAGED WORK TEAMS?

Q We are considering the development of self-managed work teams on my clinical unit. What problems can I anticipate in the development of self-managed work teams so that I can begin to plan to address them?

A The success of self-directed work teams (SDWTs) depends on management's support and the team's willingness to work together for a common goal. Switching from directing to influencing is a major change for a manager who has spent years telling people what to do. This transition from manager to coach is probably the most difficult of all individual changes that must occur to bring work teams into being.

The critical elements that SDWTs must address are
1. Internal management and coordination. What management functions will the SDWT take over?
2. Boundary management. How far can the SDWT go in its problem solving?
3. Access to information. How will the SDWT get feedback and necessary information from the organization?

S

4. How will the SDWT obtain the training necessary to get involved in the appropriate compensation system?

For a team to be productive and cohesive, its members must establish ground rules together and then agree to abide by them. The ground rules will include focusing on such issues as how to deal with individuals not doing their job, the decision-making process, how to deal with tardiness and overly critical behavior, and how to select a problem-solving procedure.

The ground rules concerning people involve team members' relationships with one another and focus on how individuals will treat each other. A fair hearing for all ideas and comments is necessary for a consensual process to exist. Team members should take the time to think of everything that could create interpersonal problems by "brainstorming" a list of items and then deciding on ground rules that members will abide by to prevent problems.

Not only is training necessary for managers as they move to a coaching style, but training is also equally necessary for the team members and should include leadership, problem solving, decision making, conflict resolution skills, facilitation skills, and administrative tasks, such as hiring, firing, and appraisal. A good exercise is to list all the different sources of decisions that teams might make and arrange them in a hierarchy. Young teams learn to make easy decisions before they make the tougher ones such as firing. Groups must go through some team-building or developmental activities to begin to function as teams. Group members will need training in areas such as self-awareness (use of the Myers-Briggs Type Indicator Assessment) and how to reach consensus in decision making ("desert survival" is a well-known consensus-building exercise).

Finally, it is important for management not to panic when productivity decreases, as it often does in the early stages of work redesign. Democratic methods are often alien to those accustomed to more authoritarian methods, and some individuals may need time to adjust to this less traditional approach. Some reports indicate as much as a 30% increase in productivity. The additional benefits of higher quality and better customer service are important in today's health care arena.

VD LACHMAN

◆ HOW DO I DEVELOP A SELF-MANAGED WORK TEAM?

Q How do I develop self-managed work teams when most of the work is individually assigned and not based on team thinking?

A First, define the leadership skills required to become an empowering leader. Take particular note of enabling skills as well as the detracting ones. Creating the environment supportive of SDWTs is a critical component and a significant role of leadership.

The new breed of leadership requires skillful coalition and consensus building, coaching, mentoring, sharing of previously held information, and a sincere acknowledgment of the new worker. Valuing, trusting, and respecting each individual encourage creative potential. Each member is given the opportunity to participate in decisions that affect how the work is done.

Leadership articulates a new vision that dissipates the notion of us/them, thereby facilitating a preferred vision of "we." The team concept "we" becomes a crucial component of the new work.

Development of empowering behaviors of leaders *and* the movement of staff members toward self-direction are a very sequential process. The leader and team advance through various stages of development, with each providing new areas of growth.

A system-wide approach acknowledging how work and staff are viewed differently begins the process of new thinking, new vision, new cultures, and thus a new future.

LM JOHNSON

Self-Scheduling

◆ CAN STAFF CREATE THEIR OWN SCHEDULE?

Q My staff is interested in creating their own schedules. How can I support them and still be sure that the unit is adequately staffed?

A Because scheduling decisions have a direct effect on the personal lives of staff members, involvement in the scheduling process gives many staff an increased sense of control of their lives. At the outset, however, few staff are aware of the multiple facets and interrelationships of scheduling decisions. You will be most supportive if you assist them in avoiding their temptation to simply plunge ahead and "write the schedule." By undertaking a process of outlining the parameters staff will use in developing the schedule, they can avoid many frustrations later. You or someone experienced in these processes can guide them in writing the necessary guidelines. These are some questions that scheduling guidelines must answer:

♦ How will the master staffing plan that outlines the required number of staff in each category (RN, LPN, NA, etc.) be used to form the foundation for the schedule?

♦ Will a master rotation plan be used? If so, who will prepare the master, and how many weeks will it cover?

♦ What will be the timing of key scheduling activities? How far in advance must requests be submitted? When will an initial draft be available? When will the final draft be posted?

♦ How will requests be handled? Consider both requests made in advance of schedule posting and requests for changes after the schedule has been posted. Will vacation requests be handled any differently than other requests? Will any situations (e.g., school schedules) receive special priority when granting requests?

♦ How will holiday time be determined? Will the normal rotation vary when major holidays occur?

♦ How many consecutive working days will normally be scheduled? What is the maximum that can be scheduled?

♦ What is expected regarding shift rotations? Is there a minimum number of hours a staff person must be off between the end of one workday and the beginning of the next?

♦ How is "weekend" defined, and what number of weekends is an individual expected to work? How will absences on weekends be handled?

Answering these and other questions in the written guidelines for schedule development ensures that advance knowledge is available to staff regarding what to expect. Management support in eliminating uncertainty while maintaining flexibility will minimize the occurrence of problems and conflicts that arise when staff develop their own schedules. Your knowledge that the parameters include meeting the requirement of the unit's master plan for number and mix of staff ensures that the unit is adequately staffed.

SA FINNIGAN

♦ **HOW CAN I FACILITATE THE TRANSITION TO SELF-SCHEDULING?**

Q What are some helpful hints in the transition to self-scheduling? My staff understand picking the days they want to work, but the accountability and negotiation for coverage are sometimes lacking.

A The process of self-scheduling needs to be explained in terms of identifying how meaningfully this change can positively affect patient care and the unit's staffing. Remember that a negative attitude toward the change can result from nurses not being well informed. Identify your goals of self-scheduling. Emphasize that the goal of providing quality care to the patients will be easier to obtain when the unit is adequately staffed. Ground rules must be set:

1. Identify staffing needs for each shift to each nurse.
2. Assign a schedule coordinator for each shift. Rotate these responsibilities to each nurse, and empower these members. Offer assistance to the coordinators to make them feel more comfortable in completing the assignment.
3. The completed schedule must be turned in to the manager.

Once every nurse has participated in negotiating the staffing, they will better understand the process and will therefore be more sensitive to the unit's needs versus the individual's needs. Throughout this process, be supportive and offer assistance when needed. Once nurses are committed, their satisfaction will increase because they will see the quality of patient care has increased, which will be sufficient reward.

K KERFOOT

S

◆ WHAT CAN I DO TO SUPPORT STAFF WHO ARE FALTERING AT SELF-SCHEDULING?

Q A unit that had implemented self-scheduling successfully has begun to turn in schedules that show overstaffing and understaffing. The charge nurse has commented that she has had to "straighten things out" to submit an acceptable schedule. What strategies would be appropriate to salvage self-scheduling in this situation?

A Several possible explanations exist as to why self-scheduling is beginning to deteriorate. The following steps should be taken to get things back on track.

1. Openly acknowledge at an upcoming staff meeting and through other communication vehicles that the staff needs to review guidelines established for self-scheduling. If a committee had originally begun this process, be sure that they are in attendance. Reassess at this point to ensure continued interest and commitment.

2. Clearly state the requirements. These should include how many Mondays and Fridays should be worked in one block schedule, the minimum and maximum amount of off-shift rotation in a work period, and how many requested days off are acceptable. Remember that your staff can better judge where to schedule themselves if you've provided additional parameters such as how many licensed and unlicensed personnel you require on each shift. Consider using a grid that shows the breakdown of patients by acuity with matching numbers of staff; as volume and acuity increase, so will staffing requirements.

3. In general, it is useful to have the evening and night staff fill in their time first so that the day shift has a sense of when they need to rotate.

4. Insist that time switches be made with "like status" employees and that this responsibility lies with the individuals involved. You should only participate here in rare instances when the staff have been unable to resolve the staffing issue.

5. If you have preceptors, their schedules should coincide with those of the preceptees, and primary and associate nurses should coordinate their schedules accordingly.

6. Be clear on how vacations will be handled. For example, you might state, "If you are beginning a vacation on a weekend that you normally are assigned to work, the vacation begins on Sunday, and you are therefore responsible for finding coverage for that Saturday if you need to take it off."

7. Restate how holidays are to be covered. For example, all employees who work more than 24 hours per week will schedule themselves to work every other holiday.

8. Remind your staff that at no time should they fill in someone else's time or make any changes after the schedule has been posted.

9. Since the staff has previously successfully implemented self-scheduling, this review should help to clarify your expectations. Remember to monitor the process closely and celebrate each month's successes. If you begin to see a decrease in turnover and nurses looking to come to your unit because they have heard of the program, be sure to congratulate your staff on a terrific job in promoting continuity in patient care through professionally handling their own schedules.

V MANCINI

Sexual Harassment

◆ WHAT STEPS SHOULD I TAKE TO RESOLVE A SEXUAL HARASSMENT COMPLAINT?

Q A vice president has repeatedly asked my secretary out on a date. She has refused each time. She reported to me that she feels harassed. What steps do I take to resolve this potentially risky issue?

A Sexual harassment is a violation of federal laws. It is a type of sex discrimination. Nurse managers must deal factually and quickly with complaints of harassment. Managers can be liable for not taking corrective actions to resolve harassment situations.

Be sure to know what your agency's policy is about harassment. The policy should clearly state that sex-

S

ual harassment will not be tolerated. The policy should be accompanied by a procedure that outlines the process to be followed to handle complaints. The process should be strictly followed. (In the instance in which an employee is being harassed by a supervisor, the employee should feel free to report the harassment to a higher authority. This should be clearly stated in the policy and procedure document.)

In the above example, the manager must obtain and document all the facts about the situation. The manager should ask:

1. Who is the harasser?
2. What happened?
3. When did the behavior occur?
4. Where did the behavior occur?
5. Who witnessed the situation?
6. How often has the behavior occurred?
7. How long has the unwelcome behavior been going on?
8. Has the harasser been confronted, and if so, what was the response?

Listen carefully while gathering the facts. Do not make any judgmental comments. Ask how the alleged recipient would like the situation dealt with. Explain to the employee how the situation will be dealt with and when you will follow up. Let the employee know that she can contact you at any time. Do follow up with the employee.

Whether it is the manager or a human resource professional that follows up on the complaint, it must be done quickly and correctly. The following must occur:

1. The allegations are investigated.
2. The alleged harasser is apprised of the specific allegations and given an opportunity to respond.
3. The alleged harasser is told clearly what action must be taken to stop the behavior immediately and that if the behavior is continued, termination may result.
4. All actions and interactions are documented.
5. The situation is monitored.
6. Decisive action is taken if the behavior does not stop.

A word about confronting the alleged harasser. Occasionally an employee just wants the supervisor to know about the harassment but does not want the harasser confronted. This is not acceptable. Incidents of harassment must be confronted and dealt with. If an employee states that she wants to confront the harasser, the manager will want to coach and counsel the employee about the confrontation. The employee should be specific about unwelcome behavior, and must state that the behavior is unwelcome and ask that the behavior stop. For example, the secretary might say to the vice president, "I find your repeated request for a date offensive and unwelcome. I expect you to stop asking me for a date. If you do not stop, I will ask my supervisor to take action to stop this behavior."

A complaint of harassment that is effectively dealt with will usually facilitate a resolution of the complaint.

LJ SHINN

Shared Governance

♦ HOW DO WE START SHARED GOVERNANCE?

Q We have shared governance started in our nursing division, and we are ready to move it to the units. What should be our first steps?

A Developing shared governance activities at the divisional level is the first step in building a solid framework for the shared governance approach. Division-wide structures provide an integrating force for shared governance and ensure that the principles being applied in the organization are consistent and appropriate. Without setting a basic and common framework, it is difficult to validate whether the principles of shared governance are being fulfilled.

Once the framework and the structure of shared governance are in place, movement to the unit is facilitated. If the principles of shared governance are to be adequately implemented, it is essential that unit-based activities be adopted. Some specific steps can ensure unit-based success at the outset.

1. Make sure all unit personnel understand what shared governance is and what it implies for changes in role expectation and staff behavior.

S

2. Be certain that the manager is able to provide leadership in making some of the initial changes. The most significant role changes will be in the manager's functions and activities.

3. Make sure the selected structure is specific to the unit's unique culture. There is no one best structure for all units. All structure must reflect the unit's character and dynamics; what may work one place does not always work every place.

4. A developmental process should be designed for staff and management to assist in the development of new leadership skills for both clinical and management leaders. A desire to implement shared governance does not mean that everyone knows the behaviors it represents. Time must be set aside to learn group process, consensus skills, and a refocusing on work outcomes.

5. Experiment with decisions and decision making. Pick low-risk decisions first and, as the staff get more skilled and more comfortable, expand the range of issues and risks addressed by staff decision-making leadership. Only through stretching skills and risking efforts can the outcomes of empowerment pay off for the staff and the organization.

T PORTER-O'GRADY

◆ WHAT DECISIONS CAN STAFF MAKE?

Q We've just implemented shared governance in our department. I've read that nurses want more involvement in decision making and responsibility; what decisions are appropriate for staff to be involved in?

A Decisions appropriate for shared governance are best determined by mutual input by staff and management. In an ideal program, all decisions would be made by the nursing staff, leaving only decisions that involve exceptions to management. In this situation, management would deal with nonroutine decisions and unique occurrences. If the nurses are not willing to undertake this level of decision making or if management is not willing to give up this level of control, boundaries can be established initially as to which decisions are covered by shared governance and which are left to management prerogative. To demonstrate the true essence of shared

governance, however, a group of managers and staff nurses must work together to establish these parameters concerning types of decisions.

For example, one area in which staff are quite often reluctant to take on decision-making responsibility is with personnel issues such as performance appraisal, hiring and firing, and discipline. If this area of decision making is one your staff may decide they want to initially leave to management, it is management's responsibility to coach the staff in the development of these skills through formal inservice training, sitting in on performance counseling sessions, and implementing programs of peer review. These activities should be completed using a time line so that staff nurses are aware in the beginning of when a system of shared decision making concerning this area will be implemented.

A similar format should be followed for all decisions until a true shared approach is achieved for all decisions. Thus, initially staff may want control of few decisions, but with appropriate coaching and time for development, they should assume responsibility for even the long-range planning decisions.

JW ALEXANDER

◆ WHAT CAN WE DO TO ENCOURAGE DECISION MAKING?

Q We are having more unit-based staff meetings in our shared governance system. However, we have a difficult time getting to decision making. Are there some techniques that we can use to be sure that we actually make decisions in these meetings rather than simply processing forever?

A All committees should follow certain guidelines to ensure success and productivity. Membership of the committee or unit-based meeting should be representative of the nursing unit. Members should be reminded that they not only represent their own personal views, but should solicit opinions and ideas from others. Individual members who compose the group should ideally include people that complement each other and provide a part for everyone: the leader, organizer, detail-oriented person, creative idea person, and so on. The chairperson should be someone who knows how to negotiate and collaborate with other staff members, the director, and other departments. Group size should be limited to groups of 12 or fewer so that consensus is not difficult.

A meeting can become more successful in several ways:

1. Set the time and place for the meeting and begin on time. People will perpetually come in late if they know that the meeting "always starts late."

2. The chairperson should be very knowledgeable about the topics on the agenda. Vague issues should be researched, facts should be obtained, and other alternatives should be ready for suggestion. This will eliminate wasting group time to investigate the issues involved, and more time can be spent on decision making and problem solving.

3. Set the agenda and think it through with a management advisor. Some issues get bogged down because the decision was never designed to be solved at that level of staff participation. Past business items should be resolved at each meeting if possible. Encourage the committee to be reasonable, and don't try to overachieve by having too much on the agenda.

4. "Hot" controversial issues that cannot be resolved immediately in the group should be postponed until the next meeting. Sometimes it is helpful to have several of the most vocal members meet separately and have them bring possible solutions to the group.

5. Take minutes, and decide which problem needs action and who is responsible for the action to be taken. Assign responsibility for follow-up or resolution.

6. Attendance at meetings should be taken seriously. Persons who are repeatedly absent should be disciplined by the manager or asked to resign from the committee. Discipline is a management issue and should not be handled by the group.

7. Encourage confidentiality about certain comments. Trust is built and members of the group will be more honest and open if they do not fear that every statement made will surface in other conversations, especially if a frustration was shared.

8. Review the minutes for clarity.

9. Celebrate the successes and accomplishments within the group and in the department. Goals should be set and time lines established.

BH DUGGER

◆ IS SHARED GOVERNANCE EXCLUSIVE TO NURSING?

Q We have had shared governance in place for 6 years in our nursing division. It has worked exceptionally well for us. We are noticing, however, that the rest of the hospital is both interested in and in need of partnering with us. We never considered shared governance outside of nursing. Is it possible? If so, how do we get started?

A Your situation is becoming more common in shared governance hospitals all over the United States and Canada. At the core of shared governance is a belief in partnership and in creating structures that support partnership. Although the concept begins within the nursing discipline, it is not exclusive to nursing services. It builds partnership behaviors between nurses but also invites partnerships between nurses and others in the organization. I have often said that if shared governance stops at nursing's door, it has failed to make a real difference. By its very design, the process invites others into the methodology and expands the circle of empowerment and partnership in the organization.

Often called "whole systems shared governance," the move to using the principles of shared governance to develop new relationships in health care is emerging in a number of settings in the United States and Canada. Often beginning in nursing, the move to include other departments and services in shared governance is becoming a vehicle for work redesign, patient-focused care, and community-based "point of service" organizational designs.

It is suggested that you begin by working with those departments or services that show interest in partnering with your service. Identifying the principles of shared governance and ways in which other services can apply those concepts and partner with others is a great first step. Another vehicle for getting others involved in shared governance is found in the effort to build multidisciplinary patient-focused care. It is a natural vehicle for incorporating learning, discussion, and service planning between the disciplines as they seek to find common ground for building a comprehensive patient care approach. Much reference material is available about implementing shared governance, and some of that should be made avail-

S

able to those interested in instituting shared governance.

Also helpful to stimulating interest in shared governance across the services is the process associated with implementing continuous quality improvement (CQI). The methodologies associated with CQI demand that relationships between workers be changed and the organizational structure be altered to support point-of-service designs. The more hospitals move to service-based designs and the more decentralized they become, the greater the opportunity to use shared governance principles in building new structures.

T PORTER-O'GRADY

♦ **WHAT'S THE BEST WAY TO EDUCATE STAFF ABOUT SHARED GOVERNANCE?**

Q What strategies have proved effective in educating the clinical staff about the new role of management in shared governance and eliciting their support for management change?

A Staff often may seem apprehensive about changes, especially if they fear the change might create more work or responsibility for them. They may feel "overworked" and stressed within their schedule, and the thoughts of adding additional decision-making demands on them may cause concern. Be honest with them, and admit that you will be asking them to participate at the decision-making level but that you will not ask more of them than they can deliver, that they usually will have a choice whether or not to actively participate in committee functions, that you will recognize and reward them for their input, and that they will benefit by having more autonomy.

The benefits of participation in a shared governance organization and the new management style to the staff nurse are numerous and need to be emphasized:

1. *Staff participation in decision making.* Staff have the opportunity to set standards by which they practice. Bedside nurses know how best to care for their patients, often setting quality and standards higher than management would expect.

Nurses are encouraged to bring possible solutions to the attention of nurse managers, not just voice complaints or identify problems.

2. *Increased self-esteem, self-confidence, and job satisfaction.* Employees are happier and more satisfied if they have a part in establishing the standards for their own practice. Nurses who are empowered to use their knowledge and experience make sound decisions and develop strong collegial relationships with their peers, physicians, and other health care team members.

3. *Enhanced personal growth.* Job satisfaction with the profession is an overflow of both major and minor accomplishments.

4. *Decision making of a higher quality.* Nurses are encouraged to read and do research to enhance patient care and communicate with physicians and other health care team members at a higher level of professionalism.

5. *Development of future nurse leaders, whether in management or at the bedside.* Not all nurses desire to be nurse managers of other employees, but most nurses want to be leaders or managers of their patients' nursing care.

BH DUGGER

♦ **HOW CAN I GET STAFF TO PARTICIPATE IN ORGANIZATIONAL COUNCILS?**

Q Our hospital nursing organization has recently adopted a council format for shared governance. In this format, each unit is to have a representative on each of the organizational councils. I have tried everything but cannot get the staff on our unit to participate. How can I help them see how important it is to participate?

A Finding the answers to various questions may assist in resolving problems that arise because of apparent lack of interest by personnel in this effort. First, review the mechanism through which shared governance was implemented. Was the shared governance structure developed as the result of a collaborative management and staff effort? If not, the participation in councils may not be viewed as important by staff. When shared governance structures are purely management driven, they are viewed as management projects and may result in failure because of suspicion and a lack of staff commitment. This is exactly what shared governance is, a governance structure that is shared between staff and management. When structures are not "shared," they are unlikely to succeed because employees are unlikely to view participation as an important part of their professional roles and responsibilities.

Second, discuss with employees the manner in which decision making by the councils will affect their jobs. When shared governance structures are initiated, not all personnel understand that councils will make decisions that will surely affect their work and professional lives. Only through time and consistent realization and operationalization of such decisions can personnel understand the importance of participation on councils. Council roles and accountabilities should have been identified before initiation of the council. If this has not occurred, identifying roles and accountabilities may assist in helping personnel appreciate the impact of participation.

Third, analyze the extent to which personnel are encouraged to participate on councils. Is it easy for staff to obtain time off to attend council meetings, or are they required to do so on "off-time"? Frequently, managers pressure personnel when they must leave their departments. Nursing staff may also criticize the nurse who participates on a council when they must "cover" that nurse's patients during the time in which she is absent from the unit. The more this pressure is placed on the nurse, the less likely the nurse is to confront conflict to attend a council meeting.

Fourth, ask how consistently council work is viewed as the work of professional nursing. Does the nurse's evaluation reflect participation in shared governance, or is this ignored during the evaluation process? Are successes in shared governance celebrated and individuals recognized for service in shared governance? One must do more than provide lip service to our belief that shared governance is a significant part of how nurses practice professionally.

As a manager, you are in a unique position to provide leadership in fostering professional growth through governance. Identifying the opportunities underlying obstacles will provide you with the tools to foster professional growth.

LM LENTENBRINK

◆ HOW CAN I OVERCOME STAFF RELUCTANCE TO PARTICIPATE IN SHARED GOVERNANCE?

Q We have adopted a council structure to build participative decision making. After 1 year, staff feelings such as "I don't have time to be a participant in the process" are still the norm. Whenever we try to invest staff, the "we don't have time" issue always arises. How do I respond to this staff reaction?

A Before you respond to the staff's comments, step back and ask yourself several questions as to what the problems could be.

- ◆ What is the norm? You have identified the "norm"; however, often the norm is the most vocal of a group and the others just "go along." Get a real sense of the issue by surveying all the group members. Are some participating more than others, and are just a few doing all the work? Get a sense of the work load.
- ◆ How were the members selected? Did they volunteer, or were they assigned? It is important to know if these group members wanted to participate and if they joined with some agenda or hopes of making a difference in their practice.
- ◆ Is there a facilitator to manage the process of the group? The group dynamics are an important feature. Any group has both a task and a process need. Paying attention to one without the other often causes a group to be unsuccessful. Who are the participants? Examine the mix of people to see if it is the most productive. An obvious problem may be that a small group of senior people within the group are monopolizing it, but other more subtle issues may need to be examined.
- ◆ Are there enough resources to facilitate participation? It takes a fair amount of time to participate in a council. Do participants get enough time to prepare, meet, and resolve issues?
- ◆ What type of responsibilities are assigned to the council? Are they tasks that can have no resolution or tasks that have been assigned to the group because someone wants to have a solution *look like* it has been a democratic process? When the committee achieves a task or resolves an issue, how is it celebrated and communicated

S

to the rest of the staff? What ways are members rewarded?

Once you have explored all these issues, you may be able to identify where the problem is. People like to feel useful, as if they are contributing, and that their resolutions are making a difference. However, they cannot make time they do not have amidst their busy schedules and will soon become discouraged if they see no changes as a result of their hard work.

JB COLTRIN ET AL.

♦ HOW CAN I MAINTAIN ENTHUSIASM FOR SHARED GOVERNANCE?

Q Our hospital has had a shared governance structure for 2 years. The staff was excited at first, but now they seem to have lost interest. What can be done to keep the enthusiasm and interest in shared governance?

A Your staff is probably experiencing the more difficult (and perhaps less glamorous) work of maintaining a system. They probably had some early successes with fairly simple problems but are now getting into more controversial matters. Often this begins to test their knowledge and skill. They may be focusing on what they haven't achieved rather than on their successes.

Several approaches may be used. With the staff leaders, set up a formal time to review the progress that has been made, knowledge and skills gained, and outcomes achieved. Celebrate these successes visibly. Have a good time. Use humor, visual tools, skits, and so on.

Second, evaluate what new skills or refinement of past skills may need to be acquired. Particular emphasis should be placed on negotiation skills, problem solving and building consensus, coaching skills, articulating clear expectations, and providing support and follow-up. Critical thinking skill building is also essential.

Finally, be sure that you are using every opportunity to recognize the staff's efforts and successes both within and outside nursing. It may be that you are receiving more credit for these than the staff is, particularly if you are recognized for these successes and fail to inform others about the staff members who are primarily responsible.

JE JENKINS

♦ IF TOP ADMINISTRATION IS NOT IN FAVOR OF SHARED GOVERNANCE, HOW CAN WE KEEP IT GOING?

Q With some recent changes in nursing administration at the hospital, in terms of both personnel and roles, the previous shared governance process seems in trouble. The decision-making process has definitely changed. Input into decisions is no longer sought; advice given is not considered in the decisions. With these changes at the top, how can those of us who firmly believe in and live shared governance continue to grow or even maintain it?

A It is administration's responsibility to make decisions that affect the hospital as a whole. This responsibility does not alter or dissolve simply because shared governance is in place. Often, time restrictions prevent obtaining input from those directly affected by these decisions. However, within the shared governance structure, we continue to have the opportunity to directly influence the implementation of these changes if we choose. Valuable time is lost in grieving over the lack of input into administrative decisions that could have been spent in creative planning and facilitation.

K KERFOOT

♦ HOW CAN WE BETTER SUPPORT OUR COUNCIL CHAIRPERSON?

Q We ask a great deal from our shared governance council chairperson in terms of commitments and time. Many times her peers do not realize or appreciate the efforts that this person is making. What are some ways that we can support the chairperson elected from our nursing unit?

A First, check in with the council chair. Does this individual think that the time and commitment are being well spent? If not, what recommendations can be brought forward to improve the process? By asking the individual directly, you will be able to clarify the issues and address them.

Second, the chairperson's responsibilities should follow guidelines established by your bylaws. You can support this individual by setting clear expectations of the role. For example, the chair may be responsible for conducting the council meeting; however, these meetings should have a preset schedule that is sent out in advance to all concerned council members. This schedule should also include who will be facilitating the meeting, that is, clarifying points, keeping the discussion focused, and being sure that closure is brought on a topic before moving to the next agenda item. It is useful as well to assign a council member to be timekeeper. This way consensus can be reached in a defined period. It is also wise to assign the task of taking minutes to one of the members. Now, all the chair needs to do is lead the meeting.

Third, to involve other staff members, set the expectation that everyone will read the minutes of meetings. This can be facilitated by having your staff check their name off or initial the minutes. Also, if the council is dealing with issues that are important to your staff, they will be more apt to appreciate the effort toward the response.

Often, staff members are less likely to appreciate the work of the chairperson and of the shared governance framework if it means that they are working short staffed on the day of the meeting. Or possibly the aloofness is actually coming from their resentment toward the council chair, who is perceived to be receiving more attention from you. It would therefore be important for you to speak with staff members to see what is underlying the behaviors you describe.

Last, if you do not have a unit-based model in place, you should give this some thought. When activities occur at the local level, they are more visible, more participative, and often more appreciated. Remember, too, that celebrations call attention to work well done. Acknowledge each piece of progress, and applaud one another regularly.

V MANCINI

◆ HOW CAN WE IMPROVE COMMUNICATIONS?

Q The other departments in the hospital sometimes find that nursing through shared governance is difficult to work with. They perceive that results take a long time and that some issues fall into a "black hole" and are never resolved. How can communication be improved?

A Determine if the other departments have a reason to complain. Although through shared governance things may sometimes appear to take longer to resolve, issues should not "fall through the cracks." Other departments must be educated regarding the nursing department's role. Nursing is a complex service and is often misunderstood by physicians and people in other departments. The Joint Commission on Accreditation of Healthcare Organizations (JCAHO) Nursing Care Standard 4 requires a written *hospital* plan for providing nursing care. Provide written updates, and keep people informed of progress or the status of a situation. Frequent feedback to the people and departments involved is critical.

Involve the other departments when possible. Invite department managers and physicians to council meetings when issues regarding their areas of interest are being addressed.

SH SMITH

◆ WHAT SHOULD THE MANAGER'S ROLE BE IN A SHARED GOVERNANCE ORGANIZATION?

Q We have a very traditional organization that is moving to shared governance. What is the manager's role in staff-driven decisions?

A As the manager, you play the key role in the transition of staff and will have the most changes to make in your own position. This combination of factors is challenging and requires planning and preparation. In a shared governance organization the authority for professional practice is shifted to the staff nurse, and the manager's role becomes one of managing the resources and facilitating the work of the unit. Staff has been oriented to look to the manager for solutions to most unit issues, so the relocation of decision making can be expected to generate mixed reactions. Although a small group may feel committed to change at the outset, resistance and skepticism of many can be expected. The tendency of staff (and managers) is to deal with issues in the traditional organizational format, since that is familiar to them.

The manager's work is to guide the process at the unit level, where the new behaviors will be played out. Although staff needs and preparation will vary from one institution to another, most staff nurses lack experience and confidence in decision making not specifically related to care at the bedside. This is especially true in traditional bureaucratic settings.

Since shared governance is difficult to understand initially, the manager should look for opportunities in practical and direct everyday activities to demonstrate its principles. Some examples of this would be to encourage staff to form a task force to deal with a unit level problem, help a staff member work through a decision that requires the use of new skills, and see that staff members are supported to attend shared governance activities off the unit. Balance your need to make the "right" decision with helping the group explore the issues and reach their own conclusion. Consistent effort on the manager's part will create an environment of trust.

B FOSTER

Skill Mix

♦ **HOW DO I MEET JOINT COMMISSION ON ACCREDITATION OF HEALTHCARE ORGANIZATIONS (JCAHO) REGULATIONS WITH REFERENCE TO PATIENT ASSIGNMENTS AND NURSING SKILL MIX?**

Q I have accepted a position as a manager on a medical-surgical unit that traditionally has used many licensed practical nurses (LPNs). I am trying to keep the unit in compliance with JCAHO regulations with reference to assignments of patients to the appropriate nursing skill mix, according to patient need. The unit practice for many years has been to divide the floor into teams—a registered nurse (RN) or an LPN conducts the team without differentiation by patient need. Some patients may not see an RN unless they need a specific procedure. The LPNs have low turnover and high tenure, so most possess greater skills and knowledge than the RNs, who are basically new graduates and who leave before gaining many skills. What suggestions do you have?

A Several issues must be addressed. JCAHO nursing standards specify requirements for nursing care. The standards do not specify numbers of staff. The standards do require the nursing department to define the delivery system, the staffing requirements, assignment process, and qualifications based on patient care needs. Therefore standards of nursing care must be clearly defined, and patient mix must be evaluated. The standards and the patient care needs then determine the staffing mix and the assignment requirements. Compliance to the standards is monitored and evaluated through the quality assessment and improvement process.

JCAHO standards (1992) require the following:
♦ NC 3.4.1 "There are sufficient qualified nursing staff members to meet the nursing care needs of patients throughout the hospital."
♦ NC 3.4.2 "Nurse staffing plans for each unit define the number and mix of nursing personnel in accordance with current patient care needs."

A critical area to be addressed involves the orientation process. Once standards are clearly defined, the orientation process should be competency based. The JCAHO standards manual includes a chapter on orientation, training, and education. The job description and the competency evaluation support the compliance to standards. Standards reflect the nursing process and are applicable to the unit's usual medical and nursing diagnoses. Standards are then individualized to meet patient needs.

Too often new graduates are placed in a situation with unclear expectations and a lack of support in the orientation period. They become frustrated and leave the organization. High turnover of RNs can be costly to the organization. Efforts must be made to determine the reason for the high turnover of RNs and to develop a plan to improve the situation. Talk to the new nurses, encourage feedback, and provide support in the adjustment period. Do not overlook the value that the LPNs offer to the unit. The LPNs should have a clear understanding of RNs' role and responsibilities and the relation of LPNs' role to state practice acts, JCAHO standards, and specific hospital nursing standards. Standards requiring RN intervention include but are not limited to patient assessments, supervision, and circulating responsibilities.

The following steps summarize suggested actions to assist you in meeting the goals for the unit:

1. Assess the unit's current status (standards of care, compliance with JCAHO standards, turnover rates, orientation process, assignment process).
2. Identify problem areas that need to be addressed.
3. Develop a plan to address each area to be improved.
4. Implement the plan.
5. Evaluate the effects of the action taken.
6. Reassess and initiate steps 1 to 5.

Involve the staff as much as possible in addressing the issues. By applying the nursing process to the care of the unit, you will demonstrate the process and its effectiveness.

SH SMITH

2. Clarify the staff nurse's accountability for designing a plan of nursing care, even though others may directly implement that plan.
3. Give the staff nurse feedback concerning her success in her new role as preceptor and advisor for paraprofessional staff.
4. Help the staff nurse identify options that may be available to her in other nursing areas. Perhaps home health or nurse practitioner roles would be more satisfying.
5. Continue to value the staff nurse's contribution to nursing care, and be supportive in helping her regain her satisfaction with nursing practice.

CE LOVERIDGE

◆ HOW CAN I HELP STAFF WHO FEEL THREATENED BY CHANGE?

Q A long-term employee has been dissatisfied with changes in operations that have occurred since the unit has redesigned the nursing care delivery system. The integration of licensed vocational nurses (LVNs) and nursing assistant "practice partners" has left this staff nurse feeling that her direct care role is vanishing and being replaced by other roles that she finds unsatisfactory. How can I be helpful?

A Many changes are occurring in today's nursing care settings. The great number and rapid pace of these changes confuse people about what is expected of them and make them uncomfortable about what is perceived as a rush to use less-expensive personnel in positions where once only RNs were employed. The integration of LVN and nursing assistant "practice partners" is often initiated without proper consultation with staff, resulting in a frustrating experience for senior staff as well as new staff.

You can take several actions to help this staff nurse and others develop their new roles.
1. Include staff nurses in the discussion of role changes that will result from the redesigned nursing care delivery system. Although resistance will still be present, there is greater acceptance of change among people who believe that their ideas were given a fair hearing even though they were not adopted.

◆ SHOULD I HIRE AVAILABLE ASSOCIATE DEGREE NURSES (ADNS) OR WAIT UNTIL A NURSE WITH A BACHELOR IN SCIENCE DEGREE (BSN) APPLIES?

Q I have been a nurse manager for 20 years and have a diploma in nursing. Generally, I see that BSN nurses on our unit have better overall skills. However, it seems to take two to three times as long to fill an RN vacancy with someone with a BSN than with an ADN. The staff does not understand why I leave a position vacant so long to search for a BSN nurse. Should I continue this practice or follow the staff's advice and fill positions with available ADNs?

A It is a luxury to be able to wait for the ideal candidate for each position, a luxury most of us never have as managers. It takes only 2 weeks to resign in most cases, whereas it may take 3 to 4 months to find eligible candidates to fill that vacancy. Bachelor-prepared nurses should bring the depth and breadth of education to a position, but using that as the only criterion may be cheating your unit of some excellent applicants. As we all know, today's nursing school graduates include many second-career moms and dads, men and women who have functioned in significant positions outside health care. Their associate degree or diploma in nursing may be simply the frosting on the cake of experience. Their work ethic, values, and life experiences may far outweigh the bachelor's degree they may pursue later.

Second, as a nurse manager, I would strongly consider the non-BSN nurse whose work history, background, interests, and ambition tell me she will pursue a bachelor's degree and help set the standard for others along the way. Expectancy theory tells us this person is already engaging in actions that lead to success. Your unit has the situational setting where a bachelor's degree is valued, and your assistance with tuition reimbursement (if possible), flexible scheduling, and encouragement will set the pace for others as well.

Third, involve the staff in the interview process so that they understand each other and the behaviors and values each brings to your section. Choosing the team then becomes a group effort, making the growth and development of each new member a goal for the whole unit.

MA SORENSEN

◆ SHOULD NURSE EXTENDERS BE INCLUDED IN THE DAILY STAFFING COUNT?

Q My unit has been staffed only by RNs. The hospital has decided to add nursing assistants and technicians. Should these staff now be excluded from the daily staffing count?

A These staff can be excluded from the staffing count. They are often regarded as nurse extenders and classified as indirect, rather than direct, care staff. Your institution needs to identify the desired staff mix, which apparently is changing, and define the expectations of each level of staff. Your institution also needs to determine its definitions of direct versus indirect care staff. That is, bed making, bathing, and gathering supplies will probably not be classified as direct care. What about taking and recording routine vital signs? Those who perform physical assessment, planning, and evaluation of care will be classified as direct care staff. Nursing assistants and technicians, if classified as indirect care staff, are counted similar to the ward clerk, unit manager, educator, charge nurse, and housekeeping personnel. With experience and valid data collection, your unit can establish a ratio of direct care staff to indirect care staff that responds to the needs of the patient population your unit serves.

J HIXON

◆ HOW CAN I MOTIVATE RELUCTANT STAFF TO WORK WITH AIDES?

Q I have been told that I have to change the skill mix on my unit to include more nonlicensed personnel. The nursing staff have already stated that they will "not work with aides." How do I gain their support to make the necessary changes?

A Much literature is available on the use and non-deleterious effects of various mixes of nonlicensed personnel on nursing staffs. Despite these facts, a predictable (although hopefully short) period of disbelief, anger, or even mourning of an actual or desired standard of care occurs when managers or staff are told of the need to change. I have noticed that at least some feelings of disappointment or worries about quality are attributed to nonlicensed staff, when actually nurses are concerned about the quality of care or sense of team spirit with their fellow RNs and manager. For example, the same concern often is stated about part-time RNs.

Thus a manager has much work to do to sift out what are real versus imagined problems. Remember, as the nurse manager, you control the use of resources by your staffing, assigning, educating, and evaluating of staff. This is a time for more staff meetings (once a week is not too many during major change) and much group creativity. Here are some suggestions:

1. Review the available literature on the subject, and talk to other nurse managers of similar units who use mixes. Learn from their successes and mistakes.
2. Consider partners-in-practice as a way to structure RN-LPN/aide mixes without "losing" professionalism (Manthey, 1989).
3. Create clear job descriptions and sample prototypes by shift for how assignments should be made given certain mixes and acuities.
4. Use off-shift times and weekends to occasionally run staff meetings and assess firsthand how the "mix" is working.
5. During your report or immediately afterward, help RNs determine how to best use the staff working with them.
6. Organize educational sessions for your staff in the skill of delegation, although I prefer to teach present delegation in the new framework of inclusion. *Inclusion* is less hierarchic, is more ac-

ceptable to women, and focuses on patient goals rather than tasks. During the shift an RN might need to include many types of personnel as well as the patient and family in helping move the patient toward desired goals.

7. Expect the RNs to make rounds, at least three per shift, on all their patients, because legally they are supervising the staff working under the RN's license.

8. Include nonlicensed personnel (including ward clerks and others) in all on-unit activities and meetings. If you want teamwork, you have to build a team. However, reserve some events only for RNs, such as peer consultation.

9. Know that staffing numbers and mixes will continue to go up and down as units open and close and as hospitals strive to stay open by restructuring.

10. If it helps, remind yourself and your staff when appropriate that being professional has nothing to do with how many other RNs surround one on a given shift. Rather, being professional involves a level of accountability for the results of one's actions. That form of professionalism comes from inside a person and should be actively sought and supported by the nurse manager.

K ZANDER

Staff Development

◆ HOW CAN STAFF DEVELOPERS HELP NURSE MANAGERS?

Q What do nurse managers see as the most helpful activities that staff developers can do to assist managers in performing their jobs as our organizations move toward the twenty-first century?

A Those in staff development have the responsibility to develop, support, and advise those in nursing management. Nurse managers have the most difficult administrative task in the hospital, and many ways exist to assess management needs on a yearly basis. Personal interviews and questionnaires can identify management and learning needs. These assessments can become the management curriculum for the nursing managers. Frequently, nurse managers

need courses in financial planning, budget development, performance evaluation systems, collective bargaining, leadership styles, motivation, communication, conflict resolution, assertiveness training, stress management, on-unit organization, staffing, and scheduling. Staff development has the responsibility of either providing these educational opportunities or bringing in experts who can provide the needed knowledge. Remember, nurse managers are often selected for their positions because they are the "best" clinical nurse. Many of these individuals are not prepared in management. Nurse managers should be given the opportunity to develop as managers and leaders.

JG O'LEARY

◆ HOW CAN I PERSUADE ADMINISTRATORS TO OFFER FINANCIAL HELP FOR EDUCATION?

Q How do I convince the nurse executive in my organization that providing and facilitating educational opportunities is essential to the growth and development of staff, especially with so many budget constraints?

A You need the numbers. Some that might help include turnover rates in your division, vacancy rates in your community, technology advances in your institution requiring advanced educators, and productivity levels of advanced practice nurses you employ. You may not have all these numbers, but you should be prepared with at least a few. When the bottom line is an institution's top priority, education and development typically fall by the wayside.

Thus the only way to argue your case, which is a good one, is to show how your recommendations fit in with the bottom line. This may mean some extra work, but in the long run it could have an enormous impact on the quality of your staff and of patient care.

P MARALDO

◆ HOW DO I DECENTRALIZE EDUCATION?

Q How do we decentralize education to the unit level and maintain an effective committed education team?

*A*Whenever an area is decentralized, two elements help maintain commitment and common purpose: goal setting/business planning and networking.

Bring all the educators together at least quarterly to design an overall business plan with a general mission statement for the group. Help them identify educational standards and common outcome goals by which to measure the effectiveness of the *group.* Then have each complete the business plan for her specific unit or area of responsibility.

Second, have educators network with each other frequently to evaluate and revise their business plans and to find ways of coordinating efforts within the business plan. This is also a good time to share success stories. Begin each session with a "win," a positive encounter or outcome an educator had on her unit. This helps focus the group on goal achievement, provides for some personal and group affirmations, and helps maintain internal motivation to the overall mission.

Although decentralized, the group may choose to develop strategies to cover for one another during absences or to use one another as expert resources on their units, similar to guest professors.

As a manager, you can help the educators balance their time between the group and the unit. They must feel full membership in both areas; commitment to just one will result in competition with the other.

RM HADDON

◆ HOW DO I DEVELOP A COMPETENCY-BASED UNIT EDUCATIONAL PROGRAM?

*Q*I need help in developing a competency-based unit educational approach for the staff. What steps do I take to accomplish this?

*A*The development of a competency-based unit educational program should be done in collaboration with the staff themselves. This is the type of a program in which a group of nurses could do an excellent job within the shared governance model. First, you should see what type of programs other units within your facility are using. Second, you should conduct a literature review and find out what other hospitals are doing in this area. When develop-

ing a program such as this, you don't need to do all the work. Many examples of competency-based educational programs should be of assistance to you. As with all good problem solvers, you should do your research, make a plan, involve the staff, and implement. Then, don't forget to evaluate and modify the program as necessary.

KJ McDONAGH

◆ HOW DO I CALCULATE THE RATIO OF STAFF DEVELOPMENT HOURS TO NURSING CARE HOURS?

*Q*What is a realistic way to calculate the appropriate ratio of staff development hours to nursing care hours?

*A*To determine the appropriate amount of education time to budget, the manager must consider that improving competence and being clinically current are obligations of both the staff person and the organization. Although the appropriate number of hours will vary from one unit to another, each organization must agree on the values and beliefs that will guide the manager in planning. Those involved must reach a common understanding of what portion of a staff member's educational development will be supported by the institution. Frequently, organizations will commit to supporting the following:

- ◆ Education required by the state, the accrediting agency, and the institution.
- ◆ Education sponsored by the institution that directly relates to accomplishment of current objectives.
- ◆ A portion of the expense for national, regional, or local programs related to a nurse's role or clinical specialty, when the nurse is willing to share the expense.

Once this agreement has been reached, an education factor, the ratio of education hours to total paid hours, can be determined using the following steps:
1. Determine the time requirement for education necessary to meet regulations. Consider such programs as cardiopulmonary resuscitation, safety, infection control, and others that may be required by your organization, and calculate the hours each staff member will spend on these.

2. Consider the objectives of your unit and the nursing department for the coming year. Decide how much education and which categories of staff must be included. Multiply the hours of education per person by the number of staff who will attend.

3. Determine the staff who will be eligible to attend conferences, seminars, or workshops outside the institution and how many conference hours will be supported by the unit. Consider staff nurses on the unit who may be officers in their professional associations, individuals who may have spent many hours of their own time achieving clinical certification, or staff members who are willing to present inservice training to their peers when they return from an outside conference. Again, determine the total number of conference hours to be paid.

4. Compute the average education hours per full-time equivalent (FTE) by dividing the unit's required education hours by the worked FTE. For example:

Required education	313 hours
(39.16 FTE × 8 hours each)	
Continuing education	100 hours
(inservice)	
Conferences/seminars	56 hours
(7 per year × 8 hours)	
	469 education hours

469 education hours ÷ 39.16 FTE = 12 education hours per FTE

5. Determine the education factor by dividing education hours per FTE by the paid hours per FTE. For example:

$$12 \div 2080 = 0.00577 \text{ (education factor)}$$

6. Use the education factor as you would the benefit (vacation, sick, holiday) factor to calculate your total required per FTE. For example:

a. Average daily census (ADC) 36 × 365 days = 13,140 patient days

b. 13,140 patient days × 6.2 hours per patient day (HPPD) = 81,468 worked hours

c. 81,468 worked hours ÷ 2080 = 39.16 worked FTEs

d. Add benefit factor   .13500
   to education factor   .00577
   _____
   0.14077 for each FTE

For example: 39.16   FTEs
            ×   1.14077
            _____
               44.67   Total paid FTEs

SA FINNIGAN

◆ HOW DO I PRICE LEARNING WORKSHOPS?

Q What are the criteria for pricing learning workshops? What is the usual percentage of markup?

A A phone survey of nurse educators and a national organization for education and training yielded no consistent guidelines for pricing workshops. Pricing is based on multiple factors that are considered in a two-step process.

The first step involves answering the following critical questions about the purpose and structure of the educational offering:

1. Do you plan on having nationally recognized speakers?

2. Will you seek co-sponsors to share the cost and profits or losses?

3. Can any of the costs be underwritten by corporate sponsors? (A word of caution: many professional groups have, or are developing, strict ethical guidelines regarding vendor donations and the influence of these donations on the information presented.)

4. Is the number of participants limited because of space and resource constraints?

5. What audience is the workshop targeting, and how will you market to this audience?

6. What are the projected attendance figures?

7. Will you offer reduced fees for students, retirees, individuals from the sponsoring organizations, or organizations who send large numbers of participants?

8. What will the length of the workshop be?

9. Are there any other major meetings or workshops on the same day or days that you are scheduling your educational offering?

10. Has the topic you are presenting been done by another provider in your geographic area recently?

11. What is the benchmark for participant fees in your area?

12. Will you cancel the workshop if a minimum number of participants have not preregistered, or are you willing to lose money to gain marketing benefits?

13. Are you capitalizing on your institutional resources and developing niche programming that promotes a reputation for quality?

S

The second step is to estimate the specific direct and indirect costs of the workshop considering the following areas:

1. Speaker honorarium and travel costs (transportation and mileage, meals, hotel, ground transportation).
2. Room rental and audiovisual equipment fees.
3. Cost of breaks and meals.
4. Design, printing, and dissemination of promotional materials.
5. Salary of the professional and support personnel who plan, implement, and evaluate.
6. Printing of handouts and evaluation forms.
7. Continuing education unit (CEU) processing.
8. Expenditures for staff development in the areas of marketing, customer relations, legal and ethical issues, and financial management.

Following your cost projection, you then set the participant fee structure based on your answers to the questions previously discussed. Decide whether you will cancel the workshop if minimum attendance is not obtained. If you decide to do this, print a statement on your brochure with an assurance that the entire fee will be refunded.

MC HANSEN

Staff Meetings

♦ HOW CAN I INCREASE STAFF ATTENDANCE AT MEETINGS?

Q Many staff nurses on our unit complain frequently but refuse to come to staff meetings. Short of making the meetings mandatory, which I know they will resent, what can I do?

A Managers are responsible for ensuring a communication avenue for staff. Staff meetings are the best tool for doing so. Ideally, staff can attend the meetings. If they are not attending, the reasons need to be ascertained. A written staff survey seems a good place to start:

1. Poll the staff as to their perception of their ability to influence decisions, voice concerns, and be willing to be a part of solutions.

2. Some questions regarding scheduling of staff meetings are also helpful. For example, does the night shift want a meeting on their shift? If so, what is the best time to hold it?
3. The survey results will provide direction regarding staff perception as well as provide you with feedback on the scheduling of meetings.
4. You may discover that staff do not believe they have the ability to influence or change policy. In that case, you will need to explore the reasons with them individually or as a group.
5. If the results show that attendance is not going to be possible for all staff, you could record minutes.
6. Post the minutes and require each absent staff member to sign them. In this way, the information that is presented is given to each staff member.

JM McMAHON

♦ HOW CAN I GENERATE ENTHUSIASM FOR STAFF MEETINGS?

Q Staff meetings are treated as a joke by the nursing staff on my unit. As a manager, what can I do to increase enthusiasm as well as attendance?

A You do not say why staff meetings are considered a joke. Some possible reasons for lack of enthusiasm are:

♦ The staff do not believe that their opinion counts for anything, and therefore meetings are a farce.
♦ Nothing ever gets achieved; things are discussed endlessly without resolution.
♦ Information only flows downward, never upward or laterally.
♦ Meetings are used by management to advise staff of nothing but bad news, such as the hospital's shaky financial status, demands that they work harder, the number of patient and physician complaints, and how many mistakes have been made.
♦ The meetings provide information that has already been noted in memos, newsletters, and so on.
♦ The meetings are dominated by a clique of staff nurses with negative attitudes.

♦ The manager is never on time or is poorly prepared, and the meetings are considered a waste of time.

In today's world of ever-increasing information overload, the unit meeting is the prime method of holding the unit together as a team and ensuring that all staff have a means of communicating with one another. Have you written a goal and objective for your unit meeting that you can publish at the top of the minutes? An example might be, "The unit meetings for Three South are seen as the principal means of discussing, as a team, our commitment to quality patient care and to each other."

Here are some other suggestions:

1. Develop a fixed agenda, 15 minutes for past business, 15 for new, 15 for clinical update news and information, 5 for report, quality assurance activities, and 10 for ad hoc groups to report back on projects. Close with honoring an employee for going the extra mile and complimenting staff for all the good things that have happened. Always stress that every negative is an opportunity in disguise.

2. Use the following guidelines for problem resolution. When a problem is brought to the group, discuss and resolve the issue, decide with the manager to do some research and bring information to the next unit meeting, or form an ad hoc group to research and bring information to the next meeting. At the next meeting, discuss and resolve, or bump up to next level for discussion. Except in rare circumstances, don't allow problems to stay on the agenda for more than three meetings without action.

3. Publish minutes in the PRAE format: problem, recommendation, action, and evaluation.

4. Start two communication books on the unit. The first one is for all memos, policy changes, and formal communications. When the communication is received, make a copy. The copy goes into the unit manuals and is posted in the book for reading and signature. The second book is for unit communication between shifts and all staff. The book is set up in three columns. Column one is the comment, column two the response, and column three the management acknowledgment or action. Do not use unit meeting time to reiterate information that has been acknowledged in the communication books.

S LENKMAN

Staffing

♦ HOW DO I PREPARE JUSTIFICATION FOR INCREASING MY UNIT'S STAFFING LEVELS?

Q Identify the beginning steps I should use to plan a documented justification for increasing the staffing levels on my unit.

A I hope your unit is not already showing the symptoms of understaffing, that is, staff turnover, poor morale, low marks on patient satisfaction, and an increase in incidence reports. Before these signs appear, a manager must be aware of trends on the unit. The first step in doing a documented justification for increasing the staffing levels would include gathering data that examine the unit's demographics:

♦ Does the patient acuity system reflect increased acuity?

♦ If an outcome monitoring system is being used, are the patient days and costs for care predictable?

♦ Has the service changed dramatically, and are the diagnosis-related groups affected, producing more revenue?

♦ What is the length of stay, and how does it compare with a previous period?

♦ What is traffic like on the unit, that is, what is the number of transfers on and off the unit compared with a previous period?

♦ What technology has been added (e.g., telemetry, autotransfusion) that affects staffing?

♦ Consider any procedural changes, new programs, or age-related factors as you gather your data.

Your documented justification must create a picture—describe what was, what is, and what needs to be. You also need to include what impact this will have on labor costs for your unit. Your justification for increased staffing may affect full-time equivalents (FTEs) but not costs because you have changed your mix to deliver quality care.

MA SORENSEN

S

◆ CAN STAFFING PATTERNS BE MADE TO FIT FIXED BUDGET PARAMETERS?

Q How can patient care needs be translated into unit-based staffing plans using budgeting methods that are preset and "baked in" to patient care needs?

A When working to set up staffing patterns within established budget parameters, it is probably best to start by determining what the "usual" work is for a period (24 hours, a week, or a month) taking into account the "usual" patient type and needs and the specific type of staff required to meet those needs. If you have an acuity system in place that you trust as accurate, the job may be easier. In this instance you have information that describes the "usual" work to be done, and the remaining task is to determine which is the most appropriate and cost-effective staff to do the work given the budget. From that position you can establish "target" staff hours for the unit or department. The target hours can be used on a regular basis to compare with the actual hours accumulated to give you an idea of your status related to the budget. Target hours, because they are based on the "usual," will at times be either over or under the actual hours accumulated depending on census; however, they should balance out if you have good information from which to derive your targets.

If you do not have an acuity system in place that will help you to obtain the data you need to determine target hours and staff mix, you will need to develop the data from scratch. In this instance it is helpful to establish a "task force" of staff (managers and first-line staff) to determine what the "usual" work is. This could be done by using an audit of a random selection of charts to uncover the usual work done by shift and type of personnel, combined with some observations of the work and/or interviews with a random selection of staff from all shifts regarding what they do on a "usual" day. Then the task force can consider whether the staffing mix is efficient considering the work to be done and can propose both target hours for the unit or department and the desired staff mix by shift and unit. The comparisons can then be made in the same way as previously described.

The budget, if preset, drives this process initially. However, the "work" is the true force to be reckoned with in that the patient's needs should be the primary consideration for what makes up the work and who (nurse aid, licensed vocational nurse, type of registered nurse) is truly the most appropriate person to do the work. You may find that this process will produce unexpected side effects. As you look at the work and who is doing it for whom, you may discover many things about the unit's efficiency and the expectations that govern work flow and distribution decisions.

M MURPHY

◆ HOW DO I RESOLVE DIFFERENCES BETWEEN MY ESTIMATES OF REQUIRED STAFFING NUMBER AND MY DIRECTOR'S ESTIMATES?

Q I am a nursing manager of a 40-bed mixed medical-surgical unit. I have been informed by my director that I am responsible for calculating my required FTEs for the coming year. She has provided me with the number of patients admitted to my unit this past year and the required hours per patient day. I have a good data base for my staffing requirement. I believe that this classification system is most accurate. Somehow, my required staffing numbers for the year disagree with my director's numbers. What is my next step?

A Staffing in today's economic environment requires changing our way of thinking. Traditionally, the nurse manager could gather acuity data and directly translate this information into required FTEs. Most often, this meant budgeting for more FTEs than the prior fiscal year, since trends in many hospitals indicated an increase in patient acuity. Unfortunately, the dollars available to fund nursing care delivery have shown the reverse trend. Less money (in millions) has been available from government and other payors each year, and present indicators suggest even tighter resources in the future. Therefore, if you continue to build your staffing levels on the acuity data alone and increase cost while revenues to your hospital are decreasing, your organization will quickly face economic demise.

In developing future years' FTE budgets, you will need to balance several data elements so that the outcomes of your staffing management system produce a level of care that will support achievement of your patient goals at a cost you can afford. Begin with the information provided by your director regarding last year's admissions and the required hours per patient day. To reach agreement on the required FTEs, you will need to reach agreement on some other factors. These are the questions you want to answer:

1. Will the number of admissions next year be the same as last year, or will the number change? Determine the projection for number of admissions to your unit for the next fiscal year.
2. What is the average length of stay (LOS) for a patient (case) on your unit? These data are probably available in medical records or data processing. Once you know the average LOS, you can determine the total number of patient days for next year: Admissions × LOS = Patient days
3. Next, you must reach agreement on the number of worked hours per patient day (HPPD). The formula is:

$$\text{Staff hours} \div \text{Patient days} = \text{HPPD}$$

To do this, you must analyze several elements, including acuity data from last year and the mode census (census occurring most often). Using your projected patient days, forecast the number of patients that will be on your unit most frequently, and consider the number of staff that will be required to care for them efficiently and effectively. Finally, examine your unit's revenue projections for next year. If your unit projects less revenue than it had last year, your staffing costs probably will need to be reduced, since personnel is your unit's most expensive resource. Compare the HPPD figures arrived at using all three parameters, and negotiate the HPPD that will be most realistic in supporting hospital goals for the coming year.

4. Once you and your director have reached agreement on the number of patient days for the next fiscal year and the HPPD, calculating your FTE will not be difficult. Here's the formula:

Patient days × Worked HPPD = Worked hours
Hours worked ÷ 2080* = Worked FTE
Worked FTE × Benefit factor† = Budget paid FTE

SA FINNIGAN

---

*Number of hours 1 FTE is paid in 1 year.

†Number that represents hours for sick time, vacation time, and holidays needed per FTE.

◆ HOW DO I CONVINCE THE CHIEF FINANCIAL OFFICER (CFO) OF OUR NEED FOR FULL-TIME EMPLOYEES?

Q Our CFO has a set of budget forms we must use that do not show the calculations needed to match staffing and skill mix to acuity. The CFO only wants to know the FTEs to occupied beds statistic. We need to change our skill mix to utilize nurse extenders and provide more care hours at less cost to meet our increased acuity. This does increase our FTEs, but not our cost. Any deviation from the accepted FTE is automatically denied. How can we present a better argument for increased FTEs?

A In general, CFOs have a better understanding of budgets and worker expenses than they do of skill mix and patient acuity. A detailed comparative cost analysis can usually persuade the CFO that increasing FTEs and worked hours may well decrease overall costs when accompanied by significant skill mix changes.

This analysis needs to reflect the need for an increase in care hours per patient day because of an increase in acuity. It should also demonstrate the cost-effectiveness of providing more care hours at a lower cost by using nurse extenders while simultaneously maintaining or improving outcomes. Additional cost savings could be demonstrated if the strategy includes part-time extenders with fewer benefits.

J O'MALLEY

◆ WHAT DO I DO WHEN ADMINISTRATION INSISTS ON INADEQUATE STAFFING?

Q As a nursing manager, I have been instructed by the vice president to staff the nursing areas I supervise at a level I consider inadequate for the delivery of safe nursing care. I have expressed my concerns and objections to these proposed staffing levels and have been told by the vice president to "just do it." I am very committed to this particular hospital, nursing staff, and the patients we serve. Although I could resign, I do not consider this a viable alternative. What strategies should I use?

S

A You may first wish to examine the roles that your staff are playing at present. Are they being used appropriately, and are they doing tasks that could easily be assigned to other less-qualified staff? Often our initial response to change is one of concern and fear that we won't be able to do what we have always done and a belief that what we have always done is the best way of doing things. However, if you have assured yourself that this is not the case, talk with the other unit managers and get their opinions regarding the staffing levels. If your concerns are validated, you are responsible and accountable as a nurse to voice your concerns to management.

This is what we recommend a nurse do, given the stated situation. A nurse is directly accountable to her patients, the public, and her employer for ensuring that standards are maintained. If you believe that you cannot maintain standards because of a situation that is beyond your control, you should proceed with the following steps.

1. *Validation.* Identify the standards that are not being met. They can be policies and procedures, ethical codes, standards for practice, standards in other agencies, or the community-accepted norm. Identify how patients could be affected.

2. *Communication.* Follow the proper channels of communication in your agency. Speak to the person you normally report to and follow up in writing. Be specific and factual, and explain what standards are not being met and the effect this is having on patient care. Document clearly, and treat all documentation as confidential. Indicate that you would like a response to your memo, and set a time frame. Sign your name and keep a copy for your records. If you do not receive a timely response and no progress is being made, send a second memo to the same person and forward copies to all levels of nursing administration. The memo should reiterate the problem, include a copy of your first memo, and request assurances that your problem be addressed quickly.

3. *Resolution.* Appropriate responses may include a verbal reply or a request for a meeting. Be open minded and be prepared to work together to solve the problem. Some compromises may be necessary as long as patient safety is not affected. If your concerns are still not being met, be prepared to carry them further. Arrange a meeting with your nursing administrator and notify her of your concerns. Although the problem is being resolved,

make certain the nurses on the affected units know how to prioritize the care they are giving so that *safe* care, but not excellent care, is being delivered.

JB COLTRIN ET AL.

♦ HOW CAN I IMPROVE REPORT TIME FOR BOTH OFF-GOING AND ON-COMING STAFF?

Q We have become confronted with a "short staffing" situation in our department. Off-going shift staff refuse to stay for report, whereas the on-coming staff refuse to start report because they claim that it is unsafe for them to assume accountability for patient care without reports. What do I do?

A Continuity of patient care requires that report occur between incoming and outgoing staff caring for the patients. There are different ways that report can be given that minimize overtime and maximize productivity. Perhaps the staff can select a few members to work with management on the resolution of this problem. Options that the group can consider include:

1. *Taped report.* The outgoing shift "tapes" report over a cassette player before the end of the shift. The oncoming shift can listen as soon as they arrive. This option doesn't require additional expense and allows each shift to do their work at their own pace and on their own time. This option seems ideal for your group, since it minimizes extra time required at the end of the shift and allows the incoming shift to start when they arrive.

2. *Group report.* The outgoing shift sits with the incoming shift and reports as a group. This option requires overlapping shifts and attendance by all to avoid repetition and seems a less ideal option for your group.

JM McMAHON

♦ WHAT DO I DO ABOUT A STAFF MEMBER WHO CANNOT TAKE NIGHT ROTATION?

Q Because of a temporary staffing shortage on our unit, it has become necessary to rotate the nursing staff on the day shift to the evening shift. Although rotation to off-shifts is outlined at point of hire, the staff has never been asked to do this before. One single parent stated that she cannot make arrangements for her child. Other staff members will not take her rotation. What should I do?

A It is always difficult to ask people to be flexible in times of temporary staffing shortages. Usually an effective nurse manager with good communication skills and an effective team will find that people will pull through in an emergency. This, however, is contingent on not having a "perpetual crisis" in staffing. In other words, people don't mind pulling an extra load for a temporary period, but if no long-term plan addresses staffing shortages, this will definitely result in demoralization, more turnover, and a refusal to be more flexible in these situations.

With this particular nurse who is not able to make child care arrangements, you should consult your human resource policies for these types of situations. You may be able to use other staff to make up for this or have this nurse do a different set of hours or schedule that may be a trade-off so that her peers do not think that they are the only ones picking up the extra load. Definitely consult your human resource staff and your nursing administrator for advice. Hospitals typically go out of their way to be flexible for nurses and others who have to work around the clock. However, the staff also has an obligation to respond to a hospital's needs. This sense of fairness or give-and-take is not always easy to define or work toward but is really necessary for an ongoing, stable environment in which excellent patient care can take place.

KJ McDONAGH

♦ **HOW CAN STAFF CONVINCE THE NURSE MANAGER THAT THEY WANT TO PARTICIPATE IN STAFFING CUTBACK DECISIONS?**

Q Our unit has been told to cut back staffing hours. The staff wants to participate in this decision. Our nurse manager has never asked us to participate in the past. How can we get her to understand that we want to help with this issue?

A Your nurse manager is fortunate to have a staff ready and willing to accept the responsibility of helping to design staffing guidelines. There may be

some constraints your manager cannot negotiate that make her hesitant to make this decision. Let your manager know that you recognize the constraints and would like to begin by better understanding the budget and then offering suggestions for consideration. You are responsible for the care you give and thus deserve to have input into maximizing effective use of resources for the best interests of all: patients, staff, management, and hospital administration.

D SHERIDAN

♦ **DO I HAVE OPTIONS WHEN EMPLOYING FULL-TIME EMPLOYEES, SUCH AS CLINICAL NURSE SPECIALISTS OR NURSE EDUCATORS?**

Q I have one exempt FTE position available to be filled. Is it appropriate to hire a clinical nurse specialist on my unit or a nurse educator?

A Today's clinical nurse specialist often studies curriculum development, and today's educator is often a specialist in some clinical area. Often either can meet your needs. Delineate your needs. What do you want this person to be able to do? Then search for the person with the appropriate education, good clinical experience and expertise in your area, and best "fit" with your unit and hospital.

D SHERIDAN

Standards of Care

♦ **WHAT IS THE DIFFERENCE BETWEEN STANDARDS OF CARE AND STANDARDS OF PRACTICE?**

Q What, if any, is the difference between standards of care and standards of practice?

A In each instance, a "standard" is a measure or expectation to which similar other things

S

should conform. It is the expected norm. *Standards of practice* are expectations of professionals regarding the competent performance of their work. These standards are established by the profession and are sometimes used as the legal parameters of practice. The American Nurses Association (ANA) publishes both general and specialty practice standards for nurses. An example of a practice standard would be, "The nurse maintains client confidentiality" (ANA, 1991).

Standards of care are expectations regarding patient treatment or outcomes. These standards may be established by an organization through such mechanisms as critical paths or CareMaps or by a group of practitioners such as patient care standards for normal deliveries set by a group of midwives. Some national standards may be accepted by a provider group or organization, such as the "clinical practice guidelines" established through the Agency for Health Care Policy and Research (U.S. Department of Health and Human Services, Public Health Service). An example of a standard of care would be, "The patient will state that he is pain free X number of days after surgery."

M MURPHY

Strategic Planning

♦ HOW CAN WE PLAN IN TIMES OF RAPID CHANGE?

Q How can my staff and I do long-term strategic planning for our departments in a rapidly changing environment, characterized by uncertainty in resource allocations, regulations, policies, and trends?

A In these challenging times, the nurse leader must abandon the notion of a fixed, linear, quantitative strategic planning model in favor of a strategic thinking model. This means to determine the future direction of your department, you need to

sit down with key stakeholders (anyone participating in or influenced by the work of your department) and *think* through the qualitative aspects of your service and the environment in which it is delivered. (Marvin Weisbord, a noted organizational theorist, has described such a qualitative process in his 1992 book *Discovering Common Ground.*)

Strategic thinking, therefore, is a process you use with your staff to formulate, communicate, and implement a vision of your service and strategies for its implementation. Most of us are so busy dealing with the day-to-day operation that we do not set aside time to think. When we do find time, we are tempted to jump right into tasks.

As the manager, you are what Roberts (1993) describes as the process owner for your department. This means that you are accountable for the facilitation of appropriate interactions and open dialogue. You also have a strong leadership role in the process itself. This means you must be visible, prepared, and engaged in giving reality-based feedback and be comfortable with debate or constructive disagreement.

You may want to consider hiring an outside facilitator to lead you and your staff in strategic thinking. This person should bring to the organization a structured process and instruments to keep the process moving toward outcomes. Beware of approaches that are highly task centered, leave little room for discussion, and are carried out by a limited number of people behind closed doors.

The difference between your role and the facilitator's role is that you own the process by your active leadership and honest appraisal of needed resources and your commitment to implementation. The facilitator, on the other hand, has a commitment to see that the process is honest, balanced, and objective. Also, this individual may be willing to train people in your organization for work within their specific departments.

Strategic thinking has many results. Sometimes it does result in a major shift in direction. In other instances, you may simply achieve greater clarity about your service and contributions or about your environment. Clarity is a powerful outcome. It leads to greater commitment of purpose and the reallocation of scarce resources to those strategic directions that really count.

CK WILSON

Stress Management

◆ HOW CAN I LEARN TO NOT "TAKE MY WORK HOME WITH ME"?

Q How do I let work issues go and be able to conduct the rest of my life, away from work, without influence from work?

A Workaholic organizations know no limits. A boundary is a limit that an individual needs to set in order to carve out a personal life. People whose lives are dominated by work will feel uneasy in the presence of someone who is doing something to change making work their primary focus. Therefore, it is important for you to remember that as you separate out your personal life from your work life, you will not necessarily receive support from your boss or other peers. Here are four suggestions on how to remove the influence of work from your personal life:

1. *Suppressing.* Suppression is when you consciously push thoughts of work out of your mind each time they enter. You make a decision to think about something else or to focus on whatever you are doing in the present. The key to getting thoughts of work out of your mind is to focus fully on what you are doing in the "now" place (e.g., talking to your children, gardening, listening to music, even housework).

2. *Planning and reflecting.* Allow yourself time at work to plan and prioritize, as well as reflection time to learn from your mistakes. It is equally important to improve your delegation of work and minimize interruptions so you can be as productive as possible while you are there.

3. *Symbolically closing the door to your workplace as you leave.* This could be done literally when you close the door to your office or as you walk out the front door of the organization itself. Each time, enact a ritual you design that indicates you are now "off duty." For example, before I finish my day, I make a "to do" list for the next day, close all drawers, and doors, turn out the lights, and say to myself, "My work is done for today. I have accomplished . . . (and I list three to five accomplishments)." This ritual puts closure to my workday. If

I do work at home during the evening, I do the same ritual, excluding the "to do" list.

4. *Scheduling decompression time between work and home.* This could include an exercise class, a walk, or simply telling your family that you need 15 to 30 minutes of alone time when you first come home. Your family's resistance will disappear over time when they learn that you are more patient and more present for them if you get the decompression time.

VD LACHMAN

◆ HOW CAN I HELP STAFF WHO ARE STRESSED OUT?

Q Are there any tried and true solutions for assisting the professional nurse when her stress level appears to be accelerating?

A The answer is a difficult one, since what may be "tried and true" for one is not so for another. The following, however, are some methods that may be used to another's advantage to decrease stress.

Sometimes it helps to have someone you trust available to talk to who will listen as you unburden your innermost feelings. It may be a co-worker, a sibling, a parent, or even a friend. Unloading your feelings and then sharing theirs may help "unload" your stress and help find a way to divert it.

Sometimes it may be helpful to be reminded of a painful or difficult memory, to reexperience it, and then let it be turned into something happier to remember. Transform that memory or experience. Remember either something good about it or something good that came about because of it. This may not be easy, but it's worth a try, especially if done with someone you trust.

Stress relief can also be experienced through activity, exercise, shopping, and playing. You could go out and be a "child" again—go roller skating, play at an amusement park, go to the beach, have a picnic, play Frisbee, or even buy some silly string to shoot someone with. Have an intimate evening with your significant other, go to a movie you've been wanting to see, or rent two or three movies on video and, along with popcorn and lemonade and your best friend, enjoy yourself. If needed, send your children

S

to visit relatives for the night or even a whole weekend. Get some time for yourself.

Start a journal with daily entries and go back and read them at a later date. You may even find that writing a letter to yourself is helpful. Mail it and read it when it arrives. It may make you realize things may not have been as bad as you remember and sometimes may even help you laugh at yourself or events around you.

Remember, too, that working through truly stressful times and events may not happen overnight. It may take some time, so find a way to relax as you work through things.

Also remember that sometimes professional help may be just what is needed. Don't be afraid to seek that help. Most hospitals have professional help available at low cost for their employees.

Don't let stress cause you strife. Fight back when and where you can. Life is serious enough, so add some fun to your life to help prevent stress buildup. Some events that cause stress may not be prevented, but they can be helped, in this manner, to be less stressful. Live, love, laugh, and be surprised.

K KERFOOT

◆ HOW CAN I HELP RELIEVE MYSELF OF STRESS?

Q As a manager, I try to set an example for the staff with positive attitudes, energy, and enthusiasm and good time management at work. Lately, my stress level at work has been increasing, and I am exhausted before the end of the day. My attitude, energy, and productivity are slipping. What are some strategies for dealing with my own stress and preventing this from stressing the staff?

A The condition you describe can be related to personal or work factors or a combination of both. Furthermore, if the stress you describe is primarily a result of the work environment, it is probably too late to prevent the staff from experiencing it. Therefore, I would recommend that you assess staff stress levels. Do not tackle this, however, until you have a better handle on your own stress.

To begin with, take adequate time to identify as many causative factors as you can. Do not assume it is one easily identified factor. Stress is usually a multifaceted problem. Examine intrapersonal, interpersonal, and environmental aspects of your stress. Use both personal and organizational resources to do this. Discuss your self-assessment with members of your personal support system, and ask them to validate or challenge your conclusions or to suggest additional stress-producing factors that you have not considered. It is hoped that this support system includes the administrator to whom you report. If needed, access the services of your human resource department to further assist you in clarifying causative factors.

Once you have a clear picture of the causes, select the appropriate strategy for positively dealing with stress and tailor it to your personality and life-style. Examples of strategies most frequently found in the literature include:

◆ Participating in a routine exercise program.
◆ Meditating.
◆ Scheduling time-outs for fun and decompression.
◆ Accessing support groups.
◆ Avoiding stressful situations.
◆ Cognitively restructuring how you view the stressful factors.
◆ Finding activities that will rekindle your professional spark (e.g., educational activities, interacting with peers who are enthused about nursing).
◆ Requesting a temporary reassignment.
◆ Redesigning your job.
◆ Collaborating with administration and staff to change the organizational culture to one that promotes an energizing versus energy-sapping environment.
◆ Keeping a journal.
◆ Seeking personal counseling.

Just as the causes of stress are multifaceted, the plan for dealing with them must also be. Therefore, use as many of the previous strategies as are appropriate to your personal way of "being" in the world.

A word of caution: unless your personal and work environments support your efforts, the changes you attempt to make will be short lived. Therefore, as you develop your own personal "care plan," be sure to use scenarios to try to predict potential barriers to effective outcomes. Then plan how you can transform your environment to overcome barriers to successful stress reduction. Finally, be sure to build in evaluation mechanisms whereby you do continuous checks on the plan's effectiveness.

MC HANSEN

Strikes

◆ WHAT ARE MY OBLIGATIONS AS A NURSE MANAGER DURING A STRIKE?

Q During a strike, what are my obligations as a nurse manager in the hospital, and what expectation should I have regarding my availability for patient care during the strike?

A A nurse managerial role can present a dilemma of "mixed loyalties." On one side of the coin is your staff who are out on the picket line, and on the other side are the sick patients who must receive care. A way to escape the dilemma is to prioritize in terms of professional role responsibility. As part of the management team of a hospital during a strike situation, your obligation is first and foremost to patient care.

In terms of availability for patient care, limits must be set. I have known many nurse managers who worked as staff during strike situations, often 12 to 16 hours a day, 6 or 7 days a week. This is not healthful for the nurse manager and is totally unsafe for patient care. Determine your limits regarding work hours. A tired, overworked nurse does not make for safe patient care. Most important, do not feel guilty about your decision.

LG VONFROLIO

◆ WHAT ADVICE CAN I GIVE TO STAFF WHO DO NOT WANT TO STRIKE?

Q Our hospital nursing staff is anticipating a strike. I have had several staff members indicate to me that they do not want to strike even though they are members of the union. What response or advice can I offer them regarding their role during the strike?

A As a recognized supervisor of employees, the manager is in a difficult position to speak about union activities with staff members. A statement from a nurse manager could carry the same consequences as if the administrator made the statement: the institution could be held responsible for the statements made.

The manager is in jeopardy when participating in such discussions and could be discharged by the institution if these discussions were viewed as involving union activity (Rowland & Rowland, 1992).

The best response in this situation would be no response or to encourage the staff members to follow their own personal convictions by using existing forums to voice their opinion and register their vote.

J O'MALLEY

◆ ARE THERE LEGAL RESTRICTIONS FOR PICKETING?

Q What are the legal restrictions regarding picketing during a union strike, and how far can picketers go to block entrances to the institution?

A Strikes frequently involve some amount of picketing. Picketing involves patrolling an employer's premises by individuals who may or may not be employees. Under the National Labor Relations Act (NLRA), strikers are guaranteed the right to engage in peaceful picketing. The NLRA does not limit the number of picketers or the manner of picketing as long as the process remains peaceful.

Picketers, however, are subject to state laws. Therefore, if picketing becomes violent or excessive to the point that the hospital entrance is blocked and prevents egress or ingress, the institution can look to state laws for a limitation on the number of picketers and their activities. In some states, such as California, when an excessive number of picketers block entrances or similarly disrupt operations, institutions may seek a temporary restraining order.

Limitations on where picketers can patrol are dictated by the institution's solicitation policy. An up-to-date solicitation policy would limit any type of solicitation, including picketing, to public sidewalks or other public areas surrounding the hospital.

GA ADAMS

♦ IS IT LEGAL TO HARASS PEOPLE WHO CROSS PICKET LINES?

Q During a recent strike in our hospital, some staff nurses crossed the picket line. As they did so, they were yelled at, cursed, and spat on by the picketers. Is this activity acceptable or legal? What can be done about it?

A Threatened or impending strikes and their resolution are extremely emotional events and represent one of the most challenging situations that a nurse manager will face. Whether we agree or not, the act of crossing a picket line is an individual decision that is not made lightly, and it is our professional and collegial responsibility to honor that decision.

Because emotions can be volatile in threatened and actual strikes, we often witness behaviors that are quite disturbing. Although yelling, cursing, and even spitting are common practices in a strike, they are nonetheless violations of professional behavior. However, they may not be violations in the strict sense of the law.

Clearly, all parties must be protected in a labor dispute. Often those nurses who wish to continue to work are transported to the workplace in a shielded vehicle and escorted across the picket line. In any case, protection from abusive behavior and protection in the workplace becomes the employer's responsibility. If the abuse becomes a major disruption to the provision of patient care, legal counsel for the agency may attempt to secure a legal injunction preventing picketers from approaching those individuals who choose to cross the picket line. The injunction may include restrictions such as how far away from entrances picketers must stay and the number of picketers allowed at any one time on the picket line.

Although emotions run high during a labor dispute, after the strike is settled the real work begins. Because the process of patient care rarely proceeds in a professional collegial manner while an undercurrent of anger and mistrust is present, the process of organizational healing is important after a strike.

Reconciliation must be planned with the objective of returning the work environment to a level of cooperation conducive to the provision of patient care. The deep-seated differences that surfaced in a strike cannot be ignored; they must be dealt with openly and honestly. We must understand that it may be weeks and even months before differences are resolved enough to return to optimal functioning as a department.

Some of the most successful attempts at reconciliation have been facilitated by an outside agent agreed on by the agency and union. It is important to contract with an external agent to avoid the charge of favoritism. The process is meant to be healing; therefore blaming behaviors must be controlled.

Dealing openly and honestly with staff who have just come through a strike is an important step in the healing process. If staff do not have a conduit to express their feelings, the workplace will not be conducive to optimal patient care.

GL CROW

Student Nurses

♦ HOW CAN I ENCOURAGE STAFF TO ACCEPT STUDENTS ON THE UNIT?

Q Whenever I have students on our unit and they are assigned patients, the staff groans about the additional responsibility in relation to the students. How can I facilitate my staff's interest and involvement in the students' clinical learning process?

A Adding students to the already busy workday of any unit's staff certainly presents challenges and opportunities. The following strategies may be useful in converting the situation from one of dread to one of positive experiences for everyone involved:
1. Ask the faculty to meet with the staff before students come to the unit to describe the reasons for selecting the unit and the specific learning outcomes on which the students will focus. In addition, the faculty and staff could determine the "routine" in a collaborative way, as well as discuss

strategies to avoid problems or unnecessary disruptions in the unit work pattern.

2. If possible, foster some formal relationships between faculty, staff, and students. Staff should be involved in the educational process as it is carried out on their unit. Make it clear that staff affect the learning situation and that they can use that opportunity to engender and nurture the values and skills they will appreciate in their future colleagues.

3. Try to appeal to the staff's professional side, reminding them that they were students at one time and some other staff hosted them while they learned. Students are the next generation of colleagues; assisting them to learn is part of our professional obligation.

4. Remind staff that a hospital's primary recruitment method is hosting students. Graduate nurses most often apply for employment at the organizations that have provided them with positive clinical experiences.

M MURPHY

♦ WHEN STUDENTS ARE ON THE UNIT, WHO SHOULD SUPERVISE?

Q We have nursing students on our unit at least weekly. However, we are concerned that the faculty instructor selects their patients, sees that they are assigned, and then disappears during the rest of the time on the unit. On questioning, she indicates that it is the staff's obligation to make sure that issues of patient safety are addressed. What should we do?

A Education of the next generation of professionals is a joint effort of faculty and staff. The faculty member is responsible for seeing that learning objectives are met while ensuring the safety of students and patients. This can be accomplished only through the close collaboration of faculty, staff, and students in understanding one another's roles and respecting those rights and responsibilities. I would suggest that you sit down with the faculty member and clarify what you expect from the faculty, what you expect from the students, and what your contribution to their education will be. If agreement cannot be reached, I would not hesitate to involve nursing administration from the hospital and the school to negotiate an acceptable solution.

CCC LEVENS

Suicide

♦ HOW CAN I HELP STAFF COPE WITH A FELLOW WORKER'S SUICIDE?

Q A beloved staff member of our unit became seriously depressed and recently committed suicide. She was well respected and appreciated by her colleagues. I want to provide time for us to deal with the loss but don't know how to approach the issue. What should I do?

A As caring human beings, when we lose those we respect and love, we are saddened. When our loved ones die by their own hand, we are full of guilt and anger, but when they are one of our own, all feelings are intensified. We ask how could we, who are trained observers, have been so blind? How could we, who know how to help, have been so helpless? The familiar and well-known reactions to death and dying can be present in all staff, even those who, by their actions and comments, may seem removed from the most obvious expressions of grief.

You could choose from several approaches in this situation. The first may be to get help in dealing with your own feelings. To help others, you need to think through your feelings and recognize your own emotions. Have you had the opportunity to talk to a peer, a friend, or other support person to establish how you are dealing with the loss? A second and obvious method of supporting your staff is to have a counselor meet with staff regularly for a few months and by request. A monthly meeting could be held on the unit at close of shift and the other meetings in the counselor's office through the employee assistance program or human resources. Some staff may request transfer off the unit. After discussion, these requests should be honored with an understanding that they could be temporary. The staff could memorialize the

S

deceased by establishing a small fund with which to buy texts, starting a yearly inservice day during which they teach the hospital staff about suicide, planting a tree on the hospital grounds in her memory, or finding other ways in which they can turn her memory into a positive one. In addition, the unique gifts that she brought to the profession could be given to all new graduates working on your unit by incorporating into the preceptorship program those ideas for which she stood.

S LENKMAN

◆ HOW DO I HELP STAFF COPE WITH A PATIENT'S SUICIDE?

Q One of the patients admitted to our unit committed suicide in his room. The staff was very upset, especially the staff member who found him. She refuses to discuss it in any way. What can I do to encourage her to be open and to deal with the issue as a part of helping her through it?

A Confronting death is an individual experience that is shaped by culture, experience, and maturity. In the nursing domain, the frequency with which nurses confront death varies according to the acuity of patients being cared for. When death is unexpected, such as in suicide, it can be a devastating experience.

Helping someone work through the experience requires sensitivity, patience, and trust. Your staff member might have an added burden of guilt associated with suicide. "What if I . . ." and "If only I . . ." are frequently thought, even if not expressed.

Some ways you can help include:
1. Calling in a consultant to provide an inservice program on suicide for all staff to attend. Offering such an opportunity for group discussion of the underlying dynamics of suicide may help all staff to examine their experiences more objectively.
2. Continuing to provide support to the staff member who found the victim. Do not force her to respond according to your expectations, but respect her privacy while being ready to help when needed.
3. Examining the group cohesion of your unit and developing some opportunities for teamwork and trust building.

CE LOVERIDGE

Team Building

◆ HOW CAN I HELP STAFF ACHIEVE TEAM MANAGEMENT?

Q How does one manage a group of nurses through team management?

A Building an effective team can be a long process with both ups and downs along the way. Nevertheless, it can also be an investment in the success of the team as a whole, with positive effects on the quality of patient care and rewards in retention of staff.

The following steps may help to simplify a complex process:
1. Lead the team in understanding and buying into the institution's overall vision. Involve the staff in creating a vision for the team and department. Focus on purpose, products, service, and quality.
2. Engage a neutral person to facilitate team-building activities. Education or human resources staff can be skilled, cost-effective facilitators. The facilitator can lead a data collection of the staff's view of priorities, summarize the data, and present it to the staff for validation. The facilitator can also lead activities in which the staff identifies the group's strengths and weaknesses and compares the characteristics of the group's functioning with the characteristics of a winning team. This activity identifies strengths and begins the process for closing the gap between the actual and the desired level of functioning.

    Some issues to be discussed are trust, adequacy of group process in feedback and critique, level of intragroup support (collaboration versus competition), and ability to celebrate successes and have fun. Can the team look to the future rather than just cope with the present? Does the team identify with the larger picture of the institution?
3. Once the data have been collected and analyzed, a development plan with time frames and check points is established. Goals should be stated in terms of task and quality outcomes.
4. The facilitator and the manager, as well as the more able team members, must be ready to guide the team through the inevitable conflicts and impasses. The team must be helped to understand

that these events are not evidence of failure but are necessary to the development of a highly functioning team.

When the process of team building is yielding results, the team expects to observe a higher level of energy, higher productivity, greater flexibility, and a forming sense of community and trust.

It is important to know that team building is neither sensitivity training nor an attempt to get everyone to be best friends. It *is* an opportunity to empower each team member through the team's effectiveness. It is also important to recognize that the team's success is largely evaluated in terms of task and project accomplishments.

In today's clinical environment, an ideal team-building situation is rare indeed. Most such efforts are carried out an hour or two at a time here and there. It is important that those hours be jealously guarded and the group's needs be respected and nurtured to as great a degree as possible.

Then, rather than the leader managing the team, the team becomes more self-managing, with problem-solving skills and resources beyond those of the most energetic leader.

J HIXON

◆ WHAT'S THE BEST WAY TO HANDLE A NEGATIVE CLIQUE?

Q I have a small yet powerful negative clique on my unit. They find fault with everything. Staff have come to me about them, but they are fearful of taking them on. How can I neutralize their negative impact?

A This small group reduces unit productivity and involves everyone on the staff. New managers can expect to be tested early to see what their response will be. Establishing leadership and setting unit direction will be challenging. If this is a long-standing problem for a manager, a different approach will be necessary, one that indicates the manager is setting a new direction.

Deal with members of the group individually. Set meetings as close to one another as reasonably possible. Frame the content of the meetings on your management perspective.
1. Discuss the observed behavior.

2. Point out that clinical activities are only one component of evaluating the effectiveness of staff performance.
3. Clearly define overall expectations, and set a time frame against which agreed-on objectives will be measured. Outline what the next steps will be if success is not achieved.
4. Evaluate behavior related to the objectives on a set schedule. Keep written individual notes as examples occur.

Your management of this small but significant group will set an example for the rest of the work group. Use the opportunity to model the appropriate behaviors.

The fear expressed by staff suggests an environment in which trust is low and there is a lack of confidence in having the skills to manage the situation. Your skills and other resources available in the organization should be used to develop the staff's ability to deal openly with conflict and to develop a sense of teamwork. Adopting a set of commitments to one another that spell out expectations and define expected behaviors can help focus their attention.

B FOSTER

◆ WHAT'S THE BEST WAY TO BREAK UP A CLIQUE?

Q I am a nursing manager on a 20-bed telemetry unit. The staff has been at the hospital for a long time and really enjoy working with each other. Recently we hired two new staff members. Now I find that the older staff are laughing about them, making fun of them, and generally making their time at work miserable. What suggestions do you have to break up this clique?

A As a manager, your leadership is needed to facilitate growth of nursing staff and ensure quality of nursing for patients on your unit. "Breaking up" this group of nurses actually calls for creating situations in which "joining" can occur. The sense of separation between the older staff members and the new nurses on the unit must be overcome. Calling the nurses together and honestly telling them your concerns and observations is one place to start. Remember that what is going on is no secret to any of the nurses. Working together in a caring environment is essential for care of your patients and development of expert nursing practice. All the nurses must share responsibility for these objectives with you. My suggestion is that you arrange for use of the Myers-Briggs Type Indicator (MBTI) for all of you and that this be followed by an exploration of values that guide practice of each nurse on the unit.

The MBTI is a safe, helpful tool that is self-administered and scored by the individual. It provides information to individuals about their preferred ways of learning, communicating, relating, and problem solving. By increased knowing of the self, each nurse can begin to gain appreciation of her own and of others' preferences. Nurses are helped to gain insight into ways of sharing and working together. Increased tolerance and humor as well as growth of individuals and the group are ensured. The MBTI is nonthreatening and fun to use. A search of nursing and related literature will yield information about a variety of uses in nursing. You may also contact Consulting Psychologists Press, 577 College Ave., Palo Alto, CA 94306 for a list of publications and general information.

Nursing values are the enduring beliefs that form the glue that unites nurses. Ways to encourage unity among nurses, no matter how diverse the individuals may seem, include exploring commonly held values about nursing and nurses. What value does each nurse hold most dear? Ask each nurse to share a story that illustrates how this value has guided nursing practice. The story may be one of conflict when the value seemed to be violated in the nursing situation. What values and beliefs do several of the nurses hold that guide the nursing on the unit? How should these values and beliefs influence working together on the unit? What talents, abilities, and ideas are needed to support the nursing values each one is committed to?

ME PARKER

◆ HOW LONG DOES IT TAKE A SELF-MANAGED WORK TEAM TO BECOME EFFECTIVE?

Q How long can I reasonably expect it will take for work teams to be effective on my unit? We have a multidisciplinary approach to clinical delivery, with nursing leadership coordinating the process. It has been a year, however, and the teams are still struggling with their relationship and role conflicts. How can I help them, and how long can we expect these conflicts to continue?

A Team building is a critical issue for the effective operation of any working unit. With the introduction of multidisciplinary teams, you have additional issues of territoriality and lack of trust to deal with. To begin with, you will be more successful in implementing teams if the people working together have some participation in developing their roles and negotiating differences rather than having solutions imposed.

How long will conflicts continue? As long as an acceptable process for resolving those conflicts cannot be found. The "finding" must be done by the participants. This requires time to develop. Teams should continue to examine their operations to find the best methods. This process of role clarification and negotiation is key to conflict resolution.

Your role is to provide continued support and encouragement during the process but turn the job of resolution back to the people in conflict.

CE LOVERIDGE

Telephone Orders

◆ ARE THERE TIMES WHEN TELEPHONE ORDERS ARE NOT APPROPRIATE?

Q When is it not appropriate for nurses to accept telephone orders?

A As a nurse manager, you need to be familiar with the nurse practice act and the state board of nursing that manages the act within the state in which you practice. Each state board of nursing has its own set of operating guidelines based on its particular nurse practice act in regard to the issue of telephone orders. The state guidelines may or may not differentiate between a licensed practical nurse (LPN) and a registered nurse (RN), but you should ask that question. Clearly this source should provide you with the most clear, succinct answer to your question for your particular geographic area.

Most hospitals are accredited by the Joint Commission on the Accreditation of Healthcare Organizations (JCAHO). JCAHO requires that all nursing departments have a policy that clarifies institutional policy on this matter. Institutional policy needs to reflect the legal parameters outlined by the state nurse practice acts. When making institutional decisions regarding telephone policy, one should next be guided by the principle of patient safety. Convenience and urgency are the two main drivers for the need for telephone orders, but both should be balanced with safety first. Within that context, most facilities allow RNs and LPNs to accept most physician orders over the telephone. Some types of orders, such as "do not resuscitate" or certain pharmaceutical orders, may not be appropriate for the telephone. Certain increased documentation issues involve receiving orders over the phone, and those should also be addressed in the institutional policy. In addition, whether nurses may receive telephone orders from the RN or LPN in a physician's office needs to be clarified both legally and institutionally. In some states an RN can accept a physician's order from a pharmacist as well. Involving staff nurses in these discussions will provide all the usual "request" scenarios that you may run into, and from there each scenario will need to be researched and evaluated within your state and institutional parameters. You and your staff nurses must know what is and is not a safe practice and will need to negotiate an acceptable balance with the organized medical staff.

CCC LEVENS

◆ IS IT LEGAL FOR NURSES TO SUGGEST TREATMENT TO A PHYSICIAN OVER THE PHONE?

Q One of our physicians, when asked for telephone orders, replies, "What do you think you would like to do?" Although the nurses appreciate the opportunity for input and advice, they are uncertain as to their liability regarding this. The physician is usually very good about incorporating the advice and frequently supports it with her telephone orders. If a problem should result, is there liability on the nursing staff for having made the suggestion?

A From your question, it sounds as though the physician's attempt to collaborate is making you uncomfortable. It would be your best interest to find a way to let her know that the manner in which she solicits input is making the staff uncomfortable.

It would also be helpful for you to review your state board rules and regulations, as well as the American Nurses Association (ANA) *Nursing: A Social Policy Statement* and *Code for Nurses with Interpretive Statements,* to better understand your professional obligations and potential for liability. The *Social Policy Statement* defines the practice of nursing and the scope of nursing practice. The *Code For Nurses* has a set of 11 statements to guide ethical decision making.

The ANA *Social Policy Statement* defines nursing as "the diagnosis and the treatment of human responses to actual or potential health problems" (ANA, 1980). This means that as professional nurses, we aim to modify, improve, or correct conditions that interfere with the patient's ability to attain a state of health. In some organizations, certain nursing actions cannot be initiated independently because of state regulations or limitations of the professional culture. In such instances, it is appropriate to remind a physician which nursing action requires an order for you to address the situation at hand.

The scope of nursing practice is also addressed in the ANA *Social Policy Statement.* Of particular relevance to the situation that you have described is the discussion of professional intersections. As a professional nurse, you intersect in your work with other disciplines. These are not rigid boundaries but fluid and flexible ones that require judgment in the collaborative process.

In collaborating with physicians, you are under obligation to discuss only those issues for which you are educated, experienced, and competent. The third and fourth statements of the ANA *Code for Nurses* address ethical accountabilities in this situation (ANA, 1985).

Statement three of the *Code for Nurses* states that you are obligated to safeguard your patients from harm. If the physician in this situation is practicing incompetent, unethical, or illegal medicine, you are under obligation to report it. You need to call to the physician's attention that a practice may have a negative impact on the patient. If there is not a response, you must then act on your organization's policy for reporting questionable medical practice. If the patient still remains at risk, you are obligated to report the physician to other appropriate authorities, such as the state board of medical examiners.

T

Statement four of the *Code for Nurses* states that you are obligated to assume accountability for your own nursing judgment and actions. In collaborating with the physician, you will meet your accountability by ensuring that your recommendations conform to the *Code for Nurses,* the standards of nursing practice, nursing theory, educational and certification requirements, or hospital policy.

CK WILSON

Termination

◆ HOW DO I FIRE A STAFF MEMBER?

Q What is the appropriate process for terminating a staff member?

A Each institution has policies regarding what a person can and cannot be terminated for. The nurse manager must follow institutional policy to protect the employee's rights as well as protect her own and the institution's rights. Assuming you have done all that is appropriate in regard to counseling and warnings regarding possible termination with no positive results, then you have an obligation to follow through with termination and should do the following:

1. Collect all your thoughts and information, anecdotal and formal documentation, and carefully review them to determine cause for termination.
2. Talk with the human resources (HR) department next. Let them review your documentation and act as a neutral reviewer and critiquer of your decision to terminate. Review the employee's personnel file and coordinate that information with your information. Let HR educate you and guide you in the process of termination specific to your institution. The forms that you use and employees' rights to grievance will need to be explained to you in detail before you approach the employee. Prepare all the documentation necessary to approach the employee, and have HR review for completeness and equity with similar employees in the past or in other departments in similar situations.

3. Rehearse with HR how you will approach the employee, what you will say, how you will respond to likely questions, and so on. Be as prepared as you possibly can be.
4. When you do approach the employee, be succinct, brief, and clear about the cause for termination, what has been attempted toward resolution in the past, and that you have decided to terminate her effective whatever date you set. Be firm, answer the employee's questions, and then end the conference.
5. After you have met with the employee, return all paperwork and information per institution policy to HR.

Your first experience with terminating an employee can be an emotionally difficult task. Don't expect perfection from yourself. Be prepared. Be fair and direct. Seek advice from HR; one of the reasons the department exists is to provide support. If you are a newer manager, you can also seek out one of your more seasoned colleagues to help you in this process. Generally speaking, you should check with HR about whether to involve your direct supervisor in the decision process because of the existence of a grievance process in most institutions.

CCC LEVENS

◆ WHAT STEPS ARE NECESSARY IN THE FIRING PROCESS?

Q After progressive discipline, what are the steps I should follow in the actual event of firing a staff member?

A Keep in mind that terminating an employee is equally stressful for three people: the employee, yourself, and any other person who works with your group (the staff will be keenly aware of your action). You'll remember every person you ever fire. After you've exhausted progressive discipline without positive results, common guidelines can be easily adapted to your situation for terminating an employee.

First, be sure to do the following:

1. Meet with human resources personnel to ensure that no legal reason exists that might prohibit you from this action and that you are proceeding within your organization's customary guidelines.

T

2. Inform the appropriate people so the employee is unable to sabotage the organization on the way out.

3. Determine any compensation or benefits due the employee and prepare a last paycheck and a letter explaining the disposition of remaining benefits (e.g., retirement funds).

4. Carry out the termination as soon as possible. Don't allow the employee to continue or return to work on the unit.

5. Make a timely appointment with the employee on your own turf. Have another person present if you have reason to believe that the employee will become agitated or aggressive or might misrepresent the termination interview at a later date.

6. Otherwise, meet privately with the employee and explain clearly and directly why you are terminating employment. Although you should try to preserve the employee's self-esteem, it is difficult for anyone not to personalize being fired. Be prepared to deal with an upset employee.

7. Make sure that the employee understands that employment has been terminated immediately. There can be no bargaining or deals. One nurse stated, "You can't do this to me; I've been here for 8 years." I had to reply, "I'm sorry, but you don't seem to understand me. You are *already* no longer employed here."

8. Reclaim official identification badges, keys, or any other authorizations; make sure that computer access codes have been revoked. Tell the employee what can be expected in the way of future references. Give the employee the final paycheck and a letter explaining remaining benefits and find out where to send a future W-2 form.

9. Someone should escort the person to retrieve personal belongings and then directly off the premises. One nurse refused to leave the office, and security had to remove her. Don't leave the employee alone or allow her to stop and talk with other employees.

10. Immediately document the encounter for possible future reference, particularly noting the employee's reaction and comments.

11. Meet with the staff to inform them that the employee will no longer be working with them. Give no other details. Explain that you must respect employee confidentiality.

12. Again, make sure that personnel who need to know about this action have been informed.

RG HESS

◆ HOW DO I RESPOND TO A FIRED PERSON'S ARGUMENTS?

Q After much documentation, the time had come for firing one of our staff members. However, during the firing session, every comment, issue, concern, and documented piece of data I had she countered with an equally persuasive argument. Before long, I thought I was unjustified, unfair, and inadequate even though I was quite convinced going into the session. What happened to me, and how do I prevent that from happening again?

A In listening to the nurse, you must examine the data you used in reaching your decision. It should be objective and validated. If you saved up data for a time without confronting the staff nurse with each incident, you may not have based your decision on accurate information. Remember, there are always two sides to every story.

Particularly when termination is imminent, the employee deserves fair notice and a right to a meaningful hearing. Presumed violations should be shared in a manner that provides a nurse with an opportunity to respond before a determination of termination is made. If your data are based on reports from others, always require documentation by them to avoid misinterpretation of what you perceive they have perceived. Depending on the severity of the violation, progressive disciplinary action may be used to ensure that the nurse has fair notice and an opportunity to respond to each presumed violation of work rules.

When the nurse leaves you with the feeling that you have been unjustified, unfair, and inadequate despite notice and appropriate progressive action, another phenomenon has probably occurred. The nurse has turned her problem into your problem. This is not uncommon with the employee who is on the verge of termination because of poor work performance. That is why she is confronted with this situation. This nurse has consistently blamed others for lack of performance and therefore never performed because she has denied the need to change behavior. In this case, it is important not to get hooked. If you do and change direction, you become part of the problem rather than the solution. Remember, the nurse's behavior, not yours, has placed her in this situation.

LM LENTENBRINK

Theory

♦ **CAN MORE THAN ONE NURSING THEORY BE USED IN A HOSPITAL?**

Q I'd like to know practical ways to develop theory-based nursing practice on this unit and perhaps in the hospital. How can we learn about nursing theories, specifically ones that can work in this setting and with our patients and our nurses? Since our services in this hospital are so various and complex, is it possible to use more than one nursing theory in this hospital? What are the benefits? What is realistic to expect in terms of time commitment, benefits, and changes in our practice?

A Your staff are already using several theories to guide their practice, including biologic (germ, communicability), psychologic (therapeutic communication, growth and development), and social (family systems, community) theories. Some nurses may be using nursing theories to guide their practice. However, it is unlikely that all the nurses use the same nursing theory. Therefore, each nurse's approach to the nursing problems of patients takes on a somewhat different emphasis or slant. The outcome of these different ways of thinking about and acting on patients' nursing problems is a lack of consistency. That lack of consistency results in the inability to evaluate nursing care effectively. Exactly what is evaluated (e.g., self-care ability, adaptive capacity) would vary, and therefore evaluation often is not based on specific nursing care issues but rather on different issues altogether (e.g., length of stay, incidence of comorbidities). Consistent use of a nursing theory would direct the emphasis of care, the documentation system, and the evaluation criteria for nursing.

Several ways exist to approach the development of the consistent use of a nursing theory. You could use an *inductive method.* That is, find out what theory or components of theory the staff are already using and match this to the nursing theory that resembles it most closely. Then you would refine and develop your knowledge of that theory and design your systems for delivering care, documentation, and evaluation around it. You could also use a *deductive method.* In this instance you would study various theories and select one that you prefer and then build your systems. In either instance, it would be helpful to tap a nursing theory "expert" or two to guide the process and assist you and the staff to raise and answer all the questions that need to be considered as you grow in knowledge and design your systems.

Since nursing theories deal with concepts such as health and illness and humanity and *not* with settings (e.g., emergency room, intensive care unit), they can be used to frame nursing care wherever nurses and patients interact. Thus you could make this either a unit-based or hospital-wide endeavor.

M MURPHY

♦ **IS THERE A PRACTICAL WAY TO STUDY NURSING THEORY FOR USE IN PRACTICE?**

Q We have a nursing study club that meets once a month for potluck supper and discussion about nursing practice. Nurses throughout the organization come, although not every time. Some of us would like to study nursing theories, but it all seems so esoteric and impractical (we don't all have nursing degrees). Is there a practical way to study nursing theories for use in practice?

A What we think about nursing directs the way we practice nursing. Thus each nurse is continually doing nursing from a conception of nursing that guides her thinking and her practice. It should not be surprising to find this thinking is consistent with one or more nursing theories. This realization is often the bridge between nursing theory and nursing practice for the nurse who wants to know more about nursing theory. Nurses in practice, regardless of their types of education, often find connections between nursing theory and nursing practice and realize nursing theory is ultimately practical. Nursing practice can be enriched by study and use of nursing theory. In the same way, nursing practice is essential for enriching nursing theory.

I expect your nursing study club to have questions similar to the ones I have often been asked by practicing nurses (Parker, 1993). Nurses have many concerns about nursing theory and want to know ways of exploring nursing theories for use in practice. The questions cover the range from fear of being overwhelmed by theoretic work to wondering if particular theories are useful in multiple clinical situations. Nurses often wonder if nursing theories will be compatible with expectations of patients, physicians, and administrators.

The study and selection of nursing theory and its use in practice must be grounded in the practice of the nurses involved in your study club and must reflect goals and realities of their nursing practice. The initial study of actual clinical nursing situations is the first step toward exploring nursing theories. Following is an brief overview to guide ideas in the nursing study group (Parker, 1993):

1. Nurses can be asked to reflect on an interaction between nurse and patient and write about this. The illustration of the nursing situation should include needs for nursing, a range of nursing responses, and possibilities for desired outcomes. Aspects of the environment should also be included.

2. From the shared illustrations of nursing situations, strongly held nursing values and beliefs can be identified and recorded. These values and beliefs will help in knowing what nurses want from a nursing theory and give direction for selection of theories for study.

3. The key ideas in the nursing situations and the identified values can direct nurses in the study group to begin searches of the literature. The concepts of caring, compassion, wholeness, self-care, health, and respect for persons are often cited in descriptions of nursing situations and can direct this initial search.

4. Nursing theories and literature about their use in practice can be studied to find the focus and purpose of nursing set forth in each theory. The theories may help nurses distinguish nursing from other helping fields in the hospital. These and

many other questions will yield information that helps with understanding of nursing on the units as described in the nursing situations, as well as ways nursing theories may be useful to that practice.

ME PARKER

◆ HOW CAN I HELP MY STAFF DEFINE THE ESSENTIALS OF NURSING PRACTICE?

Q I'd like to know ways to help my staff explore what is really important to us in our practice and to work toward ways we can support our ideas about the essential nature of nursing. How can I assist the staff I work with to refresh their commitment to these parts of our nursing practice?

A There may be differing thoughts on what constitutes the essential nature of nursing. Creating a forum where these ideas can be presented, discussed, and categorized could be very helpful to your staff. Several options could be considered for action:

1. Identify or ask your staff to identify those who would like to meet for an all-day retreat to create a framework to describe the essence of professional nursing for your unit. This could be similar to the development of a mission statement that acts as a guide for everyone as they conduct their activities as a professional nurse. Once this framework and essential components are identified, your staff should present the ideas to their peers for their input and/or critique. Once the final framework is complete, it should be posted where all can refer to it. Having the document professionally printed and framed is symbolic of its value. Communication should refer to the "essence framework," and behaviors, plans, and professional decisions need to consider the elements included in it. By having it immediately available visually, the concepts included in the framework are continually reinforced in everyone's mind.

2. Schedule a series of inservice education sessions that address the topic of the professional practice of nursing to refresh the staff's thinking about how they conceptualize nursing. Videotapes on the history and evolution of nursing practice, the art and science of nursing, the development of nursing

T

theory, and the caring aspects of nursing can awaken the emotional commitment to nursing and patient care that often becomes tarnished with use or bruised in the strife of everyday work life. Discussion sessions should be offered with your staff after the continuing education sessions to provide them opportunity to identify elements that they believe are essential components to nursing and steps to preserve the essence of nursing on your unit.

3. Identify behaviors that you and other staff leaders on your unit believe are characteristic to the essential nature of nursing. Talk of these behaviors in staff forums, and identify how they can be enhanced in everyone's daily practice. Remember to reward and recognize nurses who emulate these ideals in their interactions with the patients and their colleagues. Most importantly, ensure that managers and other staff leaders are role-modeling these behaviors as well.

4. Help the nursing staff to identify the uniqueness of nursing as contrasted to other helping professions to assist them in understanding the essence of nursing. The use of a theoretic framework as a guide for nursing practice can facilitate the process of nurses' identifying the essential components of nursing. A theoretic framework can direct the thinking and behavior of nurses from a nursing perspective to a medical perspective. Once a conceptual model is chosen to guide nursing practice, it can be used as the framework for nursing philosophy, development of documentation forms, standards of care, quality indicators, and critical paths. By integrating the model into the very fabric of nursing practice, it becomes integrated into the conscious awareness of the nurses as they begin to use the model to explain phenomena to themselves and others. The nursing conceptual framework provides a way for nurses to organize their thinking about the patient, the environment, the patient's state of health, and the nursing actions taken in the patient's behalf. The conceptual framework can also provide the foundation for nursing research and inquiry into phenomena of interest to your staff, a continuity and unity in the language used to describe the observations and interpretations about the patient, and clarification about the responsibility and accountability of nursing practice.

It is important to research the various nursing theories for one that "fits" the organization's philosophy and values. Different hospitals use different methods for choosing a nursing theory. In some organizations the nursing executive group chooses the nursing conceptual model to serve as a framework for all nursing activities. Other organizations encourage staff involvement at the clinical unit level in choosing a model that will guide their practice. Whatever method is used to select the model, theory-based nursing practice can make a significant difference in how nurses view their profession from a nursing perspective.

JF STICHLER

Time Management

♦ WHAT ARE SOME TIPS FOR SUCCESSFULLY MANAGING MY TIME?

Q How do I manage my time effectively, that is, setting priorities, saying no, delegating, and so on?

A Probably as many effective styles of time management exist as effective managers. You must choose approaches that fit for you. It can be most helpful to observe and interview other managers you admire. Ask one to be your mentor.

Here are some tips and strategies that may work for you:

1. Start or end each day by reviewing long-term priorities (upcoming deadlines, commitments) and establishing short-term priorities (what you want to accomplish today and tomorrow). If you skip this step, you can fall into the trap of becoming the "hired gun" to accomplish the priorities of others, leaving your own goals to hang over your head like a cloud.

2. Keep an informal record of how you spend your time for an entire day. This will help you know what time-consuming but unproductive tasks and interactions are slowing you down. Guard against putting too much energy into the "squeaky wheels." Let it be known that you expect at least one possible solution to be identified for every problem reported to you.

3. Remember that projects that have operational detail involved are more amenable to delegation than those that involve planning and organization.

4. Delegate gradually, increasing the scope of projects as staff members show competence to handle them. Follow-up on each project on a regular predictable basis so that you are well informed and can offer support and advice when needed.

J HIXON

◆ HOW CAN I KEEP FROM BEING OVERWHELMED WITH WORK PROBLEMS?

Q My job as a manager is overwhelming. Staff expect me to care for patients, but my management responsibilities require full-time attention. Budgets have to be kept up-to-date, appropriate cuts must be made, supplies need to be ordered, and so on. How can I possibly get this all done?

A The inevitable response to trying to meet the needs of a lot of people is a sense of frustration, anger, and helplessness as the pressure increases and no white knights seem to be riding to the rescue. Essentially the answer lies within yourself to determine how you will manage your responsibilities.

1. Frequently, managers are expected to pick up a full patient assignment by their staff and by physicians. This is particularly true if they once were staff nurses on their unit and total patient care assignments are the norm. Refuse to do this, and when your work load permits, pick up certain functions (e.g., start all intravenous lines, admit/transfer patients).

2. Be the second person assisting with challenging patients but do not take a full assignment. Write policies relative to staffing on your unit; have a special place to note requests with clear dates and time lines. Construct a basic 4- or 6-week schedule of normal staff workdays; copy this to use as a base format rather than hand write each time.

3. Take the time, even if it takes you a week of 12-hour days, to get organized. Use a 3 × 5 file box to hold cards on each staff member with pertinent information, birth date, anniversary date, quarterly counseling, and updating sessions. Color code cards for each skill mix. Invest in a large calendar/planner. Write in all committees and meetings for the year at one time. Highlight with different colors for different purposes. Match the colors with folders, and keep minutes or other materials in those folders.

4. Lay three piles on your desk: committees/meetings, current, and review and pass on. Go through your mail when you are at low-energy ebb, force yourself to scan all mail, put it into one of the three piles, and discard the rest. Close out your current file each day, close out your review, and disseminate files once a week. Never go through mail when you are full of energy; you will have unrealistic expectations of yourself and keep too large a pile for working or reading.

5. Delegate as much supply inventory and ordering as you can, and review average levels once a month for appropriateness.

6. Look at how you are explaining variances in budget. Do you have a good system? Design a format that works for you, either a "write-on" board on the office wall in which you keep a running track of hours or a form on which you write daily the reason for variances.

7. Last, you need to pull out your job description and highlight all the functions that you need to do to function satisfactorily. If you find very few highlighted areas and yet you know of expectations you must fill, your job description may need updating. Once this is established, make a list of all that you see as expectations, and request to update your job description so that you have a legitimate base from which to start to control your time.

S LENKMAN

◆ HOW CAN I DO ALL I NEED TO DO?

Q As a manager, it seems as though I never have time to do all that needs to be done. Staff want me to be available to care for patients, yet they are angry when staffing and supplies are not up to par. My supervisor wants me to keep budgets up-to-date and make appropriate cuts. It seems as though everyone manages my life rather than allowing me to manage my own time. What are some techniques I can use to take control of my overtime and get the job done?

T

*A*The role of the middle manager can seem never ending. The demands and expectations from staff and from administration often are disproportionate to the number of hours in a day. Fortunately, some excellent resources are available to develop time management skills. Seminars, articles, and entire books have been devoted to this topic. Although these resources can help, your time management skills will improve only with daily practice.

A few suggested techniques that can help include:

1. Take time to review the job description specific to the role of nurse manager at your institution. Make sure that the written description matches the real work load of the job. Verify this with other managers in the role. If this seems out of proportion, work needs to be done at a different level than just on your unit.

2. Discuss role expectations with your supervisor, and be sure that both of you are in agreement as to job details.

3. Spend time with your staff outlining the role of nurse manager. Be sure that they understand the responsibilities. Staff will continue to demand your assistance in direct patient care unless you make other expectations clear. Repeat as necessary. It may be beneficial to post a monthly updated calendar for staff to refer to, with your schedule including meetings and so on.

4. Budgetary measures are important but should not consume all your time. Technical assistance for reports, computers, and personnel needs to be available to ensure the most efficient, effective methods of budgetary control.

5. List priorities on a weekly basis, and spend time updating that list.

MT SINNEN

Trust

◆ HOW DO I CULTIVATE TRUST?

*Q*As a result of a major organizational restructuring, I have been assigned an additional nursing unit that was lacking a nurse manager. The unit's focus is not my usual nursing specialty, and I have heard that this is an issue with the nursing staff. How do I gain their trust?

*A*Perhaps the key is to not overreact to this situation. Both you and the staff need some time to get to know each other. If you make this too major an issue, you may place more emphasis on it than is required. You must be honest, respect staff's contributions, be clear about your expectations of them, ask them what they expect of you, articulate what they can expect from you, be consistent and fair, and use a sense of humor.

One of the first actions to take is to find what is common between you. Have some sessions discussing what all of you feel is important about relationships, communication, and patient care. Put these on flip charts. Pictures can be very helpful, as can mind maps. Where differences exist, discuss why each of you sees the situation differently and agree to work toward a consensus (not that day, but later). Capture these differences on flip charts as well, and refer to them over the next year as you get to know each other better. Some of these will resolve themselves simply by all of you working together and getting to know each other better. Others will be worked on as they are relevant to other projects. Some will be dropped.

As you begin to work with the staff, be open to learning from them. Also, teach them about your job by showing them how your work helps them be successful. For example, you might say during a staff meeting, "I want to thank you for covering staffing last Wednesday night. Because you were able to handle it yourselves, I was able to get a good night's sleep and be fresh for the budget meeting on Thursday. As a result of that meeting, I will be processing a purchase order for additional thermometers that you identified as necessary for improved efficiency and quality of care. Thank you." This demonstrates your respect for their contribution and for taking care of their business so you can do your job. In doing that, they helped you support them.

If you take action or say something you later regret, acknowledge it to them and apologize. Where appropriate, laugh with your staff about your mistake and move on.

JE JENKINS

Unions

◆ WHAT IS THE FUTURE FOR UNIONS?

Q Are unions declining in America? What is the future of the union?

A Nurses have been using collective bargaining for more than 40 years to address practice and economic issues. Organizing activity is on the rise in health care. The trend in health care is the opposite of trends in other economic sectors. The proportion of unionized health care workers is rising, and reports in labor news and industry journals indicate that unions increasingly will be looking to health care as a potential source of members.

Since this is a time of organizational upheaval because of restructuring, mergers, and takeovers, the growing interest among health care workers in collective bargaining is symptomatic of an industry undergoing tremendous change. An increasingly tight labor market and pressures for cost containment are conditions that make collective bargaining a viable option for improving work conditions within a hospital.

Workers today are confronted with the challenge to achieve more with less. This translates into doing more with fewer dollars and less staff and minimal support systems while the numbers and acuity levels of patients continue to rise. The results may be compromises in quality of care. Within this environment, nurses in particular are discovering the need for a reliable means for:

- ◆ Maintaining a voice in decision making that affects their practice.
- ◆ Acquiring the resources necessary to carry out their responsibilities effectively.
- ◆ Safeguarding the standards of practice set by the profession.
- ◆ Protecting their employment right under the law.
- ◆ Securing terms and conditions of employment that will attract and retain qualified personnel.

Nurses are turning to collective bargaining to directly shape the workplace and control their practice. Nurses know that working conditions are inextricably linked with standards of care. Collective bargaining creates the power base and provides a legally enforceable mechanism to address employment conditions that prevent nurses from delivering high-quality nursing care.

Professionalism and autonomy are control over both the performance of professional tasks and the immediate environment in which such tasks are performed. Collective bargaining has contributed substantially to nursing's evolution as a profession in the past and will continue to increase nursing's power in meeting present and future challenges. To improve the environment for nursing, nurses will turn increasingly to collective bargaining, demonstrating their commitment to improving practice where they work.

Collective bargaining is proving to be a viable mechanism for addressing a broad range of issues. The American Nurses Association (ANA) supports and encourages the use of collective bargaining by nurses. By supporting workplace advocacy, including collective bargaining activities, the ANA seeks to fulfill its responsibility to represent the interest and concerns of the profession and to ensure the public's access to quality nursing care.

LG VONFROLIO

◆ WHAT SHOULD I DO IF MY NURSES WANT TO ORGANIZE?

Q The nurses I manage informed me that they want to unionize. How should I respond?

A When a staff expresses an interest in unionization, it is usually a clear message that they are not happy with the current hospital working environment. Nurses are apt to see unionization as an alternative to what is often perceived as the hospital's indifference or refusal to deal with their concerns. Nurses' decision to seek collective bargaining is complex. Some primary sources of dissatisfaction are concerned with limited autonomy in the nursing role, lack of communication with management, exclusion from participation in organizational decision making, and dissatisfaction with compensation. Other factors may include the fact that nurses are coming from families of higher socioeconomic backgrounds. This type of background usually fosters individuals who

U

are more self-directed and desiring of autonomy. Such characteristics predispose younger nurses to conflict with a system that has traditionally reinforced nonassertive, uncritical following of orders on the part of nurses. Another trend can be attributed to the increase in educational background of nurses. This has led nurses to view themselves more as professionals, capable of assuming broad responsibility and acting autonomously.

As a nurse manager, ask yourself the following questions:

♦ Is attention given to economic incentives to practice nursing?

♦ Are there efforts to control the implementation of practice in the workplace?

♦ Does your staff control or have significant input into the practice environment?

You need to explore with your staff issues that are of concern to them. Most important, as a group, act on them.

LG VONFROLIO

♦ HOW DO I RETAIN COMPETENT STAFF DURING LAYOFF PERIODS AND NOT RUN AFOUL OF THE UNION?

Q In a union environment, what can a nurse manager do to retain nursing staff with excellent clinical skills during a time when nurses are being laid off?

A This is an issue that has major implications for unionized hospitals, particularly when the contract may allow for hospital-wide seniority placement during layoffs. Building the best possible relationship on both a unit-wide and a division-wide basis is in the best interest of both the union and the hospital. Both represent the staff nurses, even though the focus of each may be somewhat different. Building these bridges is not a matter easily accomplished in a crisis, when anxiety levels are high and trust levels are low. Staff representatives can be expected to have an interest in professional aspects of patient care.

Elements of professionalism are not the same as wages, hours, and working conditions, which are subject to collective bargaining. Look for areas of common agreement in the issues. Addressing the issue of

how to keep professional practice at the forefront in a time of tension, as occurs with downsizing, is an important and timely topic for discussion with unit, staff, and union representatives.

The union is the sole representative of its members on wages, hours, and conditions of employment, so discussion on these issues should be handled through an official bargaining committee. Exploration of how to maintain staff in areas where they have advanced skills or closely related areas can be discussed in relation to contract language that speaks to layoff and seniority. Balancing the concepts of retaining nurses with high levels of skills and seniority is difficult. Building trust and open relationships is in everyone's best interest.

B FOSTER

♦ WHAT IS THE RELATIONSHIP BETWEEN EMPOWERED STAFF AND A MANAGER IN A UNIONIZED HOSPITAL?

Q What is the relationship between staff nurses and the nurse manager in an empowered nursing organization that is also in a collective bargaining/union hospital?

A With the empowerment of nursing staff, which includes the transfer of legitimate decision making, the norm of labor versus management in unionized settings has been challenged. Since this relationship has generally been fraught with conflict or at best mistrust, breaking the tradition will affect relationships between management and staff.

The change process involved in moving union and management to an empowered organization is complex and carries many concerns from both a management and union point of view. In analysis, both have similar concerns: will this represent a "caving in" to the interest of the other group? Will there be a lack of mutual cooperation with hidden agendas? Should so much decision-making authority be given to staff?

Actions of the unit manager will be a key in getting solid support for activities associated with an empowered organization. Acknowledging long-standing concerns of staff is helpful when it is understood

U

these issues will only be resolved over time as a new working relationship develops.

Professional practice issues do not lend themselves to the collective bargaining process, which tends to be static and restrictive in focus. Recognizing that nurse managers and unionized staff are part of the same profession, although fulfilling different roles, can focus the necessary energy to agree on approaches to resolving professional issues.

Resistance and testing can be expected as staff begin dealing directly with the manager. The manager should avoid making decisions for the staff or giving other indications of lack of confidence in staff empowerment, or trust will be eroded. Much developmental work must occur with staff who have not usually developed collaborative professional relationships. The manager plays a critical leadership role in this development.

B FOSTER

♦ WHAT SHOULD I DO IF STAFF CONTINUALLY RUN TO THE UNION FOR HELP?

Q I am a new nurse manager and new to this organization. I have noticed that whenever a problem exists, the staff "run to the union." When I question the staff, it is clear that they do not trust us to help them with problems. How can this cycle be broken?

A Trust is having a firm belief or confidence in the integrity, reliability, and justice of another person or thing. Trust makes it unnecessary to examine motives, to "have it in writing," to have someone intervene between two parties so they can understand each other, or to be sure that neither is going to hurt the other.

When this condition of fear and distrust exists, it takes time, patience, and specific behaviors to help the other regain trust. The following four behaviors are necessary for a trusting environment to exist:

1. *Honesty.* Tell no lies, make no exaggerations, and don't be afraid to speak because you are afraid the other might be upset or get angry. Honesty is a frank, straightforward statement of the truth. Honesty is free from deceit; it is being what you are.

2. *Openness.* In communication, individuals demonstrate openness when they permit a clear view of themselves through self-disclosure and nondefensive responses. Open individuals are not closed to new ideas and are free from discrimination restrictions.

3. *Consistency.* An individual who is consistent in her behavior holds to the same principles or actions repeatedly. Such an individual is perceived as predictable, reliable, and dependable. When an individual varies in her emotional response or management style, she is seen as unpredictable. Therefore, consistency versus variable responses sets the stage for renewed trust.

4. *Respect.* When you treat an individual with dignity and fairness, you foster trust because you show the individual consideration. Showing respect means you are courteous and polite and demonstrate regard for the other's feelings, thoughts, and opinions. It means you don't talk negatively to an individual in front of other people, that you do not show favoritism, and that you avoid intruding into the individual's privacy.

To break the cycle of distrust, you will need to demonstrate these behaviors over time. The more times the trust has been broken for your employees, the longer it will take to repair. Since you are not perfect, it is important for you to also acknowledge any time you do not demonstrate these behaviors.

VD LACHMAN

♦ WHAT CAN I DO IF THE UNION RESISTS CHANGE?

Q If I find our union resists almost any innovation, what can I do?

A Innovation automatically implies change. In today's world a new health care delivery system is evolving, and the traditional hospital environment is being forced to change its service characteristics. The resistance you are experiencing is likely related to fear of change and what that may bring. Most health care workers are very aware of the downsizings that have become so common in the industry.

In many union environments an adversarial relationship exists between staff and management. This is

U

especially true when management still plays the traditional role of decision maker for all issues. If staff involvement is minimal, a lack of trust can be expected.

The manager's role is to create an environment where workers want to be involved in creating successful models of care. Involving the staff in planning and freely sharing information to make their contributions meaningful will be fundamental to getting their participation. Concerns should be addressed openly and support and information given to reach a realistic understanding of the issues. Acknowledge participation generously, and let staff own their successes. Attempts that fail to achieve goals should be analyzed for learning purposes, establishing an atmosphere that supports taking risks. Positive outcomes created by staff involvement will reflect success for the manager.

B FOSTER

◆ WHAT SHOULD I DO IF ONE DEPARTMENT IN THE HOSPITAL BEGINS RECRUITING FOR THE UNION?

Q I came to work this morning and saw that the emergency room staff was passing out information outside the hospital encouraging all the nursing staff to sign a card joining the union. I am a nursing manager on the critical care unit. What should I do now?

A The first thing you should do is to contact your human resources department and ensure that the hospital's legal counsel is informed of this effort. In collaboration with these groups, a strategy should be developed to determine how personnel will be approached because of an apparent union-organizing campaign.

One cannot prevent staff from signing cards requesting that a union shop be organized. Staff members have a right to organize under current law. However, managers can take several actions to ensure that personnel have all the pertinent information before making the determination whether they choose to join a union:

1. Meet with your personnel department and appropriate legal counsel. Identify do's and don'ts under applicable federal and state law.
2. Call a meeting of all management staff. Make a determination on how extensive the union-organizing effort is.
3. Meet with your staff. During these meetings:
   a. Identify issues and alternatives to resolution.
   b. Inform personnel of their rights during such a campaign. Frequently, personnel are not aware that they do not have to sign cards or allow union organizers to approach them.
4. Usually campaigns are not permitted during work hours or in such a way as to create interference with the facility's operation. If this is occurring, it is likely that you can request that union organizers leave the premises.
5. Do not discipline those who are passing out cards unless their effort creates an interference with operations.

Personnel often unionize when they perceive that their issues and requirements cannot be resolved in any way but through solidarity. When managers are able to address issues in a manner that staff perceive provides them control over resolution, a union-organizing effort is less likely to be successful.

LM LENTENBRINK

Vacations

◆ HOW CAN I ENCOURAGE STAFF TO TAKE LONG-OVERDUE VACATIONS?

Q We have a member of our nursing staff who has accrued a great deal of vacation time; however, even though she is eligible, she never takes it. Although she does not appear to be stressed or disadvantaged by it, we are concerned regarding the balance in her life. What can I do to encourage her to take vacation time, or should I do anything?

A Yes, the employee should be encouraged to take vacation. This encouragement is based on current human resource policy in most institutions

V

whereby vacation leave is a benefit provided for the purpose of rest and relaxation. In addition, vacation time, if accrued and not taken, is subject to forfeiture once the limit is reached. Strategies for the encouragement of staff personnel to take advantage of vacation time may be approached in the following ways:

♦ The supervisor and employee can sit down together and review accumulated hours, review the vacation book to see what times are available, and establish a time when vacation may be taken.

♦ Leave vacation brochures on the employee's desk or in her mailbox in an effort to make the process friendly and less threatening.

♦ Discuss the importance of time away from work even though the employee may not be aware of the need.

It is well documented that burnout can be attributed to increased job mobility and temporary or permanent withdrawal.

K KERFOOT

♦ HOW CAN I MAKE MY VACATION TIME MORE PROFITABLE?

Q As a nurse manager, I take regular vacations of at least 1 week every 3 months. The problem is that I find I cannot relax; I am always thinking about work. By the time the week is over, I don't feel I've had a vacation. What can I do about this?

A A personal assessment or inventory of your feelings and attitude about your "quality of life" and work is a beginning. Seek honest answers to potentially difficult questions, such as: Am I in the right job at the right time? Am I qualified for this job? How is my self-esteem?

In other words, a personal inventory of who, what, and why is in order. Various resources are available to help you seek the most honest analysis. Candid discussions with your superior, peers, employee assistance staff, and so on will help you delineate the root causes of your behavior.

Insights obtained from this process may identify companion issues that are correctable with addi-

tional skills development. Issues surrounding managerial proficiency such as the art of delegating; human resource managerial skills; valuing, trusting, and respecting your staff; and skills in defining expectations for self and others are all areas for further exploration that can be developed and will aid you in becoming more comfortable and proficient as a nurse manager. *If* you conclude after the self-appraisal, with or without external advice, that you are in the right job for you at this time, you should make a personal commitment to alter your perception.

LM JOHNSON

Violence

♦ WHAT SHOULD BE DONE IF A PATIENT HITS A STAFF MEMBER?

Q One of our patients struck a member of the nursing staff several times during a recent stay. Hospital administration was informed of this, and the patient was counseled. However, the patient continued to act out and to physically abuse nurses. How should this situation be handled, and what are the rights and responsibilities related to physical violence between patients and staff?

A It is difficult to answer these questions without further information about this particular situation. Physical violence from a patient always warrants further investigation into details of the given case. As with police work, all leads must be reviewed. For example, patients can act out because of stimuli in the environment that provoke anger. Certain medications can adversely affect patients and cause physically violent reactions. Patients with histories of certain mental diseases will act out if not controlled with their prescribed medications.

If the situation described is not related to environmental stimuli and all given leads are ruled out, the hospital is responsible for examining the situation within a context of patient and staff rights. The hospital does have the obligation to create a proper, safe

V

environment for the practice of patient care. Counseling the patient may not be enough. The physician prescribing the care, the staff providing the care, and the patient receiving the care must be involved in the dialogue. Strategies such as limit setting have been used successfully in similar situations, with the ultimate result being patient discharge when all else fails.

Most human resources or personnel departments are able to provide further information and guidance in this matter. They also can share any legal ramifications related to physically violent acts by patients.

MT SINNEN

◆ HOW CAN I PREVENT VIOLENCE FROM ERUPTING?

Q A patient's boyfriend struck her physician for using abusive language toward him. This physician has a history of abusive language and has almost been struck in the past. One of our orderlies approached the patient's boyfriend, pulled him away from the physician, wrestled him to the floor, then was soundly beaten by the boyfriend, who then left the unit. How could we have handled this situation better?

A This situation sounds both frightening and complex. There are really two issues here: the physician's history of abusive language and the situational violence generated by a visitor. Each needed to be handled differently and preferably at different times.

First, the situation you described happened so quickly that it is difficult to define just how it could have been better handled after the fact. If the potential for violence was anticipated, some proactive planning for it could have occurred. However, for the most part these events cannot be anticipated, and reaction to them is usually based on the circumstance. A plan for handling acting-out behavior such as you describe is helpful. It gives the staff a framework for undertaking an appropriate response. Working out the details of such a plan with your security service is also helpful. Devising a public call code for a security alert or response can also be helpful to obtain immediate and full response.

It appears in this case that two very volatile personalities tangled. If it could be anticipated that the

patient or her friend would "trip" certain switches for acting out in the physician, the patient's nurse could have addressed the possibility with either the patient or physician. Separating the two players is always much easier before the altercation than afterward.

We can admire the heroism of your orderly but not his wisdom. It was a high-risk experiment on his part, and he barely escaped. The tension here certainly was between waiting for security to arrive and preventing further damage to the physician, although we cannot know exactly what would have happened if something else had been attempted. The physician should certainly be thankful. I am told by my police friends that it is generally better for two persons to work together in stopping an altercation to help prevent what happened when your orderly was beaten by the patient's visitor.

Second, it is necessary to address the physician's verbal volatility to prevent such possibilities for conflict in the future. This acting out may alert him to the need for counseling. If it doesn't, the nursing leadership should report his behavior in person and in writing to the medical staff leadership. Clearly, an investigation of this matter needs to be undertaken by those responsible for risk management. Here again, anticipating the possibility of reaction to the physician's verbal indiscretions (and you should have acted earlier, since his mouth has gotten him in trouble in the past) and preventing them is better than dealing with the aftereffects of a violent altercation.

T PORTER-O'GRADY

Witnessing

◆ AM I LEGALLY LIABLE IF I WITNESS A LIVING WILL?

Q On our unit, nurses are frequently asked to provide witness to living wills and other legal documents on behalf of patients. Should nurses provide witnessing services? Is there some legal liability involved if they do?

A It is not unusual for nurses to be asked to provide witnessing services for living wills and other legal documents on behalf of patients. Although it is frequently the nurse's nature to try to help the patient in any way possible, it is not always wise for nurses to provide witnessing services. They may be subject to charges of coercion if anyone questions the patient's state of mind when signing documents. Much depends on the type of document signed and the institution's policy on such practices.

Nurses are in a unique role of control over the patient. Some patients may sign a document under the misunderstanding that to do so will please a nurse while to refuse to do so would make the nurse less likely to care for that patient. Nurses better serve as patient advocates by ensuring that patients receive an explanation of the documents being signed, ensuring access to documents, and ensuring choice while protecting the patient from being inappropriately influenced by other sources.

Although it may be unlikely that nurses will be accused of coercion or undue influence because of their unique role in controlling the patient's care, many hospitals and other medical institutions prefer that the nurse assist the patient in obtaining witnesses to legal documentation rather than witnessing such documents. Since practices may vary among institutions, the nurse should always request instructions from legal counsel and review personnel policies before proceeding.

LM LENTENBRINK

Work Redesign

◆ WHAT IS REDESIGNING, AND WHAT DIFFERENCE CAN IT MAKE?

Q Redesigning health care organizations with patient-focused care models is rapidly becoming the top priority for the 1990s. Why are hospitals redesigning and operationally restructuring patient care? What is redesign? What issues does redesign address? What outcomes does it achieve?

A Hospitals are redesigning and restructuring patient care because the traditional way is just not working any longer. Patient care was developed in a very cumbersome and inefficient fashion. This was not done intentionally; it resulted from a financial system that reimbursed us based on charges for services provided. In the 1960s the federal government began reimbursing hospitals based on charges. The more we charged, the more we made. We were never able to charge for nursing care, so this payment structure encouraged us to develop reimbursable "revenue centers." As a result, we began to see various departments develop that either delivered care to the patient or brought the patient to the department for some form of care. Over time, we moved more and more away from the patient and designed our organizations around highly specialized departments.

During the 1980s, in an effort to reduce the rising cost of health care, the government changed the reimbursement structure to a predetermined amount based on the patient's diagnosis (diagnosis-related group, DRG). Soon after Medicare switched to a DRG payment system, other forms of payment models came on the market—health maintenance organizations, preferred provider organizations, independent practice associations, and so on (HMOs, PPOs, IPAs, etc.). We saw a reversal of how hospitals were being reimbursed. Suddenly, the more we spent, the more we lost.

If you look at other industries, they restructure their work every 10 to 15 years. Health care continues to provide its service in the way it was designed 70 to 80 years ago. We have continued to build on top of the existing structure. However, the fundamental way we are reimbursed has radically changed, providing us an excellent opportunity to look carefully at the way we provide our services and to change the way in which we are structured. Health care needs to be structured around the patient, not departments; the patient is the reason we exist. Redesign is fundamentally changing the way we do business. It is totally rethinking how we deliver care, putting the patient at the center of the business and designing the organization around the patient's wants and needs. It is tearing down the walls that have been built between and within the organization, getting all disciplines focused on working together to design the organization in such a way that the patient becomes the focal point.

W

Historically, the only people who came to work for the patient were the individuals assigned to the patient care unit. Everyone else came to work for a department. Over time, this created a number of turfs, conflict, lack of continuity of care, and lack of camaraderie. Little teamwork existed because people interacted only when they needed something from other people, such as a call to the pharmacy to get medications or to indicate that someone had not done her job (e.g., the medication never arrived). Redesign has everyone working together for a common goal, meeting the patient's needs. It creates a paradigm shift in the organization's focus and becomes one of a common purpose, the patient. The structure in the past focused on departments versus patients, with each department built as a minibusiness with its own staff, structure, and policies. This created tremendous complexities, inefficiencies, and duplication within the organization.

In addition, staff had limited flexibility because of a narrow focus of what was included in their area of responsibility. This narrow focus contributed to a wide variety of people coming in contact with and asking the patient very similar, if not repeated, questions. This created patient confusion, frustration, and concern about the potential for us to miss something or make a mistake, which we have done. This structure of inefficiency created many non–value-added tasks and multiple "handoffs" within the organization.

Patient-focused redesign has four outcomes: service, quality, satisfaction, and cost. First, an immediate upgrade in service: redesigning the organization around the patient immediately affects the patient's experience and increases satisfaction with the care received. Reducing the number of handoffs increases the efficiency and effectiveness of the care delivered. Moving all services and caregivers to the patient care unit increases the amount of time the caregivers spend with the patient and enhances patients' satisfaction with the time caregivers physically spend with them.

Second, an increased level of quality is provided. Clinical indicators such as nosocomial infections, patient falls, and errors (e.g., medication, missed treatments, wrong patient) are greatly reduced because fewer people are providing the care, and everyone who is providing the care is assigned to the patient care area, working together as a team.

Third, satisfaction levels are increased from patient, staff, and physician standpoints. Patients are given care more frequently by fewer caregivers. The care provided has enhanced consistency, is less fragmented, and is better communicated. Patient-centered care creates an environment supported by the value of teamwork. Staff work as a team and have enhanced support by all disciplines working for the common purpose, the patient. Caregivers experience an increased level of knowledge because they are centered around and assigned to the patient care area sharing information and knowledge with each other. Staff, in their expanded, cross-trained role, sense greater satisfaction because they are allowed to do more and feel as if they really do make a difference. Physicians appreciate having all the professional disciplines on the floor providing readily available resources, information, and much more efficient turnaround times. The ability to talk to the pharmacist on the spot has a direct effect on what the physician may order for the patient to ensure drug compatibility or drug effectiveness.

The fourth outcome is financial impact. By decreasing the number of process steps, handoffs, department interactions, and people delivering the care, the number of individuals needed is reduced. Whenever efficiency can be increased, the effect is higher productivity. In addition, by having all multidisciplinary caregivers assigned to the patient care area and under the leadership of one individual, the number of supervisory people is reduced. It is no longer necessary to have multiple patient care areas because these individuals are now working for a patient care business unit and under the direction of one person. Reducing handoffs and cross-training individuals who do most of the tests the patient requires (laboratory, electrocardiogram, respiratory) decreases the need for clerical or secretarial staff to coordinate or schedule those procedures.

The reason it is critical for hospitals to aggressively redesign is to ensure an environment in which caregivers can be continually responsive to patient needs; to increase patient, staff, and physician satisfaction; to improve the efficiency and effectiveness of the care delivered; and to foster an environment that is innovative and eager for change. This can be successful only when an environment exists where empowerment is valued and supported. Risk taking must be supported and encouraged, meaning that mistakes are welcomed and viewed as learning opportunities. It is critical that the redesign efforts are ongoing, continually changing, and improving. The true success of redesign rests with the organization's understanding, commitment, and perseverance in the philosophy of continuous quality improvement. Only if the organization recognizes the need to continue to enhance and modify the structure through the staff will this strategy have long-term success.

J TORNABENI

◆ DOES REDESIGNING DISEMPOWER NURSES?

Q It seems as if the efforts to redesign work and change nursing relationships are really a subtle attempt to disempower nursing in the interest of raising productivity and lowering costs. What is really going on here?

A There is a real and important emphasis on cost-effective delivery of health care services in the United States. The health system has been driven by ever-accelerating costs for at least 30 years. The current financial condition of the United States and continuation of business as usual simply do not pass the cost/benefit analysis test. The system itself has been weakened by the ever-spiraling costs of service and technology.

Redesign is a legitimate effort to experiment and address newer ways of providing health care services in a cost-effective and quality-reflective manner. As always, attendant risks exist during a change as major as this. Inadequate processes and uncertain methodologies contribute to the uncertainty, confusion, and "noise" of implementing needed change. It is also consistent with transformation that some strategies used to make change are questionable in both intent and design. Some people have an agenda for change that threatens the integrity of the professions, impedes balanced and equitable relationships, and fails to recognize the need for a strong balance between concept and implementation. Also, some people want to create work groups that are homogenized and amorphous with no discernible distinction between the expectations for one team member and another. These are clearly misguided intentions and are fairly easy to recognize.

For the most part, leaders do respect the need for diversity and culturally specific change. They also know that real change must be driven by those on whom it has the greatest impact. Some elements of redesign at first appear strange and inappropriate when compared with the template of our past expe-

riences. The challenge of sorting through newer realities and different ways of working and the recognition of economic constraint can sometimes be very threatening. It is imperative that we sort through what is happening and discern whether it is our response to change with which we are uncertain or whether it is a legitimate reaction to inappropriate strategies for change. The one option not available is to go back to the way things were.

T PORTER-O'GRADY

◆ HOW CAN I ENSURE STAFF COOPERATION WITH WORK REDESIGN?

Q In planning for work redesign, what needs to be anticipated to deal with those who would undermine redesign or not entirely "buy into" it?

A Whenever work structures change and staff must buy in, some basic principles should be addressed.

It is more successful to have the staff participate from the beginning rather than have the changes revealed to them later. Initially, you would want to bring together the people involved and present the need for changing their jobs, the rationale, and the necessary outcome. At that point, you may introduce the available options. It is important that all the staff understand and buy into the need for change and the rationale for it. They need to participate fully in the discussion of the options for resolving the problem. If you are not willing to accept alternate solutions for the problem, and if you are using staff participation to achieve these ends, you will likely not be successful, and the staff will feel tricked or betrayed. You must be willing to modify your plans to accommodate the staff's needs. If you have been given parameters for the decision making, inform the staff of the limitations. If it will not be a totally democratic process and you must have the final veto, clarify that as well. If the change has been dictated to you and you have no choices, ask the staff how you can make it work and what they need to do to be effective and protect patient safety. The staff must be involved in determining what work is being done and in discussing whether each task or activity is necessary and appropriate, and if it is, who could or should be doing it. As new roles are being created, staff need to participate so they clearly understand how the role is being defined.

Communication regarding the effectiveness of the staff's actions as the project progresses is vital. Ongoing discussions and group meetings need to be held to iron out the problems and identify issues that may have the potential for problems. If the staff participate in designing and carrying out the evaluation process, more attention will be paid to those staff who return to past methods of doing things.

Attaining a positive attitude regarding the change can be achieved with clear communication, participation, much staff input, and good feedback.

JB COLTRIN ET AL.

◆ HOW CAN I USE DIFFERENTIATED PRACTICE IN MANAGING?

Q What are some specific strategies for managing individuals with varying educational backgrounds and varying attitudes toward their work through the use of differentiating practice?

A *Differentiated practice* denotes a variety of meanings to different nurses. For example, for some it means a differentiation in practice by entry level into the profession. This still remains an emotionally charged issue in some circles. Research done on the topic of educational preparation, however, differentiates certain criteria regarding the educational experience.

More important factors are the role design and clarification that occur within an institution as the care delivery system is built. Certain roles lend themselves to specific qualifications, including educational level. For example, the role of the clinical nurse specialist in most facilities is specific in addressing advanced practitioners.

Specific strategies of implementation with staff include:

1. Whenever possible, involve staff in the decisions associated with patient care. This includes care delivery system design.
2. Clarify role delineations and role expectations within the system.
3. Work within the context of a team approach. It takes a team to complete the work flow process.

4. Clarify the outcome of the work to be done, making sure that everyone realizes that the *patient* is the primary customer.
5. Match the most qualified staff with the appropriate roles. Take into account educational preparation, experience, and attitudes toward work.

MT SINNEN

◆ HOW DO I BALANCE TEACHING NEEDS AND ADMINISTRATIVE RESPONSIBILITIES IN TIMES OF CHANGE?

Q How do I balance my administrative responsibilities and the staff's teaching needs as we transform to patient-focused care?

A There are both short-term and long-term responses to this concern. The short-term solution is to use organizational resources (e.g., health education, clinical specialists) or hire outside consultants to do the teaching. Given current resource constraints, this is often not feasible.

Another short-term strategy is to collaborate with your peers to develop a plan to share teaching responsibilities. Consider creative teaching modalities that foster learner accountability (e.g., self-paced learning modules, reading assignments followed by discussion groups, guided interdisciplinary case study groups).

These short-term strategies are stopgap measures. The current health care environment demands system redesign in *both* the care delivery and the structures that facilitate this delivery. Although this seems obvious, system redesign frequently ignores the need to change the way the nurse manager functions. This can lead to the nurse manager feeling left out and fragmented.

One way to avoid this job fragmentation is transformation of your governance structure. The purpose of this is to engender a sense of mutual accountability for meeting organizational and unit goals. It then becomes everyone's responsibility to see that administrative and learning needs are attained. However, this long-term strategy requires a major shift in how you and your staff view your complementary roles and responsibilities.

To plan for this long-term strategy, review the literature on shared governance, transformational leadership, and learning organizations. In addition, contact other nurse managers who have experience in these areas and ask for their suggestions. Do not hesitate to call authors of articles on these topics. These individuals can act as resources and refer you to other experts.

The following is a brief summary of the major components of a transformational governance model:

1. The organization is committed to quality care for the patient and a quality work environment for the employee.
2. All employees are committed to and live the agreed organizational vision. This commitment is exemplified by continuous proactive efforts to improve their own and the organization's performance.
3. The staff are empowered to participate in the educational process.
4. The administrative team members are the mentors, teachers, and resource coordinators.

After researching these topics, engage other critical members of the organization in a discussion of administrative structure redesign tailored to your organization. Suggested participants in this dialogue include the nursing administration team, staff representatives, and managers of the other professionals who will be members of the interdisciplinary patient-focused care team.

Be aware that this transformation takes time, usually 3 to 5 years. However, only through careful, proactive planning will the process remain flexible and not be stretched to the breaking point. I believe that keeping the new design flexible and whole is the key to organizational survival.

MC HANSEN

◆ IN A WORK REDESIGN PROGRAM, HOW CAN WE MAINTAIN CONTINUITY?

Q In a large (600 bed) hospital where work redesign is being implemented and where each manager has free rein of unit activities, how do we develop some form of continuity for the organization?

A The key to organizational survival in today's environment is to know where you are going and how you'll get there. Workplace redesign is a tool many businesses are using to position an organization to be efficient, effective, and competitive. Organizational continuity in workplace redesign can be ensured by focus on a common goal or desired result.

In the example given, each manager must be clear about the organization's and nursing department's goals. The nursing department's goals must clearly fit with the organization's goals.

Work redesign should be a planned, coordinated effort across the organization. It cannot be done in a vacuum. The chief of the nursing department will want to bring the managers together to identify common ground rules or guidelines within which redesign can occur. Training of managers together in redesign strategies can set the stage for common understanding of terminology, processes, and procedures. Ample time will be devoted to obtaining agreement and understanding design techniques under consideration. Ongoing networking among nurse managers and the chief nurse executive will assist in keeping efforts focused and coordinated. Continuous communication ensures all are in touch with strategies that work and those that should be discarded.

Managers must be encouraged to include staff in the redesign efforts, since they are in daily contact with the patient. Staff know the strengths and weaknesses of the nursing product. Staff are likely to have good ideas for work redesign. Involvement of staff in work redesign across the organization at the beginning sets the stage for a smoother implementation of workplace changes.

The "free rein" described in the question undoubtedly is meant to promote creativity, risk taking, and innovation. The work under way must be communicated up, down, and laterally to ensure coordination. Such communication also ensures that new ways of doing business are shared.

LJ SHINN

◆ HOW MANY LEVELS OF NURSE MANAGEMENT SHOULD THERE BE?

Q Is there really a role for any managerial level other than nurse executive and first-line manager in health care organizations of the future?

W

As hospitals continue to restructure and empower staff, the number of layers between staff and the chief executive officer (CEO) will continue to decrease. The number of managers will also continue to decline as costs are streamlined and empowered front-line staff assume greater responsibility and accountability for their work.

The traditional first-line manager role is rapidly evolving to a role of leader. The front-line manager's role in the environment is one of supporting, coaching, advising, championing, and leading change. This calls for a new type of individual who is willing to let go and step back to allow the professional staff to manage themselves. The new role of the front-line manager is to ensure that support, information, and resources exist for the bedside nurse to carry out her work. The front-line manager's role also becomes one of strategist and visionary. She must be continually learning, growing, and evolving as her staff continue to grow and evolve. She needs to continue to move to the next level to stay at least one step ahead of her staff. If she doesn't, the staff will pass her up and grow up around her, leaving her behind, and probably out of a job.

The professional nurse at the bedside is really the manager. She must view herself as the person both responsible for and accountable for managing the patients' care. Coordination and delegation of care to the most appropriate team member are the responsibility of the bedside nurse. As we continue to restructure our patient care delivery model, the nurse at the bedside must change the way she has traditionally viewed her role. Nurses should no longer view their role as total caregiver, but rather as the manager or coordinator of care. Nursing must clearly understand which tasks only a nurse can do and which can be delegated to others. In an era of limited resources, both financially and in available numbers, nursing must at last truly define what is and is not nursing. Nursing must give up the need to hang on to tasks. Being task oriented has occurred at the expense of fully using the knowledge and skills only nursing can bring to patient care. Nursing time needs to be spent on assessing, planning, educating, implementing, and evaluating patient care. A conscious move must be made to focus on patient outcomes. Nurses must spend their time only on nursing, not on performing tasks that other disciplines can and should be doing.

No manager level exists per se other than the nurse executive and the first-line manager. However, as the number of managers continues to decrease and the span of control expands, a support system needs to evolve for the nurse manager. This support system will need to have business and financial skills that can assist the nurse manager in managing multimillion dollar operations and in project planning and information system support.

J TORNABENI

◆ HOW CAN I REDESIGN A SMALL HOSPITAL UNIT TO BE EFFICIENT AND PRODUCTIVE?

Q What is needed to redesign small hospital units with a census of 15 or fewer and still achieve productive targets?

A It is clear from your question that you recognize the difficulty of efficiently operating a unit of less than 15 patients. Both physical redesign of the unit and work redesign can be used to achieve the greater efficiency you desire.

First, if you must maintain a unit this small, be sure the unit is not located in an isolated area of the hospital. You will be able to staff the unit with a minimum core of nurses only if backup support is available close by. Preferably, place two or more of these small units together, locating the nurses' station between the units so that one station will serve both. This will provide an opportunity for greater efficiency through sharing staff, such as a unit clerk or a nursing assistant on night shift. The same applies to location of supplies and equipment. The center station design is particularly useful in mental health, where adult, adolescent, and child programs must be separated and volumes for all three can be low.

For other types of units, or when a common station connecting two small units is not possible, the important consideration in physical design remains flexibility. This can be accomplished by wiring the communication equipment (e.g., call lights, telephones, emergency buttons) to an adjacent nursing unit in addition to the nurses' station on the unit. By installing communication systems in two places, the small unit can function as a "swing" unit. When the census drops to an inefficient level, the patients can be handled by the adjacent unit without having to be physically moved.

W

In designing the staffing pattern for the unit, the same rule applies. Design the roles and responsibilities for the positions that will be needed to staff the unit so that the greatest flexibility can be achieved. Consider combining the responsibilities of the nursing assistant and the unit clerk into a broader-scope position of patient services associate. In doing this, the unit ensures not only that the ancillary staff will be kept busy when census is low, but also that continuity of care will be provided. When a nurse and a patient services associate together provide all the services, including professional nursing, hygiene and comfort measures, nutrition, clinical documentation, and maintenance of an up-to-date clinical record, quality service can be provided in a cost-effective manner.

Finally, recognize that frequently shifts will be staffed at the minimum core level. When this occurs, simple tasks such as answering the telephone may become frustrations if not considered in advance. Pocket pagers for staff on a unit this small can make a major difference. With pagers the staff can be anywhere on the unit and communicate with each other as well as answer incoming telephone calls promptly.

SA FINNIGAN

◆ HOW DO I CONVINCE AN ADMINISTRATOR TO RESTRUCTURE?

Q How do I sell work restructuring to an administrator who thinks a full-time equivalent (FTE) is only an FTE?

A To imply that those administrators who consistently raise issues of productivity, labor costs, and expense control are persons who do not or will not discriminate among the different categories of workers in considering costs is patently unfair to all concerned. More than at any time in the history of health care, hospitals today are under increasing pressure to reduce expenses, improve outcomes, and become more productive. Organizations throughout the United States are struggling to identify and implement survival strategies in this new, hostile environment.

Managers may respond prematurely with, "We can't reduce any more!" when administrators continue to challenge them to excel in cost-reduction efforts. These frustrated managers sometimes perceive their administrators as thinking "an FTE is only that, an FTE," when in reality the administrators are simply appealing to them to alter their paradigm and to look for new answers. Perform a few tasks differently; for example, alter or enhance systems so they are less labor intensive. In short, "restructure the work."

To sell or present work restructuring in your organization, I would suggest you consider the following actions:

1. Set goals and objectives and review them regularly for currentness, deletions, and additions. Make them specific and clear so everyone understands them.
2. To identify and evaluate work processes for possible improvement or outright elimination, spell out "who, what, when, where, why, and how" for each process.
3. Determine the current cost of each process as accurately as possible in terms of time and the "3 Ms": manpower, materials, and money, as well as any cost history.
4. Determine both real and perceived benefits to the organization and patients if a work process is restructured. Likewise, list and validate any disadvantages that restructuring could cause.
5. Bear in mind in developing and presenting your findings to your administrator that maintaining quality outcome is a must. However, the bottom-line issue in today's health care environment is DOLLARS; give your administrator the benefit of the doubt that she does not think "an FTE is an FTE is an FTE."

GA ADAMS

Writing for Publication

◆ HOW SHOULD I SELECT A JOURNAL TO WRITE FOR?

Q I am interested in submitting an article for publication, but I don't know the process for select-

W

ing a journal. There are so many out there. What criteria should I use?

A Before writing your manuscript but after you have (1) reviewed the literature, (2) decided what the purpose of your paper is, and (3) decided who needs to hear your message, you need to identify all the *potential* journals that might be right for your idea. For example, perhaps your topic is financial management in the hospital. Depending on how you want to focus, your manuscript might be appropriate for journals read by nurse executives or first-line managers, staff development directors or clinical nurse specialists, or staff nurses. When you know who you want to write for, select journals read by that group.

After identifying journals appropriate for your ideas, you can write letters to the editors of those journals, asking their interest in your topic. Your first-choice journal for financial management might be *The Journal of Nursing Administration.* However, if that journal is not interested in your idea but a journal for first-level managers is, you are ready to refocus your information to a different level of nurse manager.

The best source for identifying potential journals is "Publishing Opportunities for Nurses: A Comparison of 92 U.S. Journals" (Swanson, McCloskey, & Bodensteiner, 1991). This article gives demographics you can use to select and prioritize journals that best match your ideas.

After selecting potential journals, obtain the most recent copy of each journal. Study the journal for its style and format. Identify the reader of the journal and the level of sophistication of the content. Make sure your topic and your experience lend themselves to writing comfortably for the journal's readership and in the journal's style.

Some other factors you might want to consider when choosing your journals: How relevant is your topic to the journal's readers? How many of the people you want to reach read the journal? Does the journal pay for articles (very few do)? How much time, on average, does review of manuscripts take? How long is the period from acceptance until publication? How soon do your ideas have to be published to be timely? What is the journal's manuscript acceptance rate? Which journal has a reputation for excellence in your specialty or among your colleagues?

The previously mentioned article by Swanson, McCloskey, and Bodensteiner provides each journal's information for authors' guidelines (usually published in every issue of the journal), and the journal itself will give you this information. If these resources do not answer all your questions, call or write the editorial office. In the end, only you can decide what combination of factors is most important to you in selecting journals.

SS BLANCETT

♦ HOW DO I GET STARTED WRITING?

Q I would like to write for publication, but the process seems overwhelming. How do I get started?

A Writing for publication is an exciting direction for nurses to pursue. The idea may seem intimidating, but the process itself can relieve much anxiety. First, you need an idea. Many times the idea for writing comes from your own experience in searching for articles to help yourself. For example, you may need to know more about a nursing intervention your hospital wants to replace with a different one. In searching the literature for a rationale for either keeping or discontinuing the practice, you may discover that little evidence exists for either course of action. Such a condition is ideal for a small study comparing the results of each intervention. Your findings will add to the literature on that topic.

Once you have formed your idea, you should select the audience that would benefit most from the information. Journals are published for clinical nurses in numerous specialties (e.g., gerontology, oncology, critical care), for nurse managers and administrators, for researchers, and for the general public. You should read several issues of the journals in your area of interest before you select your target. Most journals contain instructions for potential authors. You should become familiar with these guidelines and follow them explicitly. After choosing your journal, write a letter of inquiry to the editor, outlining your idea and asking if there is interest in publishing an article on that topic. The editor's response will direct you further.

Remember, every published author has received her share of rejection letters. Do not become discouraged. Just because you swing and miss the ball a few times doesn't mean that the next one won't be a home run!

CE LOVERIDGE

♦ MAY I SUBMIT MY ARTICLE TO MORE THAN ONE JOURNAL AT THE SAME TIME?

Q Eager to share an innovative management ideas with others, I wrote a manuscript and sent copies to all the major nursing administration journals. I have already heard from two editors who want to publish my paper. However, both editors asked me to sign a copyright transfer form, which says in part my manuscript is being published by no one else. Did I make a mistake in sending my manuscript to so many journals at the same time?

A It is customary when submitting manuscripts to include a copyright transfer. My experience is that most manuscript guidelines from publishers will request this. Provisions of the Copyright Act of 1976 became effective on January 1, 1978. Therefore, manuscripts should be accompanied by the following written statement and signed by one author: "The undersigned author transfers all copyright ownership of the manuscript to _____ in the event the work is published. The undersigned author warrants that the article is original, *is not under consideration by another journal,* and has not been previously published. . . ."

If you did not have manuscript guidelines before submitting your manuscript, or if this is your first time submitting a manuscript for consideration for publication, no intentional mistake was made. Since you have two editors interested in your manuscript, pick the journal that has the following elements: refereed journal, indexed journal, and largest circulation. Sign the copyright transfer form and send in your manuscript. Wait for a letter from the editor either accepting or rejecting your manuscript. If your manuscript is rejected, it is usually accompanied by reasons why. This is an opportunity to perfect your

manuscript. After the rewrite, send it in to the second interested editor.

LG VONFROLIO

♦ SHOULD I LIST AS CO-AUTHOR SOMEONE WHO ONLY CONTRIBUTED IDEAS?

Q I am co-authoring with a colleague. Although she has developed most of the ideas, I have done most of the writing. I'm having a difficult time working with her because she wants to take equal credit with me. How do I deal with a situation like this?

A I have to side with your colleague. Based on the little you have told me, she does seem entitled to authorship.

Authorship entitlement is based on several factors. According to the International Committee for Medical Journal Editors (1988), authorship credit is based on substantial contributions:

- ♦ Conception and design or analysis and interpretation of data.
- ♦ Drafting the article or revising it critically for important intellectual content.
- ♦ Final approval of the version to be published.

To be a legitimate author, you must meet all three criteria. Participation solely in acquiring funding, collecting data, or general supervision of a group is not sufficient for authorship. People doing these types of activities certainly make your work and manuscript possible; they should not be forgotten. The appropriate way to thank them is in an acknowledgment, not by giving them honorary authorship. Honorary authorship gives credit where credit is not due and dilutes the work of the real authors.

Many journals now require authors to sign a statement saying not only that they have seen and approved the final manuscript, but also that they have taken due care to ensure the work's integrity. This last requirement means that all authors are familiar with the data from which the manuscript arose, so if this is called into question, they could publicly defend the content (Glass, 1992).

Your problem raises an important issue related to collaborative work with your colleagues. Before you

W

start any project, discuss publishing possibilities. Decide who will do what and what will entitle a person in the group to be an author versus being acknowledged for a contribution. This will help avoid the feelings now occurring between you and your colleague.

For now, I encourage you to relax and work in equal partnership with your colleague. I suspect you could not have written the manuscript without your colleague's great ideas. Likewise, you were the motivating force that captured those ideas in writing. You two may be the perfect team.

SS BLANCETT

◆ WHY SHOULD WRITING BE A CRITERION FOR CAREER ADVANCEMENT?

Q I resent that writing for publication has just been made a criterion for career advancement in my institution. I don't have time, I can't be bothered, and too many other critical activities demand my attention. How can writing for publication benefit me, the staff, patients, or the institution?

A For nursing to advance as a profession, we must continue to add to the body of knowledge related to the art and science of nursing. This literature must include theoretic and applied knowledge related to the practice of nursing. Nursing is a practice discipline. Most of us are in that practice arena and thus need to share in the validation of, as well as creation of, new and/or expanded literature.

Lack of time is a valid reason for not writing. Time management principles can be applied to daily work to make room for writing. Because you are fortunate enough to be practicing in a nursing division that values publishing, you can be assured that assistance would be provided.

Lack of skill in writing is another common reason for not publishing. Many very good seminars are available to assist with this aspect.

As for the benefits to be gained by publishing, here are just a few:

1. The thinking processes involved in writing assists in clarifying your own thoughts about a given topic.
2. Writing helps with verbal skill development.
3. Staff involvement with a research project that ends up in print is most rewarding. As staff read your name in print, it is conceivable that they also will publish.
4. Beyond your specific staff, many practicing nurses will benefit from reading about new interventions and so on.
5. As staff become more knowledgeable, practice levels are elevated and patient care is enhanced.
6. As members of a given staff publish, the institution's professionalism becomes recognized. This benefits the reputation of the organization in the eyes of other nurses, physicians, administrators, and the public.

MT SINNEN

◆ SHOULD A COLLEAGUE WHO ONLY EDITED A MANUSCRIPT BE INCLUDED AS AUTHOR?

Q Two of us have been involved in preparing a manuscript for publication. Our division of responsibility required that I did most of the writing and my colleague did most of the editing. Although my colleague did no writing, can we still include her as an author for her contribution?

A Substantial contribution and public defense of content are hallmarks of authorship. The division of tasks you mention certainly means both of you could be intimately familiar with the content and thus entitled to authorship.

The answer to your question rests on what you mean by "involved" and "editing." If your colleague simply edited for grammar, punctuation, and clarity, she is not entitled to authorship. If, in addition to those activities, she analyzed the accuracy of the content, identified areas that were incomplete, added missing information, and generally contributed to the manuscript's intellectual ideas, she is entitled to be an author.

SS BLANCETT

◆ WHAT SHOULD I INCLUDE IN A QUERY LETTER TO A JOURNAL'S EDITOR?

Q A colleague who has published extensively said that I should write an initial query to the editor before sending a manuscript. What is the purpose of a query, and what information should the letter contain?

A The purpose of a query letter is to acquaint the editor with your topic in a concise, interesting way and ascertain the editor's interest. A query letter allows the editor to give you advice about developing your topic and addressing the readers' information needs. This increases your chance of having your paper accepted for publication. However, remember that a positive response from the editor only indicates an interest in your topic; it is not a commitment to publish.

A query letter also lets the editor tell you he or she is not interested in your topic. Reasons for lack of interest may be that the journal has recently published or is soon to publish an article similar to yours, that your ideas add nothing new to what is already available in the literature, or that the topic is not a high priority for the journal. If the editor is not interested in your topic, your query letter will have saved you time and energy in not developing and formatting your manuscript for the wrong journal.

Take great care in writing your query letter. It is the editor's first introduction to you, your thinking, and your ideas. The physical appearance and the content of your letter tell the editor many things about you. For example, your ability to express your ideas clearly and logically, your attention to details, the pride you take in your work, your grasp of the topic, and your knowledge of what is important to the readership can all be judged. When a query letter does not address the editor by name, has spelling and grammatical errors, is a photocopy rather than an original printout, and is not personalized to the specific journal and its readers' needs, the editor might assume you won't give much attention to your manuscript either.

A query letter should be no longer than one typed page. The first paragraph should get the editor's attention by discussing an issue or problem the reader faces and how your work will address that issue. For example, "Nurse managers face unprecedented changes in the workplace. These changes are forcing them to reconsider how they allocate human resources. To help them with this issue, I would like to write a manuscript that describes a unique approach to staffing."

The next paragraph should give a thumbnail sketch of the major points you will make. Use an example if it will highlight your point. The third paragraph should discuss how your approach differs from what is already published and how the journal's readers will benefit from reading your paper. If your institutional letterhead and your job title do not implicitly indicate why you are qualified to write on this topic (perhaps you are a nurse manager wanting to write on a clinical topic), explain your expertise.

End your query by asking the editor's interest in your topic. If you want to set a submission deadline for yourself, tell the editor how soon you can submit a manuscript after receiving a positive response. If you don't indicate a submission date and the editor is eager to receive a paper on your topic, the editor will suggest a date.

Your query letter should be sent after you have reviewed the literature and know the purpose and focus of your topic. You may have an initial outline or draft of the paper. This allows you to discuss the main points of your topic and its relationship to current literature. After receiving a positive response, you can then tailor the paper's content to that journal's readers.

It is appropriate to send query letters to all journals you think might be interested in your topic. However, legal and ethical principles allow you to send your completed paper to only one journal at a time. If that journal rejects your manuscript, you are free to send the paper to another one.

SS BLANCETT

◆ WHAT DOES THE COPY EDITOR DO?

Q What is the role of the publisher's copy editor? What obligations and rights does that person have with regard to changing the content or character of a submitted manuscript?

W

A The copy editor's role varies from publisher to publisher. Traditionally, a copy editor's job was to review a manuscript for spelling, grammar, punctuation, consistency, and conformity to style. Today, many copy editors' roles have expanded to include substantive editing. In addition to copy editing, substantive editing involves reviewing content for accuracy and logic, often rewriting ideas, reorganizing content, writing transitions and summaries, eliminating wordiness and jargon, clarifying meaning, and consulting with authors.

The goal of all editing is to improve the authors' expression of their ideas, not to change their intent or mask their unique "voice." Most authors have no problem with an editor who is copy editing in the traditional sense; it's easy to see how their manuscript has been changed and improved.

However, substantive editing can change an author's meaning, often without the editor realizing it. The careful editor will always insert a query to the author pointing out major changes and asking the author's approval. Although an author should not quibble over traditional copy editing changes, such as changing the word "utilization" to "use," they have an obligation and a right to contest editing that changes their intent.

Most nursing journals have an editor or editor-in-chief who works with authors to arrive at satisfactory content after peer review of the manuscript. When the editor and author agree the paper's content is acceptable, the paper is sent to the journal's copy or production editor for copy editing. The copy-edited paper is sent to the author for approval. As an author, you should always feel free to call the editor and discuss editing changes with which you disagree. Since authors and editors have the same goal—conveying information to the reader in the best way possible—negotiate until an agreement on the expression of the idea is reached. Always remember, and remind the editor if necessary, that it is your paper, and how your ideas are expressed will "live forever in print."

SS BLANCETT

♦ IS USING THE FIRST PERSON ACCEPTABLE IN PROFESSIONAL JOURNALS?

Q When is it appropriate to use first-person references in a professional article?

A As with many aspects of the publishing process, the answer to this question varies by journal and publisher. Some editors think it is unprofessional to insert the "self" into a manuscript. Other editors believe it personalizes the content, letting the author speak as an expert. Generally, it is never appropriate to use the first person in a formal research report, seldom appropriate to use it in a highly conceptual or scholarly journal, and often appropriate in a clinical journal. However, you will see exceptions.

Two factors influence your choice of first-person or third-person voice. The first is the nature of your content. If you are writing about the impact a patient's death had on staff, the more personal first-person voice seems appropriate. On the other hand, if you are writing about how you chose a statistical test to analyze data, a more formal, third-person style is appropriate.

The second factor is the usual style of your target journal. Examine recent issues to see if you can use the first-person voice. Although there are always exceptions to the rule, if your style does not match that of the journal, you may want to find another journal.

SS BLANCETT

♦ WHAT SHOULD I DO IF A COLLEAGUE HAS USED CREDENTIALS SHE DOES NOT HAVE?

Q Reading a journal article recently, I noticed a colleague had listed credentials after her name that she does not have. Is this ethical? Should I do anything about it?

A First, a remote possibility exists that your colleague did not commit the error. In some journals, almost all authors have the same credentials. If your colleague did not list the credentials, an overzealous copy editor might have added them, assuming their omission was an oversight. Whether deliberate misrepresentation or an unintentional mistake, you do have to confront your colleague with your knowledge. Your colleague needs to write or call the editor, explaining the error and asking that a correction notice be printed in the next available issue of the journal.

If your colleague is not willing to do this, you have a moral obligation to tell your colleague's boss and/or the editor. The next step will be the boss' or the editor's; you will have discharged your obligation. Confronting your colleague and perhaps having to expose the unethical behavior publicly will not be easy. However, the profession's integrity rests on not allowing people to get away with unethical behavior.

SS BLANCETT

◆ IF I WRITE ABOUT MY HOSPITAL, DOES THE ARTICLE BELONG TO THE HOSPITAL?

Q I have written a manuscript describing how the staff has overcome some frustrations and concerns on our nursing unit. It has been accepted for publication; however, my supervisor indicated that I did not obtain the necessary permission from her and the hospital public relations department. Should I have done that? If so, isn't that a constraint on my freedom to write? My supervisor also indicated that since I'm employed by the hospital, anything I write that reflects on my employment belongs to the hospital. Is this true?

A This is a sticky situation. It involves ownership of ideas, contract law, copyright law, and perhaps most important, employer-employee relations. First, you need to look at your employment agreement. Was creation of your manuscript and the product you discussed within the scope of your employment responsibilities? Is writing for publication part of your written employment contract? If so, copyright law gives your employer the right to control the content and dissemination of your written work. Your manuscript would be called a work for hire. However, even in works for hire, the author can sometimes retain copyright if no written agreement exists between the employer and author about who will hold copyright. Therefore, in answer to one of your questions, your employer does not automatically own your manuscript. However, this is a complex legal issue; if you really want to proceed against your employer's wishes, see an attorney first.

A more practical issue involves your relationship with your supervisor. Politically, a first step whenever you write something related to your employment is discussing your intent with your supervisor

and colleagues. Tell them you are writing a manuscript related to an aspect of your work, and ask their permission to mention your unit and hospital in the manuscript and acknowledge their support and contribution to your work. This simple courtesy will probably please your colleagues and boss. It is also a nice public relations vehicle for any institution and staff.

If your supervisor will not give you literary freedom, you could write the paper, on your own time, without identifying the institution, the unit, or any of its people. Copyright law protects only the actual form the expression of an idea takes, not the idea itself. Therefore, writing about how you solved problems on the unit is acceptable. You would not be able to use any materials, such as a unit evaluation form or personnel policy, in your manuscript since they were written as "works for hire" and belong to the institution.

SS BLANCETT

◆ WHAT CRITERIA DO JOURNAL EDITORS USE FOR SELECTING ARTICLES TO BE PUBLISHED?

Q I often read a professional journal and think, "We've been doing that for years." What criteria do editors use to decide what they publish? How can I use that information to identify and develop a manuscript worthy of publication?

A Most journals in nursing that are refereed journals (i.e., manuscripts are reviewed and recommended for selection by editorial advisors) publish their criteria for selection. This information can tell you whether the article's content should be research based, a description, case study, or qualitative approach. The manuscript's content is evaluated for its relevancy to the journal's purpose. Accuracy of the content, timeliness of the data, and its usefulness for the readers of the journal are also criteria. These criteria are not necessarily published in each journal, but usually you can find them in at least one journal published during the year. Along with the information on the selection process, there is usually information concerning the journal's purpose, authorship responsibility, manuscript preparation, permissions, and manuscript submission.

W

In addition to this process, reading journals in the area that you are interested in can be helpful. Many nursing journals are available, and a visit to a library containing nursing journals would be enlightening. Reading a selection of articles could help you decide whether that specific journal would seem to be receptive to the content of your manuscript.

Before you decide, a call to the editors of the journal that you think may be suitable to your topic of interest can also assist you. I have found editors most willing to answer questions. They would probably suggest you send them a letter outlining the manuscript's content. This type of letter could be sent whether you called before or not. However you decide to go about the means of submitting a manuscript, do not become discouraged. Writing is a skill that can be mastered, and editors are usually very helpful.

SR. M FINNICK

◆ WHAT ARE THE MOST COMMON MISTAKES AUTHORS MAKE?

Q I'm thinking about writing a manuscript. What are some of the most frequent mistakes made by authors?

A Most journals publish guidelines for authors in every issue. If they are not published in the journal, you can request them from the editorial office. Every detail for submitting a technically correct manuscript is included in these guidelines, but authors consistently do not follow the instructions.

Here are some of the most frequently violated rules: submitting too few copies, using incorrect referencing, providing no abstract, writing an incorrect biographic statement, submitting too many manuscript pages, not spelling out abbreviations the first time they are used, using jargon, using outdated references, and single spacing. No author should make any of these technical mistakes. Pay close attention to and follow every procedural detail mentioned in the guidelines for authors. Also, have a friend read your paper, not for content, but for grammatical composition, spelling, and style and format consistency.

Computer software programs can help you write better and avoid composition errors. Two of the bet-

ter known applications are RightWriter (RightSoft, Inc., 4545 Samuel St., Sarasota, FL 34233) and Grammatik 5 (Reference Software, 330 Townsend St., Suite 123, San Francisco, CA 94107). These types of programs analyze your manuscript and point out problem areas in grammar, style, usage, spelling, and punctuation. They also analyze the readability of your material using several formulas. Although I do not always like or agree with the style changes these programs suggest, they do make me conscious of my writing style. Even a good writer benefits from having the computer program's critique; one becomes a more deliberate and intentional, and thus better, writer.

Another mistake authors make is not tailoring the manuscript's content to address the information needs of the journal's readers. Authors fail to answer the "So what?" question. Make sure you don't just tell a story in your manuscript. Have a specific point to make, and make it to a specific reader. For example, both first-line and top-level nurse administrators need financial information; however, the depth and type of information each needs on that same topic are different. Know your journal's prime reader.

SS BLANCETT

◆ WHEN SHOULD ET AL. BE USED?

Q Sometimes in professional publications, I see the names of two authors followed by et al. What does that mean, and when should it be used?

A *Et al.* is Latin for "and others." It is used in text, reference lists, and bibliographies to indicate that there are more authors of the work than those mentioned specifically by name. Use of et al. saves space and improves readability of text by not having long lists of authors.

The *Manual of Style of the American Medical Association* (1989) states that all authors should be listed by name unless there are more than six, in which case the names of the first three authors are used, followed by et al. When mentioned in the text, only the first author's surname is used, followed by et al.

The *Chicago Manual of Style* (1982) states if there are three or more authors, use the first author's name only and then et al. *A Publication Manual of the American Psychological Association* (1991) recommends citing all authors, the first time mentioned, if there are more than two but less than six. When there are six or more authors, only the first author is listed, followed by et al.

Although you now know what et al. means, you don't automatically know how to use it in a manuscript until you know what style manual your target journal uses. You can find out by looking at how references are formatted in a recent issue or by reading the journal's guidelines for authors.

SS BLANCETT

References and Bibliography

No reference book would be complete without providing an opportunity for the reader to explore further specific information that would be helpful in both personal and professional development. This book could not possibly respond to all of the issues that could confront the manager at any given time. Further, the format of responses in this book does not permit extensive exploration of any one topic or issue.

The purpose of this extensive bibliography and reference list of current literature is to permit the manager to find and access other reading that relates to the growing number of issues of management in a changing leadership environment. Every effort has been made to select the most current and helpful resources from a number of disciplines reflecting the broad range of current management topics. It is hoped that the reader will use these resources when her own problem solving draws her to seek additional sources for reflection and planning.

Aguayo, R. (1990). *Dr. Demming.* New York: Lyle Stuart.

Albert, M. (1993). *Capitalism vs. capitalism: How America's obsession with individual achievement and short term profit has led it to the brink of collapse.* New York: Four Walls Eight Windows Press.

Allen, D., Calkin, J., & Marlis, P. (1988). Making shared governance work. *Journal of Nursing Administration, 18*(1), 37-43.

Altman, S. (1990, April). Health care in the nineties: No more of the same. *Hospitals, 64.*

American Medical Association. *Manual of style.* (8th ed.) (1989). Baltimore: Williams & Wilkins.

American Nurses Association. (1980). *Nursing. A social policy statement.* Kansas City: Author.

American Nurses Association. (1985). *Code for nurses with interpretive statements.* Kansas City: Author.

American Nurses Association. (1988). *Peer review guidelines.* Kansas City: Author.

American Nurses Association. (1989, September). Misuse of RN's spurs shortage. *American Journal of Nursing,* pp. 1223, 1231.

American Nurses Association. (1991a). *Clinical standards of nursing practice.* Kansas City: Author.

American Nurses Association. (1991b). *Nursing's agenda for health care reform.* Washington, DC: Author.

American Psychological Association. (3rd ed.) (1991). *Publication manual of the American Psychological Association.* Washington, DC: Author.

Anderson, D., & Poe, R. (1992). A culture of achievement. *39*(5), 35-39.

Anderson, H. (1992). Hospitals seek new ways to integrate health care. *Hospitals, 66*(7), 26-36.

Anderson, R. (1993). Nursing leadership and healthcare reform. *Journal of Nursing Administration, 23*(12), 8-9.

Argyris, C. (1993). *Knowledge for action.* San Francisco: Jossey-Bass.

Arnold, W. (1993, March). The leader's role in implementing quality improvement: Walking the talk. *Quality Review Bulletin,* pp. 79-82.

Arnold, W., & Plas, J. (1993). *The human touch.* New York: John Wiley & Sons.

Artinian, B. (1991). The development of the intersystem model. *Journal of Advanced Nursing (GB), 16,* 194-205.

Ashley, J.A. (1976). *Hospitals, paternalism, and the role of the nurse.* New York: Teachers College Press.

Atchison, T. (1990). *Turning health care leadership around: Cultivating, inspiring, empowered, and loyal followers.* San Francisco: Jossey-Bass.

Atkinson, P. (1990). *Creating culture change: The key to successful total quality management.* San Diego: Pfeiffer & Co.

Attali, J. (1991). *Millenium: Winners and losers in the coming world order.* New York: Times Books.

Baggs, J., & Ryan, S. (1990). ICU nurse physician collaboration and nursing satisfaction. *Nursing Economic$, 8*(6), 386-392.

Barbara, B. (1991). Shortage as shorthand for the crisis in caring. *Nursing & Health Care, 13*(9), 480-483.

Barger, S., & Rosenfeld, P. (1993). Models in community health: Findings from a national study of community nursing centers. *Nursing & Health Care, 14*(8), 426-429.

Barrentine, P., et al. (1993). *When the canary stops singing: Women's perspectives on transforming business.* San Francisco: Berrett-Koehler.

Beatty, J. (1990, February). A post cold war budget. *The Atlantic Monthly,* pp. 74-82.

Beck, M. (1990, May 14). Not enough for all: The Oregon experiment with rationing. *Time,* pp. 53-55.

Beck, M., et al. (1993, April 5). Doctors under the knife. *Newsweek,* pp. 28-40.

Beckham, D. (1993). The longest wave—Fad surfing. *Healthcare Forum Journal, 36*(6), 78-82.

Beckhard, R., & Pritchard, W. (1992). *Changing the essence: The art of creating and leading fundamental change in organizations.* San Francisco: Jossey-Bass.

Beecroft, P. (1988). A contractual model for the department of nursing. *Journal of Nursing Administration, 18*(9), 20-24.

Belcher, J.G. (1991). *Gain sharing.* Houston: Gulf Publishing.

Bell, E. & Bart, B. (1991, March-April). Pay for performance: Motivating the chief nurse executive. *Nursing Economic$. 9*(20), 92.

Belli, P. (1991). Globalizing the rest of the world. *Harvard Business Review, 69*(4), 50-55.

Bennett, A. (1990, November 12). Making the grade with the customer. *The Wall Street Journal,* p. 1.

Bennis, W. (1989a). *On becoming a leader.* Reading, MA: Addison Wesley.

Bennis, W. (1989b). *Why leaders can't lead.* San Francisco, CA: Jossey-Bass.

Bennis, W. (1993). *Beyond bureaucracy.* San Francisco: Jossey-Bass.

Bentov, I. (1988). *Stalking the wild pendulum.* Rochester, Vt.: Destiny Books.

Bergquist, W. (1993b). *The postmodern organization: Mastering the art of irreversible change.* San Francisco: Jossey-Bass.

Berman, M. (1989). *The reenchantment of the world.* New York: Bantam Books.

Berstein, A. (1990). *Grounded: Frank Lorenzo and the destruction of Eastern Air Lines.* New York: General Publishers.

Berwich, D., Godfrey, B.A., & Roessner, J. (1990). *Curing health care: New strategies for quality improvement. A report on the National Demonstration Project on Quality Improvement in Health Care.* San Francisco: Jossey-Bass.

Berwick, D., Blanton, G., & Roessner, J. (1990). *Curing health care: New strategies for quality improvement.* San Francisco: Jossey-Bass.

Bing, S. (1992). *Crazy bosses.* New York: William Morrow.

Blanchard, K. & Peale, N.V. (1988). *The power of ethical management,* New York: Fawcett Crest.

Blegan, M., Gardner, D., & McCloskey, J. (1992). Who helps you with your work. *American Journal of Nursing, 92*(1), 26-31.

Block, P. (1991). *The empowered manager.* San Francisco: Jossey-Bass.

Block, P. (1993). *Stewardship: Choosing service over self interest.* San Francisco: Berrett-Koehler.

Bluestone, B., & Bluestone, I. (1993). *Negotiating the future: A labor perspective on American business.* New York: Basic Books.

Bogdanich, W. (1991). *The great white lie: How America's hospitals betray our trust and endanger our lives.* New York: Simon & Schuster.

Bok, D. (1993). *The cost of talent.* New York: The Free Press.

Bolman, L., & Terrance, D. (1991). *Reframing organizations.* San Francisco: Jossey-Bass.

Bower, K.A. (1992). *Case management by nurses.* Washington, DC: American Nurses Publishing.

Brider, P. (1992, September). The move to patient-focused care. *American Journal of Nursing,* pp. 26-33.

Brodbeck, K. (1992). Professional practice actualized through an integrated shared governance and quality assurance model. *Journal of Nursing Care Quality, 6*(2), 20-31.

Brown, K.C. (1991). Strategies for effective communication. *American Association of Occupational Health Nursing Journal, 39*(6), 292-293.

Brown, K.C. (1990). Written communication: A key management skill. *American Association of Occupational Health Nursing Journal, 38*(9), 455-456.

Brown, L. (1991). Crime and management. *Harvard Business Review, 69*(3), 111-126.

Brown, M., & McCool, B. (1990). Health care systems: Predictions for the future. *Health Care Management Review, 15*(3), 87-94.

Bunkers, S. (1992). The healing web, Part I: *Nursing & Health Care, 13*(2), 68-73.

Burda, D. (1990, April 23). A simmering perception of inequality. *Modern Healthcare,* pp. 30-31.

Burda, D. (1991). Learn from fallen leaders: Don't neglect your constituency. *Modern Healthcare, 21*(4), 24.

Buresh, B., Gordon, S., & Bell, N. (1991). Who counts in news coverage of health care? *American Journal of Nursing, 39*(3), 204-208.

Byham, W. (1991). *Zapp! The lightning of empowerment.* New York: Harmony Books.

Byrne, J. (1993, December 20). The horizontal corporation. *Business Week, 3351,* 76-81.

Byrne, J., Brandt, R., & Port, O. (1993, February 8). The virtual corporation. *Business Week,* pp. 98-103.

Cairncross, F. (1992). *Costing the Earth.* Boston: Harvard Business School Press.

Calder, K. (1991). Quality improvement: A new approach to quality assurance. *Alberta Association of Registered Nurses Newsletter, 47*(5), 10-12.

Califano, J. (1993). The nurse as a revolutionary. *Revolution: The Journal of Nurse Empowerment, 3*(3), 67-68, 108-110.

Calleo, D. (1992). *The bankrupting of America.* New York: William Morrow.

Cantor, M. (1991). Family and community: Changing roles in an aging society. *The Gerontologist, 31*(3), 337-346.

Capuano, T.A., Fox, M.A., & Gresh, B. (1992). Staffing according to episodic census variations. *Nursing Management, 23*(10).

Castro, J. (1991). Condition: Critical. *Time, 138*(21), 34-42.

Cetron, M., & Davies, O. (1991). *Crystal globe: The haves and have-nots of the new world order.* New York: St. Martin's Press.

Chavigny, K. (1993). AMA's policies and nursing's role in emerging systems. *Nursing Management, 24*(12), 30-34.

Chicago manual of style (13th ed.). (1982). Chicago, IL: University of Chicago Press.

Choate, P. (1990, September-October). Political advantage: Japan's campaign for America. *Harvard Business Review,* pp. 87-103.

Choosing a clinical information system. (1990). Hewlett-Packard.

Christopher, F., & Mandell, M. (1992, April 6). *Industrial policy. 3260,* 70-76.

Clark, R. (1991). What do you know? *Health Management Quarterly, 13*(4), 14-17.

Cleveland, H. (1993). *Birth of a new world.* San Francisco: Jossey-Bass.

Clifford, J.E. & Horvath, K.J. (1990a). *Advancing professional nursing practice: Innovations at Boston's Beth Israel Hospital.* New York: Springer.

Clifford, J.E. & Horvath, K.J. (1990b). Professionalizing a nursing service: An integrated approach for the management of patient care. In J. Clifford (Ed.). *Advancing professional nursing practice: Innovations at Boston's Beth Israel Hospital.* New York: Springer.

Coile, R. (1989). *The new medicine: Reshaping medical practice and health care management.* Rockville, Md.: Aspen.

Cole, J. (1992). From the heart. *Modern Health Care, 21*(4), 18-20.

Collier, T. (1990). The medical staff in the financially distressed hospital. *Topics in Health Care Finance, 17*(2), 26-38.

Conrad, D. (1993). Coordinating patient care services in regional health systems: The challenge of clinical integration. *Hospitals & Health Services Administration, 38*(4), 491-508.

Cox, H. (1987, November). Verbal abuse in nursing: Report of a study. *Nursing Management, 18*(11), 47-50.

Cox, H. (1991a). Verbal abuse in nursing: Report of a study. *Nursing Management, 22*(2), 47-50.

Cox, H. (1991b). Verbal abuse nationwide, Part II: Impact and modifications. *Nursing Management, 22*(3), 66-69.

Cox, T. Jr. (1993). *Cultural diversity in organizations.* San Francisco: Berrett-Koehler.

Crosby, P.B. (1990). *Leading: The art of becoming an executive.* New York: McGraw Hill.

Culbert, S., & McDonough, J. (1985). *Radical management.* New York: The Free Press.

Cummings, S., & O'Malley, J. (1993). Designing outcome models for patient-focused care. *Seminars for Nurse Managers, 1*(1), 16-21.

Curtin, L. (1991). Moving toward unity. *Nursing Management, 22*(8), 7-8.

Curtin, L. & Flaherty, J.M. (1982). *Nursing ethics: Theories and pragmatics.* Bowie, MD: Robert J. Brady Company.

Cushing, M. (1988). *Nursing jurisprudence.* Norwalk, CT: Appleton & Lange.

Daigh, R. (1991). Financial implications of a quality improvement process. *Topics in Health Care Finance, 17*(3), 42-52.

Davenport, T. (1993). *Process innovation.* Boston: Harvard Business School Press.

Davidow, W., & Malone, M. (1993). *The virtual corporation.* New York: Times Warner Books.

Dawson, R. (1993). *The confident decision maker.* New York: William Morrow.

Deal, T.E. & Kennedy, A.A. (1982). *Corporate cultures.* Reading, MA: Addison-Wesley.

DeBaca, V., Jones, K., & Tornbeni, J. (1993, July/August). A cost-benefit analysis of shared governance. *Journal of Nursing Administration, 23,* 50-57.

del Bueno, D. (1990). Evaluation: Myths, mystiques, and obsessions. *Journal of Nursing Administration, 20*(11), 4-7.

del Bueno, D. (1991). Rational irrationality: An organizational alternative. *Journal of Nursing Administration, 21*(1), 7, 24.

del Bueno, D. (1993). Visions, hallucinations, and wannabes. *Journal of Nursing Administration, 23*(12), 10-11, 48.

Deming, W.E. (1990). *Total quality management.* New York: Warner Books.

DePree, M. (1989). *Leadership is an art.* New York: Dell.

Dienemann, J., & Gessner, T. (1992). Restructuring nursing care delivery systems. *Nursing Administration Quarterly, 10*(4), 253-256.

Diers, D. (1993). Advanced practice. *Health Management Quarterly, 15*(2), 16-20.

Dobyns, L., & Crawford-Mason, C. (1991). *Quality or else: The revolution in world business.* New York: Houghton Mifflin.

Donker, R., & Ogilvy, J. (1993). The iron triangle and the chrome pentagon. *Healthcare Forum Journal, 36*(6), 72-77.

Dougherty, C. (1992, January/February). The excesses of individualism. *Health Progress,* pp. 22-28.

Driver, M., Brouseau, K., & Hunsaker, P. (1993). *The dynamic decision maker.* San Francisco: Jossey-Bass.

Drucker, P. (1985). The discipline of innovation. *Harvard Business Review, 43*(3), 43-53.

Drucker, P. (1989). *The new realities.* New York: Harper & Row.

Drucker, P. (1991). The new productivity challenge. *Harvard Business Review, 69*(6), 69-79,

Drucker, P. (1992a). *Managing for the future: The 1990's and beyond.* New York: Truman Tally Books/Dutton.

Drucker, P. (1992b, September/October). The new society of organizations. *Harvard Business Review,* pp. 95-104.

Drucker, P. (1993). *Post-capitalist society.* New York: Harper-Collins.

Duck, J. (1993). Managing change: The art of balancing. *Harvard Business Review, 71*(6), 109-118.

Dumaine, B. (1990, May 7). Who needs a boss? *Fortune,* 52-60.

Dumaine, B. (1991). Closing the innovation gap. *Fortune, 124*(13), 56-62.

Dumaine, B. (1993). The new non-manager managers. *Fortune, 127*(4), 80-84.

Dunham, J., & Klafehn, K. (1990). Transformational leadership and the nurse executive. *Journal of Nursing Administration, 20*(4), 28-33.

Dupuis, P., & Connington, M.E. (1990). *Unit based nursing quality assurance.* Rockville, Md.: Aspen.

Dwyer, D., Schwartz, R., & Fox, M. (1992). Decisionmaking autonomy in nursing. *Journal of Nursing Administration, 22*(2), 17-21.

Easterbrook, G. (1993, September 6). The national health care phobia. *Newsweek,* pp. 22-25.

Eckhart, J. (1993). Costing out nursing service: Examining the research. *Nursing Economic$, 11* (2), 91-98.

Ehrenreich, B. (1990, October 15). The warrior culture. *Time,* p. 100.

Eisner, R. (1993). Sense and nonsense about budget deficits. *Harvard Business Review, 71*(3), 99-111.

Elliott, E. (1989). The discourse of nursing: A case of silencing. *Nursing & Health Care, 10*(10), 539-543.

Elpern, E., Yellen, S., & Burton, A. (1992). Patient self determination: Sharing the power. *Hospitals, 66*(6), 96.

Estaugh, S. (1990). Hospital nursing technical efficiency: Nurse extenders and enhanced productivity. *Hospital & Health Services Administration, 35*(4), 561-573.

Ethridge, P. & Rusch, S.C. (1989). The professional nurse/case manager in changing organizational structures. *Changing Organizational Structures, Series on Nursing Administration* (Vol 2). Redwood City, CA: Addison-Wesley.

Ethridge, P. (1991). A nursing HMO: Carondelet St. Mary's experience. *Nursing Management, 22*(7), 22-27.

Etzioni, A. (1991). *A responsive society: Collected essays on guiding deliberate social change.* San Francisco: Jossey-Bass.

Etzioni, A. (1993). *The spirit of community.* New York: Crown.

Evans, H. (1989, February 19). Old birth idea reborn in the Bronx. *New York Daily News,* pp. 7, 44.

Fagin, C. (1990, October). Nursing's value proves itself. *American Journal of Nursing,* pp. 17-30.

Fagin, C. (1992). Collaboration between nurses and physicians: No longer a choice. *Nursing & Health Care, 13*(7), 354-363.

Faludi, S. (1991). *Backlash: The undeclared war against American women.* New York: Crown Publishers.

Farnham, A. (1989, December 4). The trust gap. *Fortune,* pp. 56-78.

Farrell, C., & Mandel, M. (1992, April 6). Industrial policy. *3260,* 70-76.

Farren, E. (1991). Effects of early discharge planning on length of hospital stay. *Nursing Economic$, 9*(1), 25-30.

Feutz-Harter, S. (1989). *Nursing and the law.* Eau Claire, WI: Professional Education Systems.

Filipczak, B. (1993). *Unions in the 90's: Cooperation or capitulation. Training, 23*(5), 25-34.

Findley, S. (1993). How new alliances are changing health care. *Business & Health, 11*(12), 28-36.

Finkler, S. (1991). Performance budgeting. *Nursing Economic$, 9*(6), 401-408.

Finkler, S. & Korner, C. (1993). *Financial management for nurse managers and executives.* Philadelphia: W.B. Saunders.

Finnegan, S. (1993, August). When patient classification systems fail. *Aspen's Advisor for Nurse Executives 8*(11), 1-3.

Flarey, D. (1990). A methodology for costing nursing service. *Nursing Administration Quarterly, 14*(3), 41-51.

Flarey, D. (1991). The nurse executive and the governing body. *Journal of Nursing Administration, 21*(12), 11-17.

Flarey, D. (1993). Quality improvement through data analysis. *Journal of Nursing Administration, 23*(12), 21-30.

Flowers, J. (1993). Getting paid to keep people healthy. *Healthcare Forum Journal, 36*(2), 51-54.

Flynn, A.M., & Kilgallen, M.E. (1993). Case management: A multidisciplinary approach to the evaluation of cost and quality standards. *Journal of Nursing Care Quality, 8*(1), 58-66.

Food and Nutrition Program. (1990). *A study of the outcomes of nutritional programs on the cost of later medicaid outlays.* US Department of Agriculture.

Forsey, L., Cleland, V., & Miller, B. (1993). Job descriptions for differentiated nursing practice and differentiated pay. *Journal of Nursing Administration, 23*(5), 33-39.

Freedman, D. (1992). Is management still a science? *Harvard Business Review, 70*(6), 26-38.

Freeman, S. (1990). *Managing lives: Corporate women and social change.* Boston: University of Massachusetts.

French, T. (1993). *South of heaven: Welcome to high school at the end of the twentieth century.* New York: Doubleday.

Friedman, E. (1991, April 5). Health care's changing face: The demographics of the 21st century. *Hospitals,* pp. 36-40.

Fries, J. (1993). Reducing need and demand. *Healthcare Forum Journal, 36*(6), 18-23.

Frohman, A., & Johnson, L. (1992). *The middle management challenge: Moving from crisis to empowerment.* New York: McGraw-Hill.

Frombrum, C. (1992). *Turning points: Creating strategic change in corporations.* New York: McGraw-Hill.

Fuchs, V., & Hahn, J. (1990, September 27). How does Canada do it? *New England Journal of Medicine, 323,* 884-890.

Fukuyama, F. (1991). *The end of history and the last man.* New York: The Free Press.

Gabor, A. (1990). *The man who discovered quality.* New York: Time Books.

Galbraith, J., & Lawler, E. III (1993). *Organizing for the future.* San Francisco: Jossey-Bass.

Gardner, D., et al. (1991). Nursing administration model for administrative practice. *Journal of Nursing Administration, 21*(3), 37-41.

Garvin, D. (1993). Building a learning organization. *Harvard Business Review, 71*(3), 78-91.

Geoghegan, T. (1991). *Which side are you on?* New York: Farrar, Straus, & Giroux.

Gerlach, M. (1993). *Alliance capitalism: The social organization of Japanese business.* San Francisco: University of California Press.

Gibb, J. (1991). *Trust.* North Hollywood: Newcastle Publishing.

Gibbs, N. (1990, October 8). Shameful bequests to the next generation. *Time,* pp. 42-46.

Gibbs, N., et al. (1990). Women: The road ahead. *Time (Special Issue), 136*(19), 10-82.

Gilbraith, J., et al. (1993). *Organizing for the future.* San Francisco: Jossey-Bass.

Gilbreath, R. (1993). *Escape from management hell.* San Francisco: Berrett-Koehler.

Gilkey R, Greenbaugh L. (1984, August). Developing effective negotiating approaches among professional women in organizations. Paper presented at the Third Annual Conference on Women and Organizations, Simmons College.

Gilligan C. (1979). Women's place in man's life cycle. *Harvard Education Review, 49*(4):431-446.

Gilmore, T. (1990). Effective leadership during organizational transitions. *Nursing Economic$, 8*(3), 135-141.

Ginzberg, E. (1990). A non conforming view. *Health Management Quarterly,* (Third Quarter), pp. 20-22.

Glass, R.M. (1992). New information for authors and readers: Group authorship, acknowledgments, and rejected manuscripts. *Journal of the American Medical Association, 268*(1), 99.

Goldsmith, J. (1989, May/June). A radical prescription for hospitals. *Harvard Business Review,* pp. 104-111.

Goldsmith, J. (1993). Driving the nitroglycerin truck: The relationship between the hospital and physician. *The Healthcare Forum Journal, 36*(2), 36-40.

Goodroe, J., & Beres, M. (1991). Network leadership and today's nurse. *Nursing Management, 22*(6), 56-62.

Gordon, S. (1991). *Prisoners of men's dreams.* Boston: Little, Brown.

Gordon, S. (1993). Healthcare reform: How the system works against nurses. *Revolution: The Journal of Nurse Empowerment, 3*(3), 12-16.

Goss, T., Pascale, R., & Athos, A. (1993). The reinvention roller coaster: Risking the present for a powerful future. *Harvard Business Review, 71*(6), 97-108.

Gould, J., DiBella, A., & Nevis, E. (1993). Organizations as learning systems. *The Systems Thinker, 4*(8), 1-3.

Gould, W. (1993). *Agenda for reform: The future of employment relationships and the law.* Boston: MIT Press.

Grace, H. (1990). Can health care costs be contained? *Nursing & Health Care, 11*(3), 125-130.

Graham, N. (1990). *Quality assurance in hospitals.* Rockville, Md.: Aspen.

Greene, J. (1991, April). System pioneers economic credentialing. *Modern Healthcare,* p. 29.

Griffith, H., Thomas, N., & Griffith, L. (1991). MDs bill for these routine nursing tasks. *American Journal of Nursing, 91*(1), 22-27.

Grimaldi, P. (1990a). Model medicare physician fee schedule. *Nursing Management, 21*(11), 26-27.

Grimaldi, P. (1990b). Will new fee system slash physician payments? *Nursing Management, 21*(8), 22-23.

Grunwald, H. (1990, October 15). The second century. *Time,* 70-75.

Gunden, E., & Crissman, S. (1992). Leadership skills for empowerment. *Nursing Administration Quarterly, 16*(3), 6-10.

Haddon, R. (1989). The final frontier: Nursing in the emerging healthcare environment. *Nursing Economic$, 7*(3), 155-161.

Haddon, R. (1990). An economic agenda for health care. *Nursing & Health Care, 11*(1), 21-26.

Hagland, M. (1991). The RBVS and hospitals: The physician payment revolution on our doorstep. *Hospitals, 65*(4), 24-31.

Halberstam, D. (1991). *The next century.* New York: William Morrow.

Hall, B. (1993). Time to nurse: Musings of an aging nurse radical. *Nursing Outlook, 41*(6), 250-252.

Hall, G., Rosenthal, J., & Wade, J. (1993). How to make engineering *really* work. *Harvard Business Review, 71*(6), 119-133.

Halle, M.J. & Blatchley, M. (1987). *Introduction to leadership & management in nursing.* Boston: Jones & Bartlett.

Hames, D. (1991). Productivity enhancing work innovations: Remedies for what ails hospitals? *Hospitals & Health Services Administration, 36*(4), 545-558.

Hammer, M., & Champy, J. (1993). *Reengineering the corporation: A manifesto for business revolution.* New York: Harper Business Books.

Handy, C. (1989). *The age of unreason.* Boston: Harvard Business School Press.

Handy, C. (1992). Balancing corporate power: A new federalist paper. *Harvard Business Review, 70*(6), 59-72.

Harris, G. (1993). The post capitalist executive: An interview with Peter Drucker. *Harvard Business Review, 71*(3), 115-122.

Harris, M. (1991). Clinical and financial outcomes in patient care in a home health agency. *Journal of Nursing Quality Assurance, 5*(2), 41-49.

Hawken, P. (1992). *The ecology of commerce.* New York: Harper/Collins.

Hawken, P. (1993). *Our future and the making of things.* New York: Harper/Collins.

Hawking, S. (1988). *A brief history of time.* London: Bantam.

Hawley, J. (1993). *Reawakening the spirit in work.* San Francisco: Berrett-Koehler.

Health Care Expert Systems. (1993). Patient care expert system. A computer-based resource for clinical nursing information and full documentation and charting at point of care. *Computers in Nursing, 11*(3), 146.

Healthweek outlook. (1990, July 30). *Healthweek,* pp. 42-63.

Heider, J. (1986). *The Tao of leadership.* New York: Bantam.

Hein, E. & Nicholson, M.J. (1993). *Contemporary leadership behavior: Selected readings* (4th ed.). Philadelphia, PA: J.B. Lippincott.

Helgesen, S. (1990). *The female advantage: Women's ways of leadership.* New York: Doubleday/Currency.

Henderson, D. (1993). *The fortune encyclopedia of economics.* New York: Warner.

Hendrickson, G. & Kovner, C. (1990). Effects of computers on nursing resource use: Do computers save time? *Computers in Nursing, 8*(1), 16-22.

Henry, B. (1990). Nightingale's perspective of nursing administration. *Nursing and Health Care, 11*(4), 201-209.

Hepner, J. (1990). Physicians unions: Any doctor can join, but who can bargain collectively? *Hospitals & Health Services Administration, 35*(3), 327-340.

Herrick, N. (1990). *Joint management and employee participation: Labor and management at the crossroad.* San Francisco: Jossey-Bass.

Herron, D., & Herron, L. (1991). Entrepreneurial nursing as a conceptual basis for in-hospital nursing practice models. *Nursing Economic$, 9*(5), 310-316.

Hersey, P. (1983). *One minute manager* [video]. Escondido, CA: Blanchard Training and Development.

Hersey, P., & Blanchard, K. (1989). *Management of organizational behavior* (6th ed.). Englewood Cliffs, NJ: Prentice-Hall.

Hersey, P. & Duldt, B. (1989). *Situational leadership in nursing.* Norwalk, CT: Appleton & Lange.

Herzlinger, R. (1991, August 8). Healthy competition. *The Atlantic Monthly,* pp. 69-81.

Hill, B. (1989). The McAuley experience with changing compensation within the context of a professional nursing practice culture. *Nursing Administration Quarterly, 14*(1), 78-82.

Hoelzel, C. (1989). Using structural power sources to increase influence. *Journal of Nursing Administration, 19*(11), 10-15.

Hoerr, J. (1991). What should unions do? *Harvard Business Review, 69*(3), 30-45.

How real is America's decline? (1992). *Harvard Business Review, 70*(5), 162-174.

Howard, R. (1993). *The learning imperative.* Boston: Harvard Business School Press.

Huckabay, M.D.L. (1991). The role of conceptual frameworks in nursing practice, administration, education and research. *Nursing Administration Quarterly, 15*(3), 17-28.

Hurley, R., Henikoff, L., Pyle, T., & Connell, S. (1993). Toward a seamless health care delivery system. *Frontiers of Health Service Management, 9*(4), 5-44.

International Committee of Medical Journal Editors (1988). Uniform requirements for manuscripts submitted to biomedical journals. *Annals of Internal Medicine 108,* 258-265.

Iyer, P. (1991, January). New trends in charting. *Nursing '91,* pp. 48-50.

Jacobs, M. (1991). *Short term America: The causes and cures of our business myopia.* Cambridge, Mass.: Harvard University Press.

Jamieson, D., & O'Mara, J. (1991). *Managing workforce 2000.* San Francisco: Jossey-Bass.

Jelinek, M., & Schoonhovan, C. (1993). *The innovation marathon.* San Francisco: Jossey-Bass.

Jellison, J. (1993). *Overcoming resistance.* New York: Simon & Schuster.

Jenkins, J. (1991). Professional governance: The missing link. *Nursing Management, 22*(8), 26-30.

Jennings, M., & Porter, M. (1991). The changing elderly market. *Topics in Health Care Financing, 17*(4), 1-8.

Johnson, R. (1992). The entrepreneurial physician. *Health Care Management Review, 17*(1), 73-79.

Johnsson, J. (1991). Collaboration: Hospitals find that working together is tough, rewarding and vital. *Hospitals, 65*(23), 24-31.

Joint Commission on Accreditation of Healthcare Organizations. (1991a). Medical staff. *Accreditation Manual for Hospitals,* pp. 99-119.

Joint Commission on Accreditation of Healthcare Organizations. (1991b). Nursing care. *Accreditation Manual for Hospitals,* pp. 131-221.

Joint Commission on Accreditation of Healthcare Organizations (1991c). *Quality improvement in health care.* Oakbrook Terrace, IL: Author.

Joint Commission on Accreditation of Healthcare Organizations. (1992). *Accreditation manual for hospitals.* Oakbrook Terrace, IL: Author.

Jones, C. (1992). Calculating and updating nursing turnover costs. *Nursing Economic$, 10*(1), 39-45.

Jones, C., et al. (1993). Shared governance and the nursing practice environment. *Nursing Economic$, 11*(4), 209-213.

Jones, C.B. (1990). Staff turnover costs. *Journal of Nursing Administration, 20*(4), 18-21.

Jones, L. (1990, July 5). Hospitals and preventive care: A good match? *Hospitals,* 42-48.

Jones, L., & Ortiz, M. (1989). Increasing nursing autonomy and recognition through shared governance. *Nursing Administration Quarterly, 13*(4), 11-16.

Jones, M.A. et al. (1990). A paradigm for effective resolution of interpersonal conflict. *Nursing Management, 21*(2), 64.

Jonsen, A. (1993). Fear of rationing. *Health Management Quarterly, 14*(2), 6-9.

Kaiser, L. (1988). The visionary manager. In T. Wilson (Ed.), *Emerging issues in health care* (pp. 99-104). Englewood, Colo.: Estes Park Institute.

Kalisch, B., & Kalisch, P. (1988). An analysis of the sources of physician-nurse conflict. In J. Muff (Ed.), *Women's issues in nursing.* Prospect Heights, Ill.: Waveland Press.

Kanter RM. 1977. *Men and women of the corporation.* New York: Basic Books.

Kanter, R.M. (1989). *When giants learn to dance.* New York: Simon & Schuster.

Katzenbach, J., & Smith, D. (1993). *The wisdom of teams.* Boston: McKinsey & Company.

Katzman, E., Holman, E., & Ashley, J. (1993). A nurse managed center's client satisfaction survey. *Nursing & Health Care, 14*(8), 414-419.

Kazemek, E. (1990, August 13). Employee involvement plan needs executive involvement. *Modern Healthcare,* p. 33.

Kenkel, P. (1990, October 15). Direct contracting: A recipe for success. *Modern Healthcare,* pp. 24-31.

Kenkel, P. (1991). DRG study shows disparity among hospitals. *Modern Healthcare, 21*(4), 34.

Kennedy, C.W., Camden, C.T., & Timmerman, G.M. (1990). Relationships among perceived supervisor communication, nurse morale and sociocultural variables. *Nursing Administration Quarterly, 14*(5), 224-226.

Kennedy, P. (1991). *Preparing for the twenty-first century.* New York: Random House.

Kerr, M., Rudy, E., & Daly, B. (1991). Human response patterns to outcomes in the critically ill patient. *Journal of Nursing Quality Assurance, 5*(2), 32-40.

Kets de Vries, M. (1993). *Leaders, fools, and imposters.* San Francisco: Jossey-Bass.

Kets de Vries, M., & Miller, D. (1984). *The neurotic organization.* San Francisco: Jossey-Bass.

Kiechel, W. (1992). The leader as servant. *Fortune, 125*(9), 121-122.

Kilmann, R. (1991). *Managing beyond the quick fix.* San Francisco: Jossey-Bass.

Kimball, M. (1991). Health spending pegged for 12%-15% growth thru '95. *HealthWeek, 5*(1), 1-34.

King, R. (1990, December). Participative management and employee committees—options and restrictions under the National Labor Relations Act. *Society for Human Resource Management,* pp. 5-8.

Kinzer, D. (1990). Twelve laws of hospital interaction. *Health Care Management Review, 15*(2), 15-19.

Koerner, J. (1993). Work redesign: A journey, not a destination. In K. McDonagh (Ed.), *Patient centered hospital care.* Chicago: American Healthcare Publishers.

Koerner, J., & Bunkers, S. (1992). Transformational leadership: The power of myth. *Nursing Administration Quarterly, 17*(1), 10-16.

Koestenbaum, P. (1991). *Leadership: The inner side of greatness.* San Francisco: Jossey-Bass.

Kofman, F., & Senge, P. (1993). Communities of commitment: The heart of the learning organization. *Organizational Dynamics, 22*(2), 5-23.

Kohn, A. (1993). *Punished by rewards.* New York: Houghton Mifflin.

Koska, M. (1990, November 5). Patient centered care: Can your hospital afford to have it? *Hospitals,* pp. 48-52.

Koska, M.T. (1989). Quality—thy name is nursing care, CEOs say. *Hospitals, 63*(3), 32.

Kotlikoff, L. (1992). *Generational accounting: Knowing who pays, and when, for what we spend.* New York: The Free Press.

Kotter, J., & Heskett, J. (1992). *Corporate culture and performance.* New York: The Free Press.

Kouzes, J., & Posner, B. (1993). *Credibility.* San Francisco: Jossey-Bass.

Kovner, A. (1991). The case of the unhealthy hospital. *Harvard Business Review, 69*(5), 12-26.

Krackhardt, D., & Hanson, J. (1993). Informal networks: The company behind the chart. *Harvard Business Review, 71*(3), 104-111.

Kramer, M. (1990). The magnet hospitals: Excellence revisited. *Journal of Nursing Administration, 20*(9), 35-44.

Kuttner, R. (1991). *The end of laissez-faire: National purpose and the global economy after the cold war.* New York: Knopf Publishers.

Labovitz, G. (1991). Beyond the total quality management mystique. *Healthcare Executive, 6*(2), 15-17.

Lamm, R. (1990). *The brave new world of health care.* Denver: University of Denver.

Lamm, R. (1991). A thousand flowers. *Health Management Quarterly, 13*(1), 7-10.

Laney, J. (1990, November). Ethics in health care: What do we have to do? What Should We Do? *Journal of the Medical Association of Georgia, 79,* 829-833.

Langeler, G. (1992). The vision trap. *Harvard Business Review, 70*(2), 46-55.

Larson, J., et al. (1992). The healing web, Part II. *Nursing & Health Care, 13*(5).

Lawler, E. III. (1986). *High involvement management.* San Francisco: Jossey-Bass.

Lawler, E. III. (1993). *The ultimate advantage: Creating the high-involvement organization.* San Francisco: Jossey-Bass.

Lawler, E. III, Mohrman, S., & Ledford, G. (1992). *Employee involvement and total quality management.* San Francisco: Jossey-Bass.

Lebov, W. (1988). *Service excellence: The customer relations strategy for health care.* Chicago, IL: American Hospital Association.

Leddy, S., & Pepper, M. (1991). *Conceptual basis of professional nursing* (2nd ed.). New York: J.B. Lippincott.

Leebov, W., & Scott, G. (1990). *Health care managers in transition: Shifting roles and changing organizations.* San Francisco: Jossey-Bass.

Levering, R. (1991). *Great place to work.* New York: Random House.

Levitt, T. (1990). The thinking manager. *Health Management Quarterly, 12*(2), 6-9.

Lewis, M. (1992). *Pacific rift.* New York: W.W. Norton.

Limerick, D., & Cunningham, B. (1993). *Managing the new organization.* San Francisco: Jossey-Bass.

Lindin, W., & Lindin, K. (1993). *The healing manager.* San Francisco: Berrett-Koehler.

Lipscomb, J.A. & Lone, C.C. (1992). Violence toward health care workers: An emerging occupational hazard. *American Association of Occupational Health Nursing Journal, 40*(5), 224-226.

Longest, B. (1990). Interorganizational linkages in the health sector. *Health Care Management Review, 15*(1), 17-28.

Lovell, M. (1988). Daddy's little girl: The lethal effects of paternalism in nursing. In J. Muff (Ed.), *Women's issues in nursing.* Prospect Heights, Ill.: Waveland Press.

Lowery, S. (1992). Qualification for the successful case manager. *The Case Manager, 3*(4), 66-72.

Ludden, J. (1993). Doctors as employees. *Health Management Quarterly, 15*(1), 7-11.

Ludemann, R., & Brown, C. (1989). Staff perceptions of shared governance. *Nursing Administration Quarterly, 13*(4), 47-56.

Lundin, W., & Lundin, K. (1993). *The healing manager.* San Francisco: Berrett-Koehler.

Lutz, S. (1990). *Hospitals stretch their creativity to motivate workers.* 20-33.

Lutz, S. (1991). Practitioners are filling in for scarce physicians. *Modern Healthcare, 21*(19), 24-29.

Lynaught, J. (1993). Yesterday and tomorrow. *Health Management Quarterly, 15*(2), 2-6.

MacStravic, S. (1990). Warfare or partnership: Which way for health care? *Health Care Management Review, 15*(1), 37-45.

Magnet, M. (1992). The truth about the American worker. *Fortune, 125*(9), 48-65.

Malkemes, L. (1989). Challenging yesterday's ideas. *Journal of Nursing Administration, 19*(10), 4-5.

Manion, J. (1993). Chaos or transformation. *Journal of Nursing Administration, 23*(5), 41-48.

Manthey, M. (1989, February). Practice partnerships: The newest concept in care delivery. *Journal of Nursing Administration, 19*(2).

Manthey, M. (1991). Delivery systems and practice models: A dynamic balance. *Nursing Management, 22*(1), 28-30.

Maraldo, P. (1990a). The aftermath of DRGs: The politics of transformation. In J. McCloskey, & H. Grace (Ed.), *Current Issues in Nursing.* St. Louis: Mosby.

Maraldo, P. (1990b). The nineties: A decade in search of meaning. *Nursing and Health Care, 11*(1), 11-14.

Marquis, B. & Huston, C. (1987). *Management decision making for nurses,* Philadelphia: J.B. Lippincott.

Marshal, R., & Tucker, M. (1992). *Thinking for a living: Education and the wealth of nations.* New York: Basic Books.

Marszalek-Gaucher, E., & Coffey, R. (1990). *Transforming healthcare organizations: How to achieve and sustain organizational excellence.* San Francisco: Jossey-Bass.

Martin, D. (1990). The planetree model hospital project: An example of the patient as partner. *Hospital and Health Services Administration, 35*(4), 591-601.

Martin, F. (1992). *Motivating humans.* San Francisco: Jossey-Bass.

Mason, D., Backer, B., & Georges, A. (1991). Toward a feminist model for the political empowerment of nurses. *Image: Journal of Nursing Scholarship, 23*(2), 72-76.

Matey, D. (1991). Significance of transactional and transformational leadership theory on the hospital manager. *Hospital & Health Services Administration, 36*(4), 600-606.

Mathews, J., & Katel, P. (1992, September 7). The cost of quality. *Newsweek,* pp. 48-49.

May, T., & Spiers, J. (1991, March). What will lead to recovery. *Fortune,* (31), 32-39.

Maynard, H., & Mehrtens, S. (1993). *The fourth wave: Business in the 21st century.* San Francisco: Berrett-Koehler.

McDaniel, C., & Wolf, G. (1992). Transformational leadership in nursing service. *Journal of Nursing Administration, 22*(2), 60-64.

McCloskey, J. (1989). Implications of costing out nursing services for reimbursment. *Nursing Management, 20*(1), 49.

McConnell, C.R. (1989). Overcoming major barriers to true two-way communication with employees. *Health Care Supervisor, 7*(4), 77-82.

McCutcheon, S. (1992). A process for service transformation in the evolving health care field. *Topics in Health Care Finance, 18*(3), 21-27.

McDonagh, K. (1991). *Nursing shared governance.* Atlanta: KJ McDonagh Associates.

McGill, M., & Slocum, J. (1993). Unlearning the organization. *Organizational Dynamics, 22*(2), 67-79.

McNamee, M., & Garland, S. (1993). A guide to health reform. *US News & World Report, 115*(12), 28-33.

Meiglan, M. (1990). The most important characteristics of nursing leaders, *Nursing Administration Quarterly, 15*(1), 63-69.

Merry, M. (1991). Illusion vs. reality: TQM beyond the yellow brick road. *Healthcare Executive, 6*(2), 18-21.

Meyer, C. (1992). Bedside computer charting: Inching toward tomorrow. *92*(4), 38-45.

Mezirow, J. (1991a). *Fostering critical reflection in adulthood.* San Francisco: Jossey-Bass.

Mezirow, J. (1991b). *Transformative dimensions of adult learning.* San Francisco: Jossey-Bass.

Mick, S., et al. (1990). *Innovations in health care delivery: Insights for organizational theory.* San Francisco: Jossey-Bass.

Minerva-Melum, M. (1990, December 5). Total quality management: Steps to success. *Hospitals,* pp. 42-44.

Mink, O., et al. (1979). *Open organizations.* Austin, Tex.: Learning Concepts.

Minnen, T., et al. (1993). Sustaining work redesign innovations through shared governance. *Journal of Nursing Administration, 23,*(7, 8), 35-40.

Mintzberg, H. (1990a). The manager's job: Folklore and fact. *Harvard Business Review, 48*(2), 163-176.

Mintzberg, H. (1990b). *Mintzburg on management.* New York: The Free Press.

Mitchell, S. (1988). *Tao Te Ching.* New York: Harper & Row.

Mitroff, I., & Pearson, C. (1993). *Crisis management.* San Francisco: Jossey-Bass.

Mitty, E. (1991). The nurse as advocate. *Nursing & Health Care, 12*(10), 520-530.

Moeller, D., & Johnson, K. (1992). Shifting the paradigm for health care leadership. *Frontiers of Health Service Management, 8*(3), 28-30.

Moffit, K, et al. (1993). Patient focused care: Key principles in restructuring. *Hospitals & Health Services Administration, 38*(4), 509-522.

Montgomery, K. (1991). Response to AIDS: Large urban and small rural hospitals. *Hospital & Health Services Administration, 36*(4), 525-536.

Moore, J. (1993). Preditors and prey: A new ecology of competition. *Harvard Business Review, 71* (3), 75-86.

Morganthau, T., & Hager, M. (1993, October 4). The Clinton cure: Reinventing health care. *Newsweek,* pp. 36-43.

Morris, C. (1990). *The coming global boom.* New York: Bantam.

Morrison, A., White, R., & Van Velsor, E. (1992). *Breaking the glass ceiling.* New York: Addison-Wesley.

Morse, J., Bottorff, W., & Neader, S. (1991). Comparative analysis of conceptualizations and theories of caring. *Image: Journal of Nursing Scholarship, 23*(2), 119126.

Muff, J. (1988). *Women's issues in nursing: Socialization sexism and stereotyping* (1st ed.). Prospect Heights, Ill.: Waveland Press.

Myers, K. (1992, June). Games companies play and how to stop them. *Training,* pp. 68-70.

Naisbett, J. (1982). *Megatrends: Ten new directions transforming our lives.* New York: Warner Books.

Naisbitt, J., & Aburdene, P. (1985). *Re-inventing the corporation.* New York: Warner Books.

Naisbitt, J., & Aburdene, P. (1990). *Megatrends 2000.* New York: Warner Books.

Nanaka, I. (1991). The knowledge creating company. *Harvard Business Review, 69*(6), 96-104.

Nauert, R. (1992). Planning an alternative delivery system. *Topics in Health Care Financing, 18*(3), 64-71.

Neubauer, J. (1993). Redesign: Managing role changes and building a new team. *Seminars for Nurse Managers, 1*(1), 26-32.

Newman, M., Lamb, G., & Michaels, K. (1991). Nursing case management: The coming together of theory and practice. *Nursing & Health Care, 12*(8), 404-408.

Niagara Institute. (1987). *Labour-management relations: The search for a better way.* Toronto: Author.

Nielson, D. (1993). *Partnering with employees.* San Francisco: Jossey-Bass.

Niven, D. (1993). When times get tough, what happens to TQM. *Harvard Business Review, 71*(3), 20-34.

Noble, B. (1993). Reinventing labor. *Harvard Business Review, 71*(3), 115-120.

Noer, D. (1993). *Healing the wounds: Overcoming the trauma of layoffs and revitalizing downsized organizations.* San Francisco: Jossey-Bass.

O'Conner, S., & Lanning, J. (1992). The end of autonomy? Reflections of the postprofessional physician. *Healthcare Management Review, 17*(1), 63-72.

Ohmae, K. (1990). *The borderless world.* New York: Harper Business Books.

Ohmae, K. (1992). *Fact and friction: Kenichi Ohmae on US-Japan relations.* Tokyo: The Japanese Times, Ltd.

Ohmae, K. (1993). *The mind of the strategist.* New York: McGraw-Hill.

Olesen, E. (1993). *12 Steps to mastering the winds of change.* New York: Rawson Associates, MacMillan.

Olivas, G., et al. (1989). Case management: A bottom line care delivery model. *Journal of Nursing Administration, 19*(11-12), 16-20, 12-17.

Omachonu, V. (1990). Quality of care and the patient: New criteria for evaluation. *Health Care Management Review, 15*(4), 43-50.

Orth, C., Wilkinson, H., & Benfari, R. (1990). The manager's role as coach and mentor. *Journal of Nursing Administration, 20*(9), 11-15.

Palca, J. (1991, April 19). The sobering geography of AIDS. *Science, 252,* 372-373.

Parker, M.E. (Ed.) (1990). *Nursing theories in practice.* New York: National League for Nursing.

Parker, M.E. (Ed.) (1993). *Patterns of nursing theories in practice.* New York: National League for Nursing.

Parker, M.E., Gordon, S.C., & Brannon, P.T. (1992, April). Involving nursing staff in research: A non-traditional approach. *Journal of Nursing Administration, 22*(4), 58-63.

Parker, R.S. (1990). Nurse stories: The search for a relational ethic of care. *Advances in Nursing Science, 13*(1), 31-40.

Passau-Buck, S. (1988). Caring vs. curing: The politics of health care. In J. Huff (Ed.), *Women's issues in nursing.* Prospect Heights, Ill.: Waveland Press.

Patti, J., McDonagh, K., & Porter-O'Grady, T. (1990). Streetside support. *Health Progress, 71*(5), 60-62.

Pauchant, T., & Mitroff, I. (1992). *Transforming the crisis prone organization.* San Francisco: Jossey-Bass.

Pearce, J. (1988). *A crack in the cosmic egg.* New York: Julian Press.

Pelletier, K. (1993). Healthy people, healthy worksites. *Healthcare Forum Journal, 36*(6), 34-39.

Pence, T. & Cantrall, J. (1990). *Ethics in nursing: An anthology.* New York: National League for Nursing (Publication 20-2294; recommended chapters 3-6).

Perkins, J., Bennett, D., & Dorman, R. (1993). Why men choose nursing. *Nursing & Health Care, 14*(1), 34-38.

Perlman, D., & Takacs, G. (1990). The 10 stages of change. *Nursing Management, 21*(4), 33-38.

Perry, L. (1990, February 12). Gainsharing plans boost productivity. *Modern Healthcare,* p. 66.

Peters, T. (1987). *Thriving on chaos.* New York: Harper & Row.

Peters, T. (1992). *Liberation management.* New York: Harper & Row.

Peters, T. & Waterman, R. (1982). *In search of excellence.* New York: Harper & Row.

Peterson, K. (1990, October 1). Caring for people not profits, brings success. *Modern Healthcare,* 34.

Pine, J., Victor, B., & Boynton, A. (1993). Making mass customization work. *Harvard Business Review, 71*(5), 23-33.

Pinkerton, S.E., & Schroeder, P. (1988). *Commitment to excellence: Developing a professional nursing staff.* Rockville, Md.: Aspen.

Porter, M., & Witek, E. (1991). The nursing home industry: Past, present, and future. *Topics in Health Care Financing, 17*(4), 42-48.

Porter-O'Grady, T. (1991). Shared governance for nursing, Part II: Putting the organization into action. *AORN Journal, 53*(3), 694-703.

Porter-O'Grady, T. (1985). Credentialing, privileging, and nursing bylaws: Assuring accountability. *Journal of Nursing Administration, 15*(10), 30-36.

Porter-O'Grady, T. (1986). *Creative nursing administration: Participatory management into the 21st century.* Rockville, Md.: Aspen.

Porter-O'Grady, T. (1987). *Nursing finance.* Rockville, Md.: Aspen.

Porter-O'Grady, T. (1988). Restructuring the nursing organization for a consumer driven marketplace. *Nursing Administration Quarterly, 12*(3), 60-65.

Porter-O'Grady, T. (1989, March). Shared governance: Reality or sham. *American Journal of Nursing,* pp. 350-351.

Porter-O'Grady, T. (1990a). *Autonomy in nursing practice* (AHA # 154185). American Nurses Association, American Organization of Nurse Executives.

Porter-O'Grady, T. (1990b). Newer compensation practices for the nurse executive. *Nursing Economic$, 8*(6), 393-403.

Porter-O'Grady, T. (1990c). *The reorganization of nursing practice: Creating the corporate venture.* Rockville, Md.: Aspen.

Porter-O'Grady, T. (1991a). A nurse on the board. *Journal of Nursing Administration, 21*(1), 40-46.

Porter-O'Grady, T. (1991b). Shared governance for nursing, Part I: Creating the new organization. *AORN Journal, 53*(2), 458-466.

Porter-O'Grady, T. (1992a). *Implementing shared governance.* St. Louis, Mosby.

Porter-O'Grady, T. (1992b). Of rabbits and turtles: A time of change for unions. *Nursing Economic$, 10*(3), 177-182.

Porter-O'Grady, T. (1992c). Transformational leadership in an age of crisis. *Nursing Administration Quarterly, 17*(1), 17-24.

Porter-O'Grady, T. (1993a). Patient focused care service models and nursing: Perils and possibilities. *Journal of Nursing Administration, 23*(3), 7-15.

Porter-O'Grady, T. (1993b). Work redesign: Fact, fiction, and foible. *Seminars for Nurse Managers, 1*(1), 8-15.

Porter-O'Grady, T., & Finnigan, S. (1984). *Shared governance for nursing.* Rockville, Md.: Aspen.

Porter-O'Grady, T., & Tornabeni, J. (1993). Outcomes of shared governance: Impact on the organization. *Seminars for Nurse Managers, 1*(2), 63-73.

Porter-O'Grady, T. (1993). Of mythspinners and mapmakers: 21st century managers. *Nursing Management, 24*(4), 52-55.

Poscarella, P. & Frokman, M. (1989). *The purpose driven organization.* San Francisco: Jossey-Bass.

Postman, N. (1992). *Technopoly: The surrender of culture to technology.* New York: Knopf Publishers.

Prescott, P. (1993). Nursing: An important part of hospital survival under a reformed health care system. *Nursing Economic$, 11*(4), 193-199.

Price Waterhouse. (1982). *Getting your point across in Washington* (274703). Author.

Prowse, M. (1992). Is America in decline? *Harvard Business Review, 70*(4), 34-45.

Putnam L. (1988). Communication and conflict style in organizations, *Management Communication Quarterly 1*(3).

Quinlan, M. (1991). How does service drive the service company? *Harvard Business Review, 69*(6), 146-157.

Quinn, R. (1991). *Beyond rational management.* San Francisco: Jossey-Bass.

Rabkin, M. (1990). Ascent from mediocrity. In J. Clifford, & K. Horvath (Ed.), *Advancing professional nursing practice: Innovation at Boston's Beth Israel Hospital.* New York: Springer.

Rankin, T. (1990). *New forms of work organization: The challenge for North American unions.* Toronto: University of Toronto Press.

Raudsepp, E. (April 1990). Seven ways to cure communication breakdowns, *Nursing '90, 20*(4), 132-142.

Redland, A.R. (1992). The key to working together successfully. *Healthcare Trends and Transition, 3*(5), 26-27, 40-41.

Reiner, A. (1991). *Manual of patient care standards.* Rockville, Md.: Aspen.

Reinhardt, U. (1992). Whither private health insurance: Self destruction or rebirth? *Frontiers of Health Service Management, 9*(1), 5-31.

Relman, A. (1988). Assessment and accountability: The third revolution in medical care. *New England Journal of Medicine, 319*(18), 1220-1222.

Relman, A. (1991). Where does all that money go? *Health Management Quarterly, 13*(4), 2-5.

Reverby, S. (1987). *Ordered to care: The dilemma of American nursing, 1850-1945.* Cambridge, Mass.: Cambridge University Press.

Rheingold, H. (1993). *The virtual community: Homesteading on the electronic frontier.* New York: Addison-Wesley.

Roberts, M. (1993). *Strategy pure and simple.* Westport, Conn.: Decision Processes International.

Robinson, N. (1991). A patient centered framework for restructuring care. *Journal of Nursing Administration, 21*(9), 29-34.

Rodgers, T. (1990). No excuses management. *Harvard Business Review, 48*(4), 84-98.

Rodgers, T., Taylor, W., & Foreman, R. (1993). *No excuses management.* New York: Doubleday Currency.

Rogers, C., & Roethlisberger, F. (1991a). Barriers and gateways to communication, (1952). *Harvard Business Review, 69*(6), 105-111.

Rogers, M.F. (1973). Instrumental and infra-resources: The basis of power. *American Journal of Sociology, 79*(6), 1418-1433.

Rooks, J., et al. (1990, December 28). Outcomes of care in birth centers. *New England Journal of Medicine, 321,* 1804-1811.

Rosen, R. (1991). *The healthy company.* New York: Tarcher Press.

Rothman, D. (1990). A house divided. *Health Management Quarterly, 12*(2), 2-5.

Rowland, H., & Rowland, B. (1993). Nursing and quality improvement, assessment & management. *Nursing Administration Manual, 2,* 36:1-37:14.2

Rowland, H.S. & Rowland, B.L. (1992). *Nursing admin-*

istration handbook (3rd ed.). Gaithersburg, MD: Aspen.

Rowland, H. & Rowland, B. (1990). *Ambulatory care quality assurance manual.* Rockville, Md.: Aspen.

Russell, B. (1938). *Power.* London: Allen & Unwin.

Russell, P., & Evans, R. (1992). *The creative manager.* San Francisco: Jossey-Bass.

Ryan, K., & Oestreich, D. (1991). *Driving fear out of the workplace.* San Francisco: Jossey-Bass.

Ryan, S., & Porter, S. (1993). Men in nursing: A cautionary comparative critique. *Nursing Outlook, 41*(6), 262-267.

Sabatino, F. (1990, November 5). The delivery challenge posed by Canada: A bilateral view. *Hospitals,* pp. 58-63.

Sakai, K. (1990). The feudal world of Japanese manufacturing. *Harvard Business Review, 48*(6), 38-49.

Sampselle, C. (1991). The influence of feminist philosophy on nursing practice. *Image: The Journal of Nursing Scholarship, 22*(4), 243-246.

Sayles, L. (1993). *The working leader.* New York: The Free Press.

Schaaf, D. (1993, May). Is quality dead? *Training Supplement,* pp. 7-11.

Schafer, P., et al. (1987). Measuring nursing costs with patient acuity data. *Topics in Health Care Finance, 13*(4), 20-31.

Schein, E. (1993). On dialogue, culture, and organizational learning. *Organizational Dynamics, 22*(2), 40-51.

Schlesinger, L., & Heskett, J. (1991). The service driven service company. *Harvard Business Review, 69*(5), 71-91.

Scholtes, P. (1992). *The TEAM handbook.* Madison, WI: Joiner Associates.

Schor, J. (1992). *The overworked American.* New York: Basic Books.

Scott, V. (1993). Living the dream: Shared governance in the role of nurse executive. *Journal of Nursing Administration, 23*(12), 44-48.

Seago, J.A. (1993). Verbal abuse of nurses. *Revolution: The Journal of Nurse Empowerment, 3*(3), 63-64, 106.

Selzer, R. (1993). On being a doctor. *Health Management Quarterly, 15*(1), 2-6.

Senge, P. (1990). *The fifth discipline.* New York: Doubleday Currency.

Sharp, N. (1991). Healthcare reform: The proposal potpourri. *Nursing Management, 22*(7), 16-18.

Shea, S. (1991). Canadian nurses under a single payer system: Advantage or disadvantage. *Nursing Economic$, 9*(5), 329-333.

Sherer, J. (1993, February). Putting patients first: Patient centered care. *Hospitals,* (5), 15-18.

Sheridan, D.R. (1993). *Nursing management skills: A modular self-assessment series, Model IV: Transcultural nursing.* New York: National League of Nursing.

Sherwood, T. (1991). A word about clinical privileging. *Nursing Management, 22*(2), 52-54.

Shipper, F., & Manz, C. (1992). Employee self-management without formally designated teams: An alternative road to empowerment. *Organizational Dynamics, 20*(3), 48-63.

Shortell, S., et al. (1993). The holographic organization. *Healthcare Forum Journal, 36*(2), 20-25.

Shortell, S., Morrison, E., & Friedman, B. (1989). *Strategic choices for America's hospitals: Managing change in turbulent times.* San Francisco: Jossey-Bass.

Shortell, S., et al. (1993). Creating organized delivery systems: The barriers and facilitators. *Hospital & Health Services Administration, 33*(4), 447-466.

Sills, J. (1993). *Excess baggage: Getting out of your own way.* New York: Viking Penguin.

Simpson, R.L. (1992). *Technology: Nursing the system.* Atlanta: HBO & Company.

Singal, D. (1991). The other crisis in American education. *The Atlantic Monthly, 268*(5), 59-74.

Solovy, A. (1989, July 20). Healthcare in the 1990s. *Hospitals,* pp. 34-46.

Stacey, R. (1992). *Managing the unknowable: Strategic boundaries between order and chaos.* San Francisco: Jossey-Bass.

Starr, P. (1992). *The logic of health care reform.* Knoxville, Tenn.: Whittle Direct Books.

Stayer, R. (1990). How I learned to let my workers lead. *Harvard Business Review, 48*(6), 66-83.

Stefan, S., Gillies, D., & Biordi, D. (1992). Nursing care costs for a DRG subgroup. *10*(4), 277-281.

Stevens, G. (1991). *The strategic health care manager.* San Francisco: Jossey-Bass.

Stewart, N. (1991). *Den of thieves.* New York: Simon & Schuster.

Stillwaggon, C. (1989). The impact of nurse managed care on the cost of nurse practice and nurse satisfaction. *Journal of Nursing Administration, 19*(11), 21-26.

Swansburg, R.C. (1990). *Management and leadership for nurse managers.* Boston: Jones & Bartlett.

Swanson, E.A., McCloskey, J.C., & Bodensteiner, A. (1991). Publishing opportunities for nurses: A comparison of 92 U.S. journals. *Image, 23*(1), 33-38.

Swartz, F. (1992). *Breaking with tradition: Women and work, the new facts of life.* New York: Time Warner Books.

Sweeney, S., & Witt, K. (1990). Does nursing have the power to change the health care system? In J. McCloskey, & H. Grace (Ed.), *Current issues in nursing.* St. Louis: Mosby.

Takati, R. (1993). *A different mirror: A history of multicultural America.* New York: Little, Brown.

Tapscott, D., & Caston, A. (1993). *Paradigm shift: The new promise of information technology.* San Francisco: Jossey-Bass.

Tebbitt, B. (1993). Demystifying organizational empowerment. *Journal of Nursing Administration, 23*(1), 18-23.

Terry, R. (1993). *Authentic leadership.* San Francisco: Jossey-Bass.

Thomas, J. (1992). *Computers in healthcare,* pp. 33-35.

Thurow, L. (1992). *Head to head: The coming economic battle between Japan, Europe and America.* New York: William Morrow.

Tichy, N., & Devanna, M.A. (1990). *The transformational leader* (2nd ed.). New York: John Wiley & Sons.

Tichy, N., & Stratford, S. (1993). *Control your own destiny or someone else will.* New York: Doubleday Currency.

Toffler, A. (1990). *Powershift.* New York: Bantam.

Tonges, M., & Lawrenz, E. (1993). Re-engineering: The work redesign technology link. *Journal of Nursing Administration, 23*(10), 15-22.

Totten, N., & Scott, V. (1993). Who's on first? Shared governance in the role of the nurse executive. *Journal of Nursing Administration, 23*(5), 28-32.

Townsend, M. (1991). Creating a better work environment. *Journal of Nursing Administration, 21*(1), 11-14.

Trofino, J. (1993). Voice activated nursing documentation: On the cutting edge. *Nursing Management, 24*(7), 40-42.

Turner, L. (1991). *Democracy at work: Changing world markets and the future of labor unions.* Ithaca, N.Y.: Cornell University Press.

Ullman, D. (1993). The mainstreaming of alternative medicine. *Healthcare Forum Journal, 36*(6), 24-30.

Vaill, P. (1991). *Management as a performing art.* San Francisco: Jossey-Bass.

Vogt, J., & Murrell, K. (1990). *Empowerment in organizations.* San Diego: University Associates.

Wagner, L. (1990, September 3). Framework for reform. *Modern Healthcare,* pp. 31-35.

Wakefield, D.S. & Wakefield, B.J. (1993, March). Overcoming the barriers to implementation of TQM/CQI in hospitals: Myths and realities. *Quality Review Bulletin,* pp. 83-88.

Walton, M. (1990). *Demming management at work.* New York: G.P. Putnam's Sons.

Watkins, K., & Marsick, V. (1993). *Sculpting the learning organization.* San Francisco: Jossey-Bass.

Watson, G. (1993). *Strategic benchmarking.* New York: John Wiley & Sons.

Watson, J. (1989). The moral failure of the patriarchy. *Proceedings: American Acadamy of Nursing Scientific Session,* (October 15-17), 15-28.

Watson, P., et al. (1991). Discovering what nurses do and what it costs. *Nursing Management, 22*(5), 38-42.

Weil, T., & Stack, M. (1993). Health reform—its potential on hospital nursing service. *Nursing Economic$, 11*(4), 200-207.

Weiler, P. (1990). *Governing the workplace: The future of labor and employment law.* Cambridge, Mass.: Harvard University Press.

Wellins, R., Byham, W., & Wilson, J. (1993). *Empowered teams.* San Francisco: Jossey-Bass.

West C, Zimmerman D. (1983). Small insults: A study of interruption in cross-sex conversations between non-aquainted persons. In Thorne B, Kramar C, Henley N, (Eds). *Language, gender, and society.* Raleigh, Mass: Newberry House.

Wexley, K., & Silverman, S. (1993). *Working scared.* San Francisco: Jossey-Bass.

Wheatley, M. (1992). *Leadership and the new science.* San Francisco: Berrett-Koehler.

Whetsell, G. (1991). Total quality management. *Topics in Health Care Finance, 18*(2), 12-20.

Whitfield, C. (1989). *Healing the child within.* Deerfield Beach, Fl.: Health Communications.

Wiens, A. (1990). Expanded nurse autonomy. *Journal of Nursing Administration, 20*(12), 15-22.

Wilson, C. (1991). *Building new nursing organizations: Visions and realities.* Gathersburg, Md.: Aspen.

Wilson, K. (1989). Shared governance: The challenge of change in the early phases of implementation. *Nursing Administration Quarterly, 13*(4), 29-34.

Wilson, N., et al. (1990). Union dynamics in nursing. *Journal of Nursing Administration, 20*(2), 35-39.

Witte, J. (1980). *Democracy, authority and alienation in work.* Chicago: University of Chicago Press.

Woods, J., & Lucas, J. (1993). *The corporate closet.* New York: The Free Press.

Writer, S. (1990, November 12). Nursing homes operating at a loss. *Modern Healthcare,* pp. 37-38.

Zalesnik, A. (1992). Managers and leaders: Are they different? *Harvard Business Review, 70*(2), 126-135.

Zuboff, S. (1984). *In the age of the smart machine: The future of work and power* (1st ed.). New York: Basic Books.

Index

A

Abandonment of patient, 7-8
Absenteeism, 1
  battered spouse and, 105
  interview questions about, 123-124
Abuse
  drug, 99-102
  of patient, 192
  of sick day policy, 87-88
  spouse, 105
  of staff, by patient, 275-276
Academic community, networking with, 167
Academic degree, certification and, 25-26
Accountability
  empowerment and, 106-110
  knowledge worker and, 133
  quality improvement and, 221
Accountability-based practice, 87
  documentation errors and, 92
Achiever, managing of, 151-152
Acquired immunodeficiency syndrome, 4-5
Act, legislative
  Americans with Disabilities
    essential functions and, 131
    job interview and, 127
  Omnibus Budget Reconciliation, 76
  Patient Self-Determination
    advance directives and, 2
    no code orders and, 171
Acting out by patient, 190, 275-276
Action planning, 115-116
Activist, peer support for, 163
Acuity-based assignments, 7
Acuity system
  budgeting and, 9-10
  patient classification and, 186, 187-188
  patient transfer and, 194
Administration
  certification in, 26, 28-29
  empowerment and, 109
  ethics and, 111
  loyalty to, 152-153
  patient care versus, 103
  quality assurance and, 217-218
  quality improvement and, 215, 219, 221

restructuring and, 283
Administrative disciplinary action, 87
Administrator
  difficult, 54
  how to become, 16-17
  participative management and, 182-183
  project evaluation and, 117
Admissions
  limits on, 114
  too many, 194-195
Advance directives, 1-2
Advanced certification, 26
Advanced degree, 13-14
  when to get, 104
Advancement, career, 13-16
  headhunter and, 224
  as reward, 161
  writing as criterion for, 286
Advocate
  patient
    encouragement of, 183-184
    managed care and, 144-145
  staff, 191
Agency, staffing, 2-4
  census fluctuations and, 24
Agenda for meeting
  preventing gossip and, 157
  shared governance and, 237
  staff meeting and, 249
Agreement
  collective bargaining, 50-51
    grievance process and, 119
  interface, 194-195
Aides, nurse, working with, 244-245
AIDS, 4-5
Alcohol abuse
  abuse of sick day policy and, 88
  by physician, 100-102
Ambulatory care standards, 129-130
American Nurses Association
  collective bargaining and, 271
  legislation and, 170
  telephone orders and, 263-264
Americans with Disabilities Act
  essential functions and, 131
  job interview and, 127
Ancillary department, case management and, 23
Anger
  at manager, 207-208
  reaction to, 146-147